Manual of Pediatric Anesthesia

Manual of Pediatric Anesthesia, Fifth Edition

David J. Steward, M.B., F.R.C.P.(C.)
Professor
Department of Anesthesiology
University of Southern California School of Medicine
Director
Department of Anesthesiology
Childrens Hospital of Los Angeles
Los Angeles, California, United States

Jerrold Lerman, M.D.
Professor
Department of Anaesthesia
University of Toronto Faculty of Medicine
Department of Anaesthesia
Hospital for Sick Children
Toronto, Ontario, Canada

Anesthesia Implications of Syndromes and Unusual Disorders revised, augmented, and updated by

Joan C. Bevan, M.D.
Associate Professor of Anaesthesia
Department of Anaesthesia
University of British Columbia
British Columbia's Children's Hospital
British Columbia, Canada

CHURCHILL LIVINGSTONE

A Harcourt Health Sciences Company
New York   Edinburgh   London   Philadelphia

CHURCHILL LIVINGSTONE
A Harcourt Health Sciences Company

The Curtis Center
Independence Square West
Philadelphia, Pennsylvania 19106

Library of Congress Cataloging-in-Publication Data

Steward, David J.
Manual of pediatric anesthesia/David J. Steward, Jerrold Lerman.–5th ed.

p.   cm.

Includes bibliographical references and index.

ISBN 0–443–06562–4

1. Pediatric anesthesia–Handbooks, manuals, etc.   I. Lerman, Jerrold.
   II. Title.   [DNLM: 1. Anesthesia–methods–Child–Handbooks.
   2. Anesthesia–methods–Infant–Handbooks.   WO 231 S849m 2001]

RD139. S84 2001   617.9′6798—dc21   00–047459

Editor-in-Chief: Richard Lampert
Acquisitions Editor: Allan Ross
Production Manager: Norman Stellander
Illustration Specialist: Robert Quinn
Book Designer: Gene Harris

MANUAL OF PEDIATRIC ANESTHESIA   ISBN 0–443–06562–4

Printed in the United States of America.

Last digit is the print number: 9   8   7   6   5   4   3   2   1

Preface

In the tradition of the previous four editions, this fifth edition of the *Manual of Pediatric Anesthesia* is written and designed to provide a concise but comprehensive pocketbook guide to pediatric anesthesia practice. It should also prove useful as a study guide for trainees in pediatric anesthesia.

The first edition published in 1979 was prepared, in part, to describe the methods of anesthesia that were successfully employed at the Hospital for Sick Children, Toronto.

By moving away from Toronto in 1984, first to Vancouver and then to Los Angeles, DJS gained valuable experience with a variety of approaches to anesthesia and perioperative care for the pediatric patient. Subsequent editions of this manual were then broadened to incorporate many of these different approaches and ideas.

In the fifth edition, the process has come full circle. Once again, benefit has been gained from the vast Toronto experience. Dr. Jerrold Lerman, as coauthor, brings the expertise derived from his experiences over the last two decades at the Hospital for Sick Children. Dr. Joan C. Bevan, most recently of the British Columbia's Children's Hospital, has joined the editorial team and has extensively augmented and revised Appendix 1, *Anesthesia Implications of Syndromes and Unusual Disorders.*

Although the manual retains a format similar to the previous editions, we have expanded some sections and trimmed others. We have included much new information that has become available as a result of the greatly increased research activity in the field of pediatric anesthesiology. We have deleted redundant material. Changes were made to the content in response to the evolution of pediatric surgery and anesthesia practices and the expanded responsibilities of the pediatric anesthesiologist outside the operating room.

The chapter dealing with pain management and sedation is enlarged. Some advice is included on relating with parents. A chapter devoted to anesthesia in areas remote from the operating room has been added. The sections of the book that deal with complex pediatric surgical conditions and minimally invasive and endoscopic surgery are expanded. In other parts of the book, we have condensed segments and, where appropriate, more concisely summarized the information by the use of tables and algorithms.

Many new references have been added, but some of the old ones remain. These references represent some of the foundations on which our subspecialty was built. In addition, they are interesting to read!

The safe practice of pediatric anesthesia demands more than a well-trained anesthesiologist. It also requires an optimal facility and comprehensive support services. In February of 1999, the American Academy of

Pediatrics published in its journal *Pediatrics* proposed guidelines for the Pediatric Perioperative Anesthesia Environment (*Pediatrics* 103:512–515, 1999).

This document details, for anesthesiologists and hospitals, the suggested requirements for various levels of anesthesia care for infants and children. It is recommended that all who care for pediatric patients read and observe the standards outlined therein.

Children are rewarding patients for the skilled anesthesiologist. There is great satisfaction in the successful management of the very small infant, the extremely reticent child, and the many other children that you care for. It is hoped that our handbook helps you to achieve this satisfaction.

David J. Steward
Jerrold Lerman

Preface to the First Edition

This manual was written with three general aims: *first,* to discuss the important differences in anatomy and physiology of children compared with adults; *second,* to present the general principles of anesthetic management of pediatric patients; and *third,* to describe techniques of anesthesia used at the Hospital for Sick Children, Toronto, for some specific procedures.

This is not a comprehensive text—some conditions receive no mention—but the subject matter, based on our experience with over 14,000 cases annually, includes most problems in pediatric anesthesia.

References have not been cited in the text; relevant references to the literature, and suggested further reading, are appended to each section. Similarly, routine doses of anesthetic drugs for general pediatric use are not given in the text; these are in Appendix III. When other than the usual dose is required, however, this is detailed in the relevant section.

Though this manual includes methods of anesthesia for complex procedures, we believe very strongly that many of these conditions can be treated satisfactorily only in a specialist unit. No matter how skilled the pediatric surgeon and anesthesiologist, the necessary facilities and skills of intensive nursing care must be available for high-risk pediatric surgical patients.

Infants, particularly neonates and especially the premature, present special problems for the anesthesiologist; they have physiological problems quite different from those of adults. In these and slightly older children there are problems associated simply with their size and the immaturity of the systems that metabolize and excrete drugs. Further, for children of all ages, consideration must be given to the psychological impact of the anesthetic procedures, which may be remembered so vividly as to overshadow other hospital experiences.

Children are rewarding patients. They will amaze you by surviving—and with few problems—the most extensive surgical procedures. However, meticulous attention to even the smallest details of anesthetic technique is imperative, as well as a facility for understanding and communicating with children of all ages.

David J. Steward

Abbreviations and Acronyms

A-aDO₂ alveolar-arterial oxygen tension gradient
A-aDN₂ alveolar-arterial nitrogen difference
ACE angiotensin-converting enzyme
ACT activated clotting time
AV arteriovenous
BP blood pressure
BSA body surface area
CBF cerebral blood flow
CF cystic fibrosis
CHD congenital heart disease
CK creatine kinase
CL lung compliance
CMRO₂ cerebral metabolic rate for oxygen
CNS central nervous system
CoHb carboxyhemoglobin
CPAP continuous positive airway pressure
CPB cardiopulmonary bypass
CPK creatine phosphokinase
CPP cerebral perfusion pressure
CSF cerebrospinal fluid
CT computed tomography
CV closing volume
CVP central venous pressure
DDAVP 1-deamino-8-D-arginine vasopressin
DIC disseminated intravascular coagulation
DN dibucaine number
2,3-DPG 2,3-diphosphoglycerate
EACA epsilon-aminocaproic acid
EBV estimated blood volume
ECG electrocardiography
ECMO extracorporeal membrane oxygenation
ED₉₅ effective dose in 95% of patients
EDTA ethylenediamine tetraacetic acid
EEG electroencephalography
EMG electromyography
EUA examination under anesthesia
FIO₂ fraction of inspired oxygen
FN fluoride number
FRC functional residual capacity
GFR glomerular filtration rate
Hb hemoglobin
HbA adult hemoglobin

HbC   hemoglobin C
3-HBDH   3-hydroxybutyrate dehydrogenase
HbF   fetal hemoglobin
HbS   sickle cell hemoglobin
Hct   hematocrit
HME   heat and moisture exchanger
HpD   hematoporphyrin derivative
ICP   intracranial pressure
ID   internal diameter
IJV   internal jugular vein
IOP   intraocular pressure
IPPB   intermittent positive-pressure breathing
IPPV   intermittent positive-pressure ventilation
IVAC   intravenous accurate control [device]
IVH   intraventricular hemorrhage
LDH   lactate dehydrogenase
LMA   laryngeal mask airway
L/S   lecithin-sphingomyelin [ratio]
LV   left ventricle
MAC   minimal alveolar concentration
MEP   motor evoked potential
MetHb   methemoglobin
MH   malignant hyperpyrexia
MHS   malignant hyperpyrexia-susceptible
MRI   magnetic resonance imaging
NEC   necrotizing enterocolitis
NO   nitric oxide
N$_2$O   nitrous oxide
NSAID   nonsteroidal anti-inflammatory drug
OR   operating room
P$_{50}$ PO_2 with 50% hemoglobin saturation
PA   pulmonary artery
PaCO$_2$ arterial carbon dioxide pressure
PaO$_2$ arterial oxygen pressure
PACU   postanesthesia care unit
PAR   postanesthesia room
PC   partition coefficient
PCA   patient-controlled analgesia
PCO$_2$ partial pressure of carbon dioxide
PDA   patent ductus arteriosus
PEEP   positive end-expiratory pressure
PGE$_1$ prostaglandin E$_1$
PIP   peak inspiratory pressure
PNF   protamine neutralization factor
PO$_2$ partial pressure of oxygen
PONV   postoperative nausea and vomiting
PPM   parts per million
PT   prothrombin time
PTT   partial thromboplastin time
PVC   polyvinyl chloride

PVOD   pulmonary vascular obstructive disease
PVR   pulmonary vascular resistance
$\dot{Q}$ perfusion
Qp:Qs   ratio of pulmonary to systemic blood flow
RA   right atrium
RAST   radioallergosorbent testing
RBC   red blood cell
RDS   respiratory distress syndrome
REM   rapid eye movement
RES   reticuloendothelial system
ROP   retinopathy of prematurity
RV   right ventricle
SaO$_2$ arterial oxygen saturation
SCIWORA   spinal cord injury without radiologic abnormality
SGOT   serum glutamic oxaloacetic transaminase
SIADH   syndrome of inappropriate antidiuretic hormone secretion
SNP   sodium nitroprusside
SpO$_2$ saturation pulse oximetry
SSEP   somatosensory evoked potentials
SVR   systemic vascular resistance
TEE   transesophageal echocardiography
TEF   tracheoesophageal fistula
TLC   total lung capacity
V$_A$ alveolar ventilation
V$_D$ dead space volume
$\dot{V}$ ventilation
$\dot{V}O_2$ rate of metabolism (or consumption) for oxygen
$\dot{V}/\dot{Q}$ ventilation-perfusion [matching]
V$_T$ tidal volume
VATER association   vertebral defects, anal atresia, tracheoesophageal fistula, esophageal atresia, radial and renal dysplasia
VACTERL association   the VATER association with added cardiac and limb defects
VIP   vasoactive intestinal polypeptide
VSD   ventricular septal defect
WBC   white blood cell

NOTICE

Anesthesiology is an ever-changing field. Standard safety precautions must be followed, but as new research and clinical experience broaden our knowledge, changes in treatment and drug therapy may become necessary or appropriate. Readers are advised to check the most current product information provided by the manufacturer of each drug to be administered to verify the recommended dose, the method and duration of administration, and the contraindications. It is the responsibility of the treating physician, relying on exprience and knowledge of the patient, to determine the dosages and the best treatments for each individual patient. Neither the Publisher nor the editor assumes any liability for any injury and/or damage to persons or property arising from this publication.

THE PUBLISHER

Contents

FOUNDATIONS OF PEDIATRIC ANESTHESIA

ANESTHESIA FOR SPECIFIC PROCEDURES

Foundations of Pediatric Anesthesia

Chapter 1

Psychological Aspects of Anesthesia in Pediatric Patients

Hospitalization and medical procedures can have profound emotional consequences for infants and children. Some patients demonstrate behavior disturbances that persist long after the event. The extent of the upset is determined by several factors, among the most important of which is the child's age.

Infants younger than 6 months of age are not upset by separation from parents and readily accept a nurse as a substitute mother. From a psychological viewpoint, this is probably a good age for major surgery, although prolonged separation may impair parent-child bonding.

Older infants and young children (6 months to 4 years) are much more upset by a hospital stay, principally because of the separation from family and home. Explanations are difficult at this age, and, not surprisingly, these children show the most severe behavior regression after hospitalization.

School-age children are usually less upset by separation and more concerned with the surgical procedure and its possible mutilating effect. Adolescents fear the process of narcosis, the loss of control, and the possibility of not being able to cope with illness. However, teenagers who can be helped by the surgery to better cope with a serious illness may gain significant self-esteem from this experience.

The type and extent of the surgical procedure is obviously a factor. Major surgery, craniofacial surgery, or amputation must be expected to have significant effects, and appropriate psychiatric support should be provided. Surgery of the genitalia may also have significant psychological implications and is probably best performed before the patient is 18 months of age.

Factors other than age also influence the child's emotional response. For example, a long hospitalization is much more disturbing than a brief admission, and day surgery has a negligible effect on most patients. Repeated hospitalizations and surgeries may cause significant disturbance and deserve special attention with regard to psychological needs. The child's ethnic origin and family background are also important. Some children are much more upset than others of similar age; this probably reflects the extent to which they have been coddled at home. Those children from higher socioeconomic groups are generally more upset, as are children whose parents are separated.

Children vary in their response to impending hospitalization or medical intervention. Some seek information and participate keenly in preparation programs; they have an active coping style. These children are likely to benefit from psychological preparation and can be expected to cooperate. Other children maintain an air of disinterest; they have an avoidant coping style (the "silent child"). Children in this latter group may not benefit and indeed may be further sensitized by efforts at psychological preparation. They may benefit more from effective sedative anxiolytic premedication.

ROLE OF THE PARENTS

"Being unable to choose parents for your patients, you must make do with those who come with the child . . . ; it would be abnormal if they showed no anxiety" *Mellish, 1969*

Parents are playing an increasingly active role in the perioperative care of their children, and many expect to be present at induction and in the recovery room. However, some parents are more anxious than others, and this is readily perceived and may further upset the child. Good preparation of the parents reduces parental anxiety and thereby indirectly helps the child.

There are many factors that influence the extent of parental anxiety when a child requires an operation. Parents of children with only minor problems may initially be very anxious. Full explanations and good communication with the medical and nursing teams usually do much to reduce their anxiety level.

The anesthesiologist is frequently placed in a difficult situation when obtaining informed consent for general anesthesia: providing information on all the potential risks before a minor surgical procedure might well be expected to increase the level of anxiety of the parents. However, parents appear to benefit from an appropriate discussion of the risks of anesthesia in that this fulfills their own needs of responsibility and understanding. The parents should be permitted to dictate the extent of the information they wish to be given. Most parents of children having minor procedures accept that there are risks, including death, and prefer to have the opportunity for discussion of these risks. Such discussions should, of course, be outside the earshot of the young child.

The overanxious parents require special consideration. Excessive anxiety is often of multifactorial origin and may not be entirely related to the child's present surgical condition. Such parents may not gain much reduction in their anxiety levels from further information regarding the forthcoming procedure.

In general, the anesthesiologist should rely on some well-established general principles in dealing with anxious parents. An approach that has been found most helpful in decreasing parental anxiety is one built on genuine warmth and friendliness, empathy, and understanding, and a cooperative plan for the child. Discussions should allow ample time for questions and for the parents to express their concerns about the child and the proposed anesthesia.

The question of the parents' accompanying the child during induction of anesthesia requires special consideration. Many parents express a strong wish to be present, and many facilities routinely allow them to stay with their child. Studies are inconclusive as to the extent to which a parent's presence can positively influence the emotional outcome for the child, but it may help the parent achieve satisfaction. Certainly many parents of older handicapped children can be of great assistance.

Many parents are calm and supportive of their child and appear to benefit from participating in the induction process. However, the anxious parent who insists on remaining with the child may do more harm than good and may increase the child's anxiety level. Such anxious parents should be counseled and excluded if possible. Adequate preoperative sedation of the child may help them to agree to this course. Every parent will be pleased if you communicate the message, "We will take very good care of your child and will be with your child all the time!"

ROLE OF THE ANESTHESIOLOGIST

Anesthesia, and particularly the induction period, is recognized to have a potential to cause psychological trauma. Studies indicate that anesthesiologists vary in their ability to minimize this upset for the child. Preoperative psychological preparation is very important and has been clearly demonstrated to be beneficial to many children. Usually this must be done by the parents, and the extent of preparation necessary is determined by the child's age. The basic objective is to explain to the child in simple, understandable, and reassuring terms what will happen at the hospital. It is even possible to institute a program to prepare the child who is admitted on an emergency basis (e.g., for appendectomy). Older children and adolescents should be prepared well in advance, as soon as hospitalization is arranged. Younger children should not be prepared too far in advance—it is unnecessary and will be a continuing source of worry for them. Rather, they should be prepared a day or so beforehand. Caution should be exercised in caring for the silent child who has an avoidant coping style, especially the child who must undergo repeat procedures, because such a child may not respond as well to routine preparation methods. Some may respond more favorably if they are allowed to continue with their avoidant coping pattern but are given a well-chosen preoperative medication.

An *empathic approach* to the child before and during medical procedures is preferred (e.g., "This may be a little uncomfortable and I know you are scared, but we are going to do all we can to help and it will soon be over. We don't mind if you cry."). The alternative *directive approach* ("Hold still and be big and brave.") is generally condemned.

Some books that may help parents to prepare their child are listed at the end of this chapter. Hospital tours, puppet shows, and audiovisual presentations are easy to arrange and have all been demonstrated to be beneficial. Videotapes are most useful and may be loaned to parents to aid in preparation of the child. In some cities it has been possible to deliver prehospital preparation programs for children via community television stations on a regular weekly basis. By this means a whole population of children can be prepared for the possibility of hospitalization, rather than just those who are already scheduled for surgery.

Premedication with an anxiolytic sedative drug, orally administered, is now recognized to confer benefits in decreasing anxiety during separation, increasing cooperation during induction, and decreasing posthospitalization behavior disturbance.

Preparing Patients for an Operation

1. Try to meet the young child with the parents so that the child can see them accept you.
2. Direct most of your attention at all times to the child, even if he is developmentally delayed. Try to maintain eye contact; it helps to sit alongside the child, on the floor if necessary!
3. Talk to the child in simple terms that the child can understand.
4. Pay special attention to the silent child and recognize that she may be very upset. Consider the use of a suitable sedative premedication if not otherwise contraindicated.
5. Truthfully explain all the procedures to be undertaken but avoid unnecessary alarming details. Some children may ask about the operation: try to help them understand what is to be done, using drawings if necessary. In many cases children grossly overestimate the extent of the procedure and must be reassured, for instance, about the small size of the incision.
6. Do not use the phrase "put you to sleep"—this may worry some children if they recall a family pet who never came back! It may also cause them to worry that they might wake up from their "sleep" when the operation starts or while it is still in progress.
7. Do not present the child with unpleasant and difficult choices. For example, avoid questions such as, "Do you want the needle or the mask?" Tell the child what you intend to do and then try to meet any special requests (e.g., "I do not want to go to sleep with the mask").
8. Avoid uncovering the child more than is necessary to complete the physical examination; many children get upset at being disrobed.
9. Allow the child to bring a favorite toy or other security object to the operating room (OR). Label the toy with the child's name; if it

is a doll, suggest that perhaps the doll should also get a cast or a dressing applied during the operation. If the child is able, let him walk to the OR rather than be carried or wheeled: children are quite independent and feel more at ease walking.

10. If possible, allow those parents who are judged to be calm and supportive to accompany their child during the induction. If this is not possible, both the child and the parents may be helped by giving the child a premedicant (e.g., midazolam, *see* page 79). The parents are much happier seeing their child disappear into the OR if he or she is well sedated. It is sometimes useful to start an intravenous infusion away from the OR with the parents present, especially for handicapped or developmentally delayed children. The intravenous route can then be used for induction as soon as the child is taken to the OR. Always use local analgesia to insert the intravenous cannula; topical anesthetic cream or "Numby Stuff" is ideal if it can be applied in advance (*see* page 111). An empathic approach should be used to prepare the child. Small children who are crying during venipuncture can often be calmed by telling them, "We will put on a Band-Aid in a minute."

11. Reassure older children and adolescents and provide them with careful explanations. They may be quite scared and have many questions. It is important to reassure them of the safety of the procedure and to emphasize that they will not wake up during the operation but will definitely wake up when it is over. Older children may also benefit from a carefully selected premedicant drug (*see* page 79).

12. Select the most appropriate induction technique for each child and proceed without delay. Do not allow a child to wait on the OR table longer than is absolutely necessary for the positioning of basic monitors.

13. Talk to the child throughout the induction period in order to explain or distract her from the procedures that are required. Ensure that all extraneous noises and conversations are excluded during this time. Only one person should be talking to the child.

14. Use premedicant drugs whenever indicated; most young children will benefit. Midazolam is the current drug of choice, and there is some evidence that its use diminishes emotional sequelae after discharge.

15. Tell the child what to expect when he wakes up, where he will be, and what discomfort he will have. Carefully explain such items as eye patches, nasogastric tubes, and catheters. A urinary catheter may look like a worm to an unprepared child!

16. Plan in advance to provide an optimal postoperative pain relief for every patient.

POSTOPERATIVE CARE

The parents should be allowed to be with their child as soon as is practical—as soon as the child awakens, if possible. Every effort should be made to provide good, but safe, analgesia. Regional nerve blocks, narcotic infusions, patient-controlled analgesia, epidural narcotics, and all ancillary techniques used for adults should be considered and provided for infants and children when appropriate.

In the intensive care unit, the pediatric patient's problems are similar to those described for adults: pain, lack of sleep, and later boredom. In addition, children have their own special concerns, such as separation from the family. Special attention should be directed to pain relief, regular visitation by the parents, and provision of toys, games, and other distractions (e.g., television) as the child's condition improves. Parents of children in the intensive care unit benefit by being kept very well informed of their child's condition and progress, and they must also be continuously updated on the treatment plans for their child.

Suggested Additional Reading

Edwinson M, Arnbjornsson E, and Ekman R: Psychologic preparation program for children undergoing acute appendectomy. Pediatrics 82:30–36, 1988.

Ferguson BF: Preparing young children for hospitalization: a comparison of two methods. Pediatrics 64:656–664, 1979.

Fernald C and Corry J: Empathic versus directive preparation of children for needles. Child Health Care 10:44–47, 1981.

Manley CB: Elective genital surgery at one year of age: psychological and surgical considerations. Surg Clin North Am 62:941, 1982.

McGraw T: Preparing children for the operating room. Can J Anaesth 41:1094–1103, 1994.

Peterson L: Coping by children undergoing stressful medical procedures: some conceptual, methodological, and therapeutic issues. J Consult Clin Psychol 57:380–387, 1989.

Peterson L, Ridley-Johnson R, Tracy K, and Mullins LL: Developing cost-effective presurgical preparation: a comparative analysis. J Pediatr Psychol 9:439–455, 1984.

Seeman RG and Rockoff MA: Preoperative anxiety: the pediatric patient. Int Anesthesiol Clin 24:1–15, 1986.

Vetter TR: The epidemiology and selective identification of children at risk for preoperative anxiety reactions. Anesth Analg 77:96–99, 1993.

Zuckerberg AL: Perioperative approach to children. Pediatr Clin North Am 41:15–29, 1994.

Parental Anxiety

Litman DO, Perkons FM, and Dawson SC: Parental knowledge and attitudes toward discussing the risk of death from anesthesia. Anesth Analg 77:256–260, 1993.

Poole SR: The "over anxious" parent. Clin Pediatr (Phila) 19:557–562, 1980.

Richtsmeier AJ and Hatcher JW: Parental anxiety and minor illness. J Dev Behav Pediatr 15:14–19, 1994.

Waisel DB and Truog RD: The benefits of explanation of the risks of anesthesia in the day surgery parent. J Clin Anesth 7:200–204, 1995.

Parental Presence During Induction of Anesthesia

Bevan JC, Johnston C, Tousignant G, et al.: Preoperative parental anxiety predicts behavioural and emotional responses to induction of anaesthesia in children. Can J Anaesth 37:177–182, 1990.

Braude N, Ridley SA, and Sumner E: Parents and paediatric anaesthesia: a prospective survey of parental attitudes to their presence at induction. Ann R Coll Surg Engl 72:41–44, 1990.

Cammeron JA, Bond MJ, and Pointer SC: Reducing the anxiety of children undergoing surgery: parental presence during anaesthetic induction. J Paediatr Child Health 32:51–56, 1996.

Hannallah RS: Who benefits when parents are present during anesthesia induction in their children. Can J Anaesth 41:271–275, 1994.

Kain ZN, Mayes LC, Want S-M, et al.: Parental presence during induction of anesthesia versus sedative premedication: which intervention is more effective? Anesthesiology 89:1147–1156, 1999.

Vessey JA, Bogetz MS, Caserza CL, et al.: Parental upset associated with participation in induction of anaesthesia in children. Can J Anaesth 41:276–280, 1994.

Parents, Recovery Rooms, and the Intensive Care Unit

Dianiaco MJ and Ingoldsby BB: Parental presence in the recovery room. AORN J 38:685, 1983.

Hall PA, Payne JF, Stack CG, and Stokes MA: Parents in the recovery room: survey of parental and staff attitudes. BMJ 310:163–164, 1995.

Kasper JW and Nyamathi AM: Parents of children in the pediatric intensive care unit: what are their needs? Heart Lung 17:574–581, 1988.

Noonan AT, Anderson P, Newlon P, et al.: Family centered care in the postanesthesia care unit: evaluation of practice. J Post Anesthesia Nursing 6:13–16, 1991.

Wilson TA and Graves SA: Pediatric considerations in a general postanesthesia care unit. J Post Anesthesia Nursing 5:16–24, 1990.

Recommended Reading for Professionals

Preparing Children and Families for Health Care Encounters. Association for the Care of Children's Health, Washington, DC.

Suggested Reading for Parents and Children

American Society of Anesthesiologists, Committee on Communications and Dr Frederick Berry: My Trip to the Hospital. [A coloring book.] ASA, Park Ridge, IL.

Howe J and Warshaw M: The Hospital Book. [For school-age children.] Crown Publishers, New York, 1981.

Jason's Hospital Adventure. [A coloring book for children.] Roche Laboratories, Nutley, NJ.

Rey M and Rey H: Curious George Goes to Hospital. [For preschool-age children.] Houghton-Mifflin, Boston, 1966.

Richter E: The Teenage Hospital Experience: You Can Handle It. [For adolescents.] Coward, McCann, and Geoghegan, New York, 1982.

Understanding Your Operation. [For teenagers.] Roche Laboratories, Nutley, NJ.

Videotapes

Understanding Your Child's Operation. Roche Laboratories, Nutley, NJ.

Your Child's Anesthesia. The Nemours Foundation, Center for Biomedical Communication, Wilmington, DE.

Chapter 2

Anatomy and Physiology in Relation to Pediatric Anesthesia

CENTRAL NERVOUS SYSTEM

The central nervous system in the newborn differs from that in the older child in several ways: the myelination of nerve fibers is incomplete, the muscle tone and reflexes are different, and the cerebral cortex is less developed (its cellular elements increase during the first years of life).

Sensitivity to Pain

Until a few years ago, little was understood of the ability of infants and small children to appreciate pain. As a result there was an unfortunate tendency to ignore the need for analgesia during painful procedures and even during and after surgical operations. It is now well established that newborn infants, even those born prematurely, may have increased sensitivity to pain and will react to it with tachycardia, hypertension, and increased intracranial pressure, together with a neuroendocrine response that exceeds that seen in adults. Infants may also demonstrate measurable behavioral responses to pain (crying, grimacing, restlessness, and so forth), and these have been used as a basis for pain scoring systems. There is evidence to suggest that infants who are subjected to painful procedures (e.g., circumcision) may experience increased sensitivity to pain as they grow older. This is postulated to be caused by persisting alterations in the infant's central processing of painful stimuli. It has also been suggested that good intraoperative and postoperative pain control, by modifying stress responses, may lead to improved survival in infants with critical illness.

This knowledge of the pain sensitivity of infants and the possible consequences of undertreated pain dictates that we provide optimal analgesia or anesthesia for all babies during *any* painful procedure with the same care as we do for adult patients. As children grow from infancy, their pain threshold remains lower than that of older children or adults.

Cranium

The intact skull is less rigid in infants than in adults. As a result, an increase in the volume of its contents—blood, cerebrospinal fluid (CSF), and brain tissue—can be accommodated to some extent by expansion of the fontanelles and separation of the suture lines. Palpation of the fontanelles can be used to assess the intracranial pressure in infants.

Cerebral Blood Flow

Autoregulation of cerebral blood flow is impaired in sick newborns; as a result, blood flow is pressure dependent. Hypotension may lead to cerebral ischemia, and any pressure fluctuations are transmitted to the capillary circulation. In the preterm infant, the cerebral vessels are very fragile, especially in the region of the germinal matrix overlying the caudate nucleus. Rupture of these vessels leads to intracerebral hemorrhage, which often extends into the ventricular system as an intraventricular hemorrhage (IVH).

Small preterm infants are very prone to IVH, which usually occurs during the first few days of life and is a leading cause of morbidity and mortality. Predisposing factors to IVH include hypoxia, hypercarbia, hypernatremia, fluctuations in arterial or venous pressure or cerebral blood flow, low hematocrit, overtransfusion, and rapid administration of hypertonic fluids (e.g., sodium bicarbonate).

The anesthesiologist should avoid precipitating these factors. Airway manipulations, including awake endotracheal intubation and suctioning, have been shown to increase blood pressure and anterior fontanelle pressure. Awake intubation should be avoided; the child should be anesthetized and paralyzed before intubation. If awake intubation is to be performed, topical analgesia to the mouth and palate may minimize the infant's response to this procedure. To further prevent blood pressure fluctuations, adequate anesthesia and analgesia should be provided for all painful procedures, and care should be taken to replace blood losses accurately. Never give rapid injections of undiluted hypertonic solutions such as dextrose or sodium bicarbonate. Severe anemia and/or coagulopathy should be corrected promptly.

Cerebrospinal Fluid

The CSF, which occupies the cerebral ventricles and the subarachnoid spaces surrounding the brain and spinal cord, is formed by choroid plexuses in the temporal horns of the lateral ventricles, the posterior portion of the third ventricle, and the roof of the fourth ventricle. Meningeal and ependymal vessels and blood vessels of the brain and spinal cord also contribute a small amount of CSF.

The choroid plexuses are cauliflower-like structures consisting of blood vessels covered by thin epithelium through which CSF continuously exudes. The rate of secretion is about 750 ml/day in the adult—that is, about five times the intracavity volume. Except for the active secretion of a few substances by the choroid plexus, CSF is similar to interstitial fluid.

CSF flow is initiated by pulsation in the choroid plexus. From the lateral ventricles the CSF passes into the third ventricle via the foramen of Monro and along the aqueduct of Sylvius into the fourth ventricle, each ventricle contributing more fluid by secretion from its choroid plexus. CSF then flows through the two lateral foramina of Luschka and the midline foramen of Magendie into the cisterna magna and throughout the subarachnoid spaces.

CSF is reabsorbed into the blood by hydrostatic filtration through the arachnoid villi, which project from the subarachnoid space into the venous sinuses.

Hydrocephalus

Hydrocephalus is an abnormal accumulation of CSF within the cranium that may be obstructive or nonobstructive.

Obstructive hydrocephalus is caused by blockage in the fluid pathway of the CSF. It may be communicating (e.g., when the CSF pathway into the subarachnoid space is open, as after chronic arachnoiditis) or noncommunicating (e.g., when the fluid's pathway proximal to the subarachnoid space is obstructed, as in aqueductal stenosis or Arnold-Chiari malformation).

Nonobstructive hydrocephalus is caused by a reduction in the volume of brain substance, with secondary dilatation of the ventricles; by overproduction of CSF (e.g., in choroid plexus papilloma); or by diminished reabsorption due to scarring.

Suggested Additional Reading

Aynsley-Green A: Pain and stress in infancy and childhood—where to now? [Editorial]. Paediatr Anaesth 6:167–172, 1996.

Fitzgerald M: Development of pain pathways and mechanisms. In Anand KJS, McGrath PJ (eds.): Pain in Neonates. Elsevier, Amsterdam, 1993, pp 19–37.

Perry EH, Bada HS, Ray JD, et al.: Blood pressure increases, birth weight dependent stability boundary, and intraventricular hemorrhage. Pediatrics 85:727–732, 1990.

Taddio A, Katz J, Ilersich AL, and Koren G: Effect of neonatal circumcision on pain response during subsequent routine vaccination. Lancet 349:599–603, 1997.

Volpe JJ: Brain injury in the premature infant. Clin Perinatol 24:567–587, 1997.

Walco GA, Cassidy RC, and Schechter NL: Pain, hurt, and harm: the ethics of pain control in infants and children. N Engl J Med 331:541–544, 1994.

EYES

In the past, visual acuity was believed to develop in infants when they were a few weeks old, but it is now recognized that full-term infants can recognize and respond to objects.

Retinopathy of Prematurity

Retinopathy of prematurity (ROP), a disease of the retinal vessels also known as retrolental fibroplasia, is a leading cause of blindness. Improved survival of very-low-birth-weight infants has resulted in an increased incidence of this condition, which is most common in those newborns weighing less than 1,500 g. Increased oxygen tension in the retinal arteries is thought to be a principal cause. Hyperoxia leads to vasoconstriction, capillary endothelial swelling, and degeneration in the peripheral region of the retina, with a visible demarcation line (stage 1 ROP). These changes are followed by the formation of a ridge at this line (stage 2 ROP), extraretinal fibrovascular proliferation (stage 3 ROP), and retinal detachment (stage 4 ROP).

The risk of developing ROP is increased in direct proportion to the duration of exposure to oxygen. It had been suggested that ROP may follow oxygen administered solely during anesthesia and postoperative recovery, but the evidence is not conclusive. Undoubtedly, many infants at risk have been given additional inspired oxygen during anesthesia and have not developed ROP.

Occasionally ROP occurs in infants who have never been given additional oxygen, and the cause in these cases is considered to be multifactorial. Other risk factors for ROP include hypoxia, hypercarbia or hypocarbia, blood transfusion, exposure to light, recurrent apnea, sepsis, and other systemic illness.

All preterm infants should be examined regularly by an ophthalmologist. However, the smallest infants, who are at greatest risk, are very difficult to assess. The inspired oxygen concentration should be carefully controlled to avoid unnecessary hyperoxia. The safe level of arterial oxygen pressure (PaO_2) is now considered to be 50–70 mmHg. Continuous monitoring of oxygen saturation at a preductal site (right hand or earlobe), maintaining the arterial oxygen saturation (SaO_2) at 90%–95%, and avoiding major fluctuations in oxygenation are recommended. Vitamin E, administered regularly while the infant is receiving oxygen therapy, may confer some protection against ROP and reduce the severity of the disease. In the operating room, the anesthesiologist should certainly avoid unnecessary hyperoxia, and systemic oxygenation should be monitored in all patients at risk for ROP. Obviously it may still be necessary, on occasion, to err on the side of safety. Major surgery does not appear to predispose patients to ROP.

Suggested Additional Reading

Betts EK, Downes JJ, Schaffer DB, and Johns R: Retrolental fibroplasia and oxygen administration during general anesthesia. Anesthesiology 47:518, 1977.

Cunningham S, Fleck BW, Elton RA, and McIntosh N: Transcutaneous oxygen levels in retinopathy of prematurity. Lancet 346:1464–1465, 1995.

Flynn JT: Oxygen and retrolental fibroplasia: update and challenge. Anesthesiology 60:397–399, 1984.

Phelps DL: Retinopathy of prematurity. Pediatr Rev 16:50–56, 1995.

RESPIRATORY SYSTEM

The respiratory system is of special interest to the anesthesiologist. It is the route of administration of inhaled anesthetic agents, and its functions may be significantly altered during and after anesthesia. Changes in the respiratory system occur continuously from infancy to about age 12 years as it grows to maturity. This section describes the respiratory system of the newborn and its subsequent development.

Anatomy

There are major anatomic differences in the neonate and small infant that are important to the anesthesiologist:

1. The head is relatively large and the neck is short.
2. The tongue is relatively large and readily blocks the pharynx during and after anesthesia: therefore, an oropharyngeal airway may be required. The large tongue may also hamper attempts to visualize the glottis at laryngoscopy.
3. The nasal passages are narrow and are readily blocked by secretions or edema. Nasal obstruction can cause serious problems because young infants may not immediately switch to mouth-breathing. Neonates were previously described as "obligate nose-breathers," but whether this is always true has been questioned. It is certain that the neonate may not immediately convert to mouth-breathing if the nasal passages are obstructed. Studies of obstructive apnea in infants suggest that upper airway obstruction is more likely to occur when the head is in a flexed position. The anesthesiologist should ensure that the infant's head is extended after extubation while the patient is still under the influence of anesthetic drugs. Insertion of a nasogastric tube (NGT) also increases airway resistance; if the nares are of unequal size, the NGT should be inserted into the smaller nostril.
4. The larynx is situated more cephalad (C4) and anteriorly, and its long axis is directed inferiorly and anteriorly. The high cervical level of the larynx in the infant means that elevation of the head to the "sniffing position" during intubation will not assist in visualization of the glottis compared with the adult patient. In the infant, if the head is elevated, the larynx also tends to move anteriorly.
5. The airway is narrowest at the level of the cricoid cartilage just below the vocal cords. Here it is lined with pseudostratified, ciliated epithelium that is loosely bound to underlying areolar tissue. Any trauma to these tissues results in edema, and even a small amount of circumferential edema significantly encroaches on the small area of the infant airway. This reduces the lumen and greatly increases the resistance to airflow, causing stridor. Insertion of an endotracheal tube similarly encroaches on this space as the internal diameter of the tube essentially becomes the area for gas flow; hence, airway resistance increases. This becomes more significant with smaller infants.
6. The epiglottis is relatively long and stiff. It is U-shaped and projects posteriorly at an angle of 45° above the glottis. Often it must be elevated by the tip of a laryngoscope blade before the glottis can be seen. For this reason, the use of a straight-blade laryngoscope is recommended for infants and children.

7. The trachea is short (approximately 5 cm in the neonate), so precise placement and firm fixation of the endotracheal tube are essential. The tracheal cartilages are soft and can easily be compressed by the fingers of an anesthetist holding a mask or collapsed by the patient's vigorous attempts to breathe against an obstructed airway.
8. The right main bronchus is larger than the left and is less acutely angled at its origin. For this reason, if the endotracheal tube is advanced too far, it almost invariably enters the right main bronchus.
9. Because the ribs are almost horizontal, ventilation is mainly diaphragmatic. The abdominal viscera are bulky and can hinder diaphragmatic excursion, especially if the gastrointestinal tract is distended.

Table 2–1 lists the approximate airway dimensions in infants and children.

Physiology

Breathing movements begin in utero and are characteristically rapid, irregular, and episodic during late pregnancy. Normally, they are present for 30% of the time in the third trimester and are subject to diurnal variation. Fetal breathing movements may play a role in development of the lungs and provide exercise for the respiratory muscles. Monitoring of these movements may provide information on fetal health: hypoxemia leads to a decrease in fetal breathing, and severe hypoxemia leads to gasping movements. The fetal lung is filled with fluid, which is moved by this respiratory activity. After 26–28 weeks of gestation, production of surface-active substances (surfactants) is established in the type II pneumocytes. Surfactant is secreted into the lung and can be detected in amniotic fluid samples, providing a diagnostic index of lung maturity and hence neonatal prognosis (*see* page 22).

Passage of the fetus through the birth canal compresses the thorax,

Table 2–1. Approximate Airway Dimensions in Infants and Children

Age (yr)	Tracheal Length (cm)	Trachea (AP)	Diameter (mm) Right Bronchus	Left Bronchus
>0.5	5.9	5.0	4.5	3.5
0.5–1	7.2	5.5	4.8	3.7
1–2	7.5	6.3	5.1	3.9
2–4	8.0	7.5	6.4	4.9
4–6	8.6	8.0	6.7	5.3
6–8	9.5	9.2	7.9	6.1
8–10	10	9.75	8.4	6.5
10–12	11.5	10.5	9.2	6.8
12–14	13.5	11.5	9.8	7.5
14–16	14.5	13.2	11.5	8.8

forcing much of the fluid from the lungs through the nose and mouth. On delivery, this compression is relieved and some air is sucked into the lungs. The onset of regular, continuous breathing has been thought to be initiated by peripheral (cold, touch, and so forth) and biochemical (respiratory and metabolic acidosis) stimuli, but this has been questioned. Other factors may be important, such as a rise in the PaO_2 or a hormonal or chemical mediator. The first few spontaneous breaths are characterized by high transpulmonary pressures (more than 50 cmH$_2$O. They establish the functional residual capacity (FRC) of the neonate's lungs. Remaining lung fluid is removed over the first few days of life by the pulmonary lymphatics and blood vessels. Infants who are delivered by cesarean section are not subjected to the same thoracic squeeze and may have more residual fluid in the lungs. This can cause them to have transient respiratory distress.

The stability of the alveolar matrix in the newborn depends on the presence of adequate amounts of surfactant, which may be deficient in the premature infant. Lack of surfactant leads to collapse of alveoli, maldistribution of ventilation, impaired gas exchange, decreased compliance, and increased work of breathing—the respiratory distress syndrome (RDS). Not surprisingly, pneumothorax occurs more commonly during the neonatal period than at any other age.

Control of Ventilation in the Newborn

Observations of neonatal control of ventilation are difficult to interpret. First, the intervention necessary to obtain measurements (e.g., placing a mask on the face) may itself induce a change in ventilation. Second, the use of measurements of ventilation to assess "respiratory drive" assumes that the respiratory muscles are performing optimally to convert this "drive" into work, and such may not be the case.

Control of ventilation, which involves biochemical and reflex mechanisms, is well developed in the healthy full-term neonate but demonstrates some differences from that in adults. Ventilation of the infant in relation to body mass is greater for any given arterial carbon dioxide pressure ($PaCO_2$), reflecting a higher metabolic rate. The ventilatory response to hypercapnia is less in the neonate than in older infants, and less still in the preterm neonate. Any increase in ventilation is not well sustained. The slope of the carbon dioxide response curve is also decreased in infants displaying episodes of apnea. Hypoxemia decreases the response of the neonate to hypercapnia.

The newborn is sensitive to changes in arterial oxygen tension (PaO_2). Administration of 100% oxygen decreases ventilation, indicating the existence of chemoreceptor activity. The ventilatory response of the newborn to hypoxia is modified by many factors, including gestational and postnatal age, body temperature, and sleep state. Preterm and full-term infants younger than 1 week of age who are awake and normothermic usually demonstrate a biphasic response—a brief period of hyperpnea followed by ventilatory depression. Hypothermic infants respond to hypoxia with ventilatory depression without initial hyperpnea. This depression of ventilation is thought to be caused by the central effects of hypoxia on the cortex and medulla. The peripheral chemoreceptors, although demonstrated to be active in newborns, are presumably unable to maintain a significant influence on this response. Infants may show a less sustained response to hypoxia during rapid eye movement (REM) sleep. During hypoxia, the ventilatory response to carbon dioxide is depressed in the newborn in contrast to that in infants and adults. Hypoxia may induce periodic breathing in infants, and this may be abolished by oxygen administration. Full-term infants older than 2–3 weeks of age demonstrate hyperpnea in response to hypoxia, probably as a result of maturing of the chemoreceptor function.

Reflexes arising from the lung and chest wall are probably more important in maintaining ventilation in the newborn, primarily determining the rate (f) and tidal volume (V_T). The Hering-Breuer inflation reflex, which is active in the newborn, is even more powerful in the premature infant. This reflex disappears during REM sleep and progressively fades during the early weeks of life. The paradoxical "head" reflex, a large inspiration triggered by a small lung inflation, is active in the newborn. It may play a role in maintaining the lung volume of the newborn, and it persists even during deep halothane anesthesia.

Periodic breathing (rapid ventilation alternating with periods of apnea lasting 5–10 seconds) occurs in many preterm and some full-term infants. It is thought to result from incoordination with the feedback loops controlling ventilation. In the preterm infant, the $PaCO_2$ level is higher than normal during these episodes of periodic breathing, but the heart rate does not change significantly. In the full-term infant, hypocapnia may be found during periodic breathing, which seems to have no serious physiologic consequences and usually ceases by 44–46 weeks of postconceptual age.

Some preterm infants demonstrate far more serious and indeed life-threatening episodes of apnea. These commonly exceed 20 seconds and are accompanied by bradycardia. The pathogenesis of apnea in preterm infants is not clearly understood. Apnea may reflect excessive physiologic demands on an immature respiratory control system. A variety of pathophysiologic mechanisms seem to be involved, however. Apneic episodes may result from a failure of central control mechanisms (central apnea); in such instances, there is no ventilatory effort. It may also be caused by airway obstruction (obstructive apnea), in which case ventilatory effort may be observed but there is no gas exchange. Obstruction usually occurs in the infant's nasopharynx or pharynx. Mixed forms of apnea may occur, and one type may progress to the other (e.g., obstructive apnea may progress to central apnea). Apnea may also result from failure of the ventilatory muscles. Many apneic episodes occur during REM sleep, when it is possible that ventilatory muscle fatigue may be an important factor. Although neonatal apnea may be idiopathic, it may also be symptomatic of an underlying disease process, such as sepsis, intracranial bleeding, anemia, or patent ductus arteriosus.

Preterm infants must be carefully monitored to detect apneic episodes. Treatment is by tactile stimulation or, if this fails, by bag-and-mask resuscitation. The incidence of apneic episodes is decreased by therapy with aminophylline (central stimulation) or by institution of continuous positive airway pressure (increased reflex activity of lung and chest wall reflexes and "splinting" of the airway).

Muscles of Ventilation

The newborn's muscles of ventilation are subject to fatigue, a tendency that is determined by the types of muscle fiber present. In preterm infants, less than 10% of the fibers in the diaphragm are type I (slow-twitch, highly oxidative, fatigue-resistant). In full-term infants, 30% of these fibers are type I, and the percentage increases to 55% (the adult level) over the first year of life. The preterm infant is therefore prone to ventilatory muscle fatigue, a predisposition that progressively disappears with maturity. Ventilation is also affected by changes that occur during changing sleep states. The preterm infant spends 50%–60% of this time in REM sleep, during which intercostal muscle activity is inhibited and paradoxic movement of the soft chest wall occurs. The lack of intercostal activity is compensated by an increase in diaphragmatic activity. Much of this activity is wasted when the ribs move paradoxically and may lead to diaphragmatic fatigue.

Mechanics of Ventilation

The specific compliance of the lung (CL) increases slowly after birth as fluid is removed from the lung. At 1 week it is high, the elastic recoil of the lungs being low. The chest wall compliance of the infant (especially the preterm infant) is very high, so that total compliance approximates CL. This highly compliant chest wall provides only a relatively weak force to maintain the FRC and to oppose the action of the diaphragm. The FRC of the small infant is thought to be maintained by the high respiratory rate, the point of termination of expiration, the controlled expiration ("laryngeal braking"), and the tonic activity of the ventilatory muscles. This being so, it is not surprising that large declines in FRC occur with apnea or during anesthesia.

These large declines in FRC are accompanied by airway closure and impaired oxygenation. Intercostal muscle inhibition during REM sleep or with the use of inhaled anesthetic agents compounds the weakness of the chest wall and results in paradoxic movement. This paradoxic chest wall movement is, of course, markedly increased by any obstruction to ventilation. It may be inferred that infants generally require controlled ventilation during anesthesia and benefit from high respiratory rates or use of positive end-expiratory pressure to maintain the lung volume and avoid airway closure. As the child grows through infancy and childhood, the rib cage stiffens so that it becomes better able to oppose the action of the diaphragm and less reliant on intercostal muscle tone.

The transpulmonary pressure needed to achieve optimal lung inflation is remarkably similar in healthy infants, children, and adults. During artificial ventilation, peak inspiratory pressures of 15–20 cmH$_2$O are normal.

The nasal air passages contribute as much as 50% of the total airway flow resistance in white infants and slightly less in black infants. Insertion of an NGT increases this resistance by as much as 50%. The nasal passages are usually of unequal size; if an NGT is inserted, it should be placed through the smaller nostril, so as to have a lesser effect on total nasal airway resistance. The resistance of the neonate's peripheral airways is now thought to be low and to increase with age.

Lung Volumes in the Newborn

In the full-term infant, total lung capacity (TLC) is approximately 160 ml; the FRC is about half this volume. The V$_T$ is approximately 16 ml, and the dead space volume (V$_D$) is about 5 ml (0.3% of the V$_T$). Relative to body size, all of these volumes are similar to adult values. Note, however, that any dead space in anesthesia or ventilator circuits is much more significant in relation to the small volumes of the infant (e.g., a 5-ml apparatus dead space would increase the total effective V$_D$ by 100%).

In contrast to the static lung volumes, alveolar ventilation (V$_A$) is proportionally much larger in the newborn (100 to 150 ml per kilogram of body weight* per minute) than in the adult (60 ml/kg/min). This high V$_A$ in the infant results in a V$_A$:FRC ratio of 5:1, compared with 1.5:1 in the adult. Consequently, the FRC is a much less effective "buffer" in the infant, so that changes in the concentration of inspired gases (including anesthetic gases) are more rapidly reflected in alveolar and arterial values.

The closing volume (CV) is higher in infants and young children than in young adults; it may exceed the FRC to encroach on the V$_T$ during normal ventilation. Airway closure during normal ventilation may explain the lower normal values for PaO$_2$ during infancy and childhood (Table 2–2). A fall in FRC, which usually occurs during general anesthesia and persists into the postoperative period, may be expected to further increase the significance of the high CV and further increase the alveolar-arterial oxygen tension gradient (A-aDO$_2$). The younger the infant or child, the larger is this fall in FRC. There is a requirement to increase

---

*Note. Hereafter, throughout this manual, "kilogram of body weight" is expressed simply as kilograms (kg).

Table 2–2. Arterial Oxygen Tension in Healthy Infants and Children

Age	Normal Arterial Oxygen (mmHg) in Room Air
0–1 wk	70
1–10 mo	85
4–8 yr	90
12–16 yr	96

the oxygen concentration of inspired gases. The perioperative fall in FRC may be less during operations with the patient prone and the abdomen hanging free, and it may be partially reversed by continuous positive airway pressure.

The total surface area of the air-tissue interface of the alveoli is small in the infant (2.8 m^2). When this area is related to the metabolic rate for oxygen ($\dot{V}O_2$), it is apparent that the ratio between surface area and rate of oxygen consumption is smaller in the infant than the adult. As a result the infant has a reduced reserve capability for gas exchange. This fact may assume great significance if congenital defects (e.g., diaphragmatic hernia) are associated with pulmonary hypoplasia or if the lungs become damaged (e.g., from meconium aspiration). In such cases, the remaining healthy lung tissue may be inadequate to sustain life.

Work of Breathing

The muscles of ventilation generate the force necessary to overcome the resistance to airflow as well as the elastic recoil of the lungs and chest wall. These two factors dictate, for each child, an optimal rate of ventilation and V_T that delivers a given V_A while expending minimal muscular energy. Because the time constant of the infant's lung is relatively short, efficient alveolar ventilation can be achieved at high respiratory rates. In the newborn, a respiratory rate of 37 breaths/min has been calculated to be most efficient; this is close to the rate observed in the healthy newborn. Full-term infants are similar to adults in that they require 1% of their metabolic energy to maintain ventilation; the oxygen cost of breathing is 0.5 ml per 0.5 L of ventilation. The preterm infant has a higher oxygen cost of breathing (0.9 ml/0.5 L), which is greatly increased if the lungs are diseased, as in RDS or bronchopulmonary dysplasia.

Ventilation-Perfusion Relationships in the Newborn Lung

Ventilation ($\dot{V}$) and perfusion ($\dot{Q}$) are imperfectly matched in the neonatal lung. This may be in part a result of gas trapping in the lungs. $\dot{V}/\dot{Q}$ mismatch is evident in the alveolar-arterial nitrogen difference (A-aDN$_2$), which is 25 mmHg immediately after birth and declines to about 10 mmHg within the first week. The normal PaO$_2$ in an infant breathing room air is about 50 mmHg just after birth and increases to 70 mmHg by 24 hours of age. The high A-aDO$_2$ in infants is mainly caused by persisting anatomic shunts (*see* page 26) and the relatively high CV.

Lung Surfactant

Surfactants in the alveolar lining layer stabilize the alveoli, preventing their collapse on expiration. Lowering of the surface tension at the air-liquid interface in the alveoli also reduces the force required for their reexpansion. The principal surfactant in the lung is lecithin, which is produced by type II pneumocytes. The quantity of lecithin produced in the fetal lung rises progressively, beginning at 22 weeks of gestation and increasing sharply at 35 to 36 weeks, as the lung matures. The lecithin production of the lung can be assessed by determining the lecithin-sphingomyelin (L/S) ratio in amniotic fluid. The L/S ratio is less than 1 until 32 weeks' gestation; it is 2 by 35 weeks and 4–6 at term.

Premature infants with inadequate pulmonary lecithin production suffer from RDS. The biochemical pathways for surfactant production may also be depressed by hypoxia, hyperoxia, acidosis, or hypothermia; therefore, early correction of these abnormalities in the sick neonate is vitally important. Inhaled anesthetic agents seem to have little effect on surfactant production. Maturation of biochemical processes in the lungs of the fetus in utero may be accelerated by the administration of corticosteroids to the mother.

Lung Growth and Development

The lungs continue to develop during the first two decades of life. The number of alveoli increases rapidly over the first 6 years, almost reaching adult levels, but growth continues into adolescence. In young children, the small size of the peripheral airways may predispose to obstructive lung diseases such as bronchiolitis.

Pulmonary Function Testing in Pediatric Patients

Children older than 6 years of age may cooperate sufficiently to enable standard tests of pulmonary function to be performed, and these may be an important part of the preoperative assessment. However, they should be interpreted to account for the degree of cooperation obtained. Maximum expiratory and inspiratory flow-volume curves may be useful in determining the site and nature of airway obstruction; for example, they can differentiate between intrathoracic and extrathoracic obstruction. Such studies may be most useful in the preoperative assessment of patients with a mediastinal mass. Spirometric studies may provide useful information as to the degree of reversible airway obstruction present in those with a disease such as asthma and may assist in preoperative planning. They also may indicate the extent of restrictive disease in patients with a disease such as scoliosis, thereby predicting the likelihood of postoperative pulmonary insufficiency.

Methods to measure passive respiratory mechanics in infants have been devised. These depend on producing expiratory flow-volume curves during a passive lung deflation. Normal values have been documented, and these studies may become important in preoperative assessment in the near future.

Changes with Anesthesia

The following is a summary of some of the major changes that occur in the respiratory system during and after anesthesia.

1. Spontaneous ventilation is decreased by the potent volatile anesthetics. This is thought to occur because of the combined effects of anesthetic drugs on the central chemical control of ventilation and on the muscles of ventilation. Intercostal muscle activity is inhibited by potent volatile anesthetic agents (e.g., halothane); consequently, diaphragmatic breathing predominates and the chest wall may move paradoxically, especially if the airway is obstructed. Surgical stimulation tends to increase ventilation back toward normal levels. The effect of intravenous agents on ventilation in children is not well documented.
2. The FRC is reduced during general inhalation anesthesia with or without neuromuscular block. This reduction is greatest in the youngest patients and is caused by elevation of the diaphragm and loss of chest wall stability. As the FRC falls, airway closure may occur during tidal ventilation, with consequent impaired oxygen transfer in the lung.
3. The ratio of dead space to tidal volume ($V_D:V_T$) remains constant in patients breathing spontaneously but may increase in those whose ventilation is controlled. During controlled ventilation, major alterations in gas distribution within the lungs occur as a result of changes in the action of the diaphragm. This effect tends to markedly unbalance the $\dot{V}/\dot{Q}$ matching of the lungs.
4. Compliance is little changed and airway resistance is generally reduced by the bronchodilator action of potent volatile anesthetic agents. Insertion of an endotracheal tube increases total flow resistance (*see* page 16), especially in patients younger than 5 years of age.
5. The efficiency of gas exchange may be impaired by the effects of anesthetic drugs on the physiologic processes that normally control the regional distribution of gases and blood throughout the lung, particularly by hypoxic pulmonary vasoconstriction.
6. Laryngospasm occurs more frequently in association with pediatric anesthesia, especially during induction and after extubation (*see* Ch. 3.) Laryngeal closure results from apposition of the vocal cords and supraglottic structures. The reason for the increased incidence of laryngospasm in children is unknown.

Suggested Additional Reading

Respiratory System: Anatomy

Crelin ES: Development of the lower respiratory system. Clin Symp 28:1, 1976.

Crelin ES: Development of the upper respiratory system. Clin Symp 29:1, 1977.

Eckenhoff JE: Some anatomic considerations of the infant larynx influencing endotracheal anesthesia. Anesthesiology 12:401, 1951.

Griscom NT and Wohl MEB: Dimensions of the growing trachea related to age and gender. AJR Am J Roentgenol 146:233–237, 1986.

Morgan GAR and Steward DJ: Linear airway dimensions in children: including those with cleft palate. Can Anaesth Soc J 29:1–8, 1982.

Westhorpe RN: The position of the larynx in children and its relationship to the ease of intubation. Anaesth Intensive Care 15:384–388, 1987.

Respiratory System: Physiology

Bryan AC and Bryan MH: Control of respiration in the newborn. Clin Perinatol 5:269, 1978.

Dawes GS, Fox HE, Leduc BM, et al.: Respiratory movements and rapid eye movement sleep in the foetal lamb. J Physiol (Lond) 220:119, 1972.

Gaultier C: Early disturbances in cardiorespiratory control. Pediatr Pulmonol Suppl 16:225–227, 1997.

Gluck L, Kulovich MV, Eidelman AL, et al.: Biochemical development of surface activity in mammalian lung: IV. Pulmonary lecithin synthesis in the human fetus and newborn and etiology of the respiratory distress syndrome. Pediatr Res 6:81, 1972.

Hatch D and Fletcher M: Anaesthesia and the ventilatory system in infants and young children. Br J Anaesth 68:398–410, 1992.

Henderson-Smart DJ, Pettygrew AG, and Campbell DJ: Clinical apnea and brainstem neural function in preterm infants. N Engl J Med 308:353, 1983.

Mansell A, Bryan C, and Levison H: Airway closure in children. J Appl Physiol 33:711, 1972.

Merkus PJ, ten Have-Opbroek AA, and Quanier PH: Human lung growth: a review. Pediatr Pulmonol 21:383–397, 1996.

Miller MJ and Martin RJ: Apnea of prematurity. Clin Perinatol 19:789–808, 1992.

Motoyama EK: Respiratory physiology in infants and children. In Motoyama EK and Davis PJ (eds.): Anesthesia for Infants and Children, 5th ed. St. Louis, Mosby, 1990, pp 11–76.

Rigatto H: Maturation of breathing. Clin Perinatol 19:739–756, 1992.

Roy WL and Lerman J: Laryngospasm in paediatric anaesthesia. Can Anaesth Soc J 35:93–98, 1987.

Stocks J: Effect of nasogastric tubes on nasal resistance during infancy. Arch Dis Child 55:17–21, 1980.

Thach BT: Neuromuscular control of upper airway patency. Clin Perinatol 19:773–788, 1992.

Woo SW, Berlin D, and Hedley-Whyte J: Surfactant function and anesthetic agents. J Appl Physiol 26:571, 1969.

CARDIOVASCULAR SYSTEM

Fetus

Much of our information has been gained from studies conducted in lambs. However, a few studies in previable human fetuses indicate that the cardiovascular systems are reasonably comparable.

The fetal cardiovascular system perfuses the low-resistance placental circulation, directing 36%–42% of the combined ventricular output to this organ; only 5%–10% goes to the lungs. Flow to the fetal lungs is limited by their high vascular resistance; as a result, blood bypasses the lungs via the foramen ovale and the ductus arteriosus. Most of the blood returning from the placenta bypasses the liver via the ductus venosus. The pattern of flow from the inferior vena cava into the right atrium (RA) ensures that about one-third of the oxygenated placental blood (partial pressure of oxygen [PO_2], 28–30 mmHg) is directed through the foramen ovale into the left atrium. This blood, which combines with the limited venous return from the lungs, is pumped by the left ventricle into the ascending aorta and thence to the coronary, cerebral, and forelimb circulations. Blood returning via the superior vena cava (PO_2, 12–14 mmHg) passes through the RA into the right ventricle, from which most of the output flows through the ductus arteriosus into the descending aorta. Thus blood supplied to the heart and upper body has a higher oxygen content (saturation, 65%; PO_2, 26–28 mmHg) than that supplied to the abdominal organs, lower limbs, and placenta (saturation, 55%–60%; PO_2, 20–22 mmHg). In utero, the right ventricle pumps about 66% of the combined ventricular output, and the left ventricle pumps the remaining 34%.

Changes at Birth

At birth pulmonary ventilation is normally established quickly, and blood flow to the lungs is greatly increased while placental flow ceases. When the lungs expand and fill with gas, pulmonary vascular resistance (PVR) falls markedly as a result of mechanical effects on the vessels and relaxation of pulmonary vasomotor tone when the PO_2 rises and the partial pressure of CO_2 falls in alveolar gas. PVR falls by 80% from prenatal levels within a few minutes after normal initiation of ventilation. As PVR falls, blood flow to the lungs and then via the pulmonary veins into the left atrium increases, increasing left atrium pressure above that in the RA and closing the atrial septum over the foramen ovale.

Simultaneously, as flow to the placenta ceases because of clamping or umbilical artery constriction, a large, low-resistance vascular bed is excluded from the systemic circulation. This activity results in a large increase in systemic vascular resistance and a decline in inferior vena cava blood flow and RA pressure. The increase in systemic vascular resistance and the simultaneous fall in PVR elevate the aortic pressure above that in the pulmonary artery. Blood flow through the ductus arteriosus reverses (i.e., becomes left to right), and the ductus fills with oxygenated blood. This increased local PO_2 (to levels greater than 50–60 mmHg) causes the muscular wall of the ductus arteriosus to constrict. The entire sequence of biochemical events leading to closure of the ductus is not known, but a prostaglandin-mediated response is involved. Shunts may persist through the ductus for some hours after birth, producing audible murmurs. Normally, however, flow through the ductus is insignificant by 15 hours. Permanent histologic closure of the ductus is usually complete within 5–7 days but may not occur until 3 weeks have passed.

The ductus venosus, which communicates between the umbilical veins, the portal vein, and the inferior vena cava, also remains patent for several days after birth. This channel provides a shunt past the hepatic circulation and therefore may delay the clearance of drugs metabolized in the liver (e.g., narcotic analgesics).

Transitional Circulation

During the early neonatal period, reversion to the fetal circulatory pattern is possible under some circumstances. If hypoxia occurs, PVR increases and the ductus arteriosus may reopen; a significant proportion of blood then again bypasses the (now high-resistance) pulmonary circulation, causing a further decline in arterial oxygenation. Impaired tissue oxygenation then results in acidosis, which causes a further increase in PVR, establishing a vicious circle of hypoxemia → acidosis → impaired pulmonary blood flow → hypoxemia. Reversion to a fetal pattern of circulation may complicate any condition that causes hypoxemia or acidemia (e.g., RDS or congenital diaphragmatic hernia).

Newborn Cardiovascular System

Heart and Cardiac Output

In healthy neonates the right ventricle exceeds the left in wall thickness. This preponderance is evident in the electrocardiogram, which shows an axis of up to +180° during the first week of life. After birth the left ventricle enlarges disproportionately. By about 3–6 months, the adult ratio of ventricular size is established (axis approximately +90°). During the immediate newborn period, the heart rate is between 100 and 170 beats/min and the rhythm is regular. As the child grows, the heart rate gradually decreases (Table 2–3).

Sinus arrhythmia is common in children. All other irregular rhythms must be considered abnormal.

Systolic blood pressure is approximately 60 mmHg in the full-term newborn, and the diastolic pressure is 35 mmHg. These pressures vary considerably and may be 10–15 mmHg higher if clamping of the cord is delayed or the cord is "stripped." In either case they fall to normal levels within 4 hours. Preterm infants have lower arterial pressures, as low as 45/25 mmHg in the 750-g baby (Table 2–4).

The myocardium of the newborn contains less contractile tissue and more supporting tissue than the adult heart. Consequently, the neonate's

Table 2–3. Normal Heart Rate

Age	Heart Rate (beats/min) Average	Range
Newborn	120	100–170
1–11 mo	120	80–160
2 yr	110	80–130
4 yr	100	80–120
6 yr	100	75–115
8 yr	90	70–110
10 yr	90	70–110
14 yr		
Boys	80	60–100
Girls	85	65–105
16 yr		
Boys	75	55–95
Girls	80	60–100

Table 2–4. Normal Blood Pressure*

| Age | Blood Pressure (mmHg) | | |
---	Systolic	Diastolic	Mean
Newborn			
Preterm (750 g)	44	24	33
Preterm (1,000 g)	49	26	34.5
Full term	60	35	45
3–10 days	70–75		
6 mo	95		
4 yr	98	57	
6 yr	110	60	
8 yr	112	60	
12 yr	115	65	
16 yr	120	65	

*Reported normal blood pressure values for infants and children must be considered in light of their methods of determination. These values should serve as a guide only (*see* Monitoring During Anesthesia, page 102).

ventricles are less compliant when relaxed and generate less tension during contraction. Because the low compliance of the relaxed ventricle tends to limit the size of the stroke volume, the cardiac output of the newborn is to a large extent rate dependent. Bradycardia is invariably accompanied by reduced cardiac output. The less compliant ventricle of the neonate is also dependent on an adequate filling pressure, so that hypovolemia is followed by a fall in cardiac output. Cardiac output is both rate dependent and volume dependent. Reduced compliance and contractility of the ventricles also predisposes the infant heart to failure with increased volume load. In the infant, failure of one ventricle rapidly compromises the function of the other, and biventricular failure results.

The reduced contractility of the neonatal heart is also thought to be secondary to the immaturity of the myofibrils and to the less developed sarcoplasmic reticulum. It is postulated that the cyclic calcium flux within the neonatal myocardium is more dependent on exchange across the cell membrane (sarcolemma) and less a function of the sarcoplasmic reticulum. As the infant grows, the myocardial sarcoplasmic reticulum expands and progressively assumes a dominant role in intracellular calcium regulation, which is typical of the adult heart. The greater role of the sarcolemma in calcium regulation within the myocyte may explain the greater sensitivity of the neonate to halothane-induced myocardial depression. It may also explain the severe cardiac depressant effects of calcium channel-blocking drugs in the neonate.

The autonomic innervation of the heart is incomplete in the newborn, and there is a relative lack of sympathetic elements. This may further compromise the ability of the less contractile neonatal myocardium to respond to stress. The differences in the newborn's myocardium are all particularly marked in the preterm infant.

In the neonate, shunts hamper the precise measurement of cardiac output, which averages two to three times that of the adult on a milliliter per kilogram of body weight basis and is appropriate to the metabolic rate. The total systemic vascular resistance is low, reflecting the high proportion of vessel-rich tissue (19%—twice that in the adult) and permitting a high cardiac output despite a low systemic blood pressure.

Pulmonary Circulation

The changes in the pulmonary circulation that occur at birth continue with a slower progressive decline in PVR over the first 3 months of life. This is associated with a parallel regression in the thickness of the medial muscle layer of the pulmonary arterioles. During the neonatal period, PVR is still high and the muscular pulmonary vessels are highly reactive. Hypoxia, acidosis, and stress (e.g., from endotracheal suctioning) may all result in rapid elevation of PVR. If elevation of the PVR is sustained by such stimuli, right-sided intracardiac pressures may exceed those on the left and right-to-left shunting may ensue via the ductus arteriosus or foramen ovale. Right ventricular failure, rapidly progressing to biventricular failure, may occur.

In some circumstances the normal regression of the muscular layer of the pulmonary vessels and the associated fall in PVR may not occur. Continued hypoxemia, caused for example by high altitude or by continued high pulmonary blood flow due to left-to-right shunts (ventricular septal defect, patent ductus arteriosus, etc.), may result in persistence of a high PVR into childhood and beyond. Initially this high PVR is reversible (e.g., with pulmonary vasodilators). Later structural changes in the pulmonary vascular bed lead to irreversible pulmonary vascular obstructive disease.

Nitric oxide has been identified as an endothelium-derived relaxing factor that is normally produced continually in the lung to regulate pulmonary vascular tone. This has led to the use of nitric oxide inhalation to treat pulmonary hypertension.

Blood Volume

Blood volume varies considerably during the immediate postnatal period and depends on the amount of blood drained from the placenta before the cord is clamped. Delay in clamping or stripping the cord may increase the blood volume by more than 20%, resulting in transient respiratory distress. Conversely, fetal hypoxia during labor causes vasoconstriction and a shift of blood to the placental circulation, and asphyxiated neonates may be hypovolemic.

The response to hypovolemia and restoration of the blood volume are of great importance to the anesthesiologist, because surgery in the newborn is often accompanied by significant blood loss. Withdrawal of blood during exchange transfusion has been demonstrated to cause a progressive parallel decline in systolic blood pressure and cardiac output. Reinfusion of an equal volume of blood restores these parameters to their original values. The changes in arterial blood pressure are proportional to the degree of hypovolemia. A newborn's capacity to adapt the intravascular volume to the available blood volume is very limited, perhaps as a result of less efficient control of capacitance vessels. The baroreflexes of the infant, especially the preterm infant, are inactive, further compromising the response to hypovolemia.

In summary, the infant's systolic arterial blood pressure is closely related to the circulating blood volume. Blood pressure is an excellent guide to the adequacy of blood replacement during anesthesia, a fact that is amply confirmed by extensive clinical experience. The hypovolemic infant is unable to maintain an adequate cardiac output; hence, accurate early volume replacement is essential.

Table 2–5 shows approximate normal values for blood volume in pediatric patients. Values may be higher, however, particularly in the preterm infant.

Response to Hypoxia

Because of the high $\dot{V}O_2$, hypoxemia can develop rapidly in the neonate. The first observed response is usually bradycardia in contrast to tachycardia in the adult. The anesthesiologist should treat any episode of unexplained bradycardia by immediately ventilating the patient with 100% oxygen. During hypoxemia, pulmonary vasoconstriction occurs and the pulmonary artery pressure increases more than that in adults. The ductus arteriosus may reopen simultaneously. Then a large right-to-left shunt develops, further decreasing SaO_2. Changes in cardiac output and systemic vascular resistance in infants also differ from those in older children and adults. During hypoxemia, the principal response in adults is systemic vasodilation, which, together with an increased cardiac output, helps to maintain oxygen transport to the tissues. The fetus and some neonates respond to hypoxemia with systemic vasoconstriction. During fetal life this directs more blood to the placenta, but after birth this response may reduce cardiac output, further limiting oxygen transport and forcing the heart to work harder. In the infant, the early and pronounced bradycardia in response to hypoxia may be caused by myocardial hypoxia and acidosis.

Neonates exposed to hypoxemia experience pulmonary and systemic vasoconstriction, bradycardia, and decreased cardiac output. Rapid intervention is necessary to prevent this state from proceeding to cardiac arrest.

Blood and Oxygen Transport

Neonatal blood volume is approximately 80 ml/kg in the term infant and about 20% higher in the preterm infant (Table 2–5). The hematocrit

Table 2–5. Normal Blood Volume of Children

Age	Blood Volume (ml/kg)
Newborn	80–85
6 wk to 2 yr	75
2 yr to puberty	72

(Hct) is 60%, and the hemoglobin content (Hb) is 18–19 g/dl. The values for blood volume, hematocrit, and Hb content vary from infant to infant, depending on the time of clamping of the umbilical cord. These values change little during the first week of life, after which the Hb level starts to fall. This change occurs more rapidly in the preterm infant.

Most (70%–90%) of the Hb present at birth in a full-term infant is of the fetal type (HbF). The affinity of HbF for oxygen is greater than that of adult hemoglobin (HbA), primarily because of a lack of effect of 2,3-diphosphoglycerate (2,3-DPG) on the HbF-O_2 interaction. HbF combines with more oxygen but releases it less readily in the tissues than does HbA. The PO_2 with 50% hemoglobin saturation (P_{50}) for HbF is approximately 20 mmHg, in contrast to 26–27 mmHg for HbA. Adequate oxygen transport to the tissues of the newborn infant demands a higher Hb concentration. Less than 12 g/dl constitutes anemia, and higher levels are very desirable in hypoxic states. However, there are many risks associated with transfusion. Current thought is that correction of anemia by blood transfusion may be indicated to maintain the Hct higher than 40% in cases of severe cardiopulmonary disease, 30% in moderate cardiopulmonary disease or major surgery, and 25% in symptomatic anemia (apnea, tachycardia, lethargy, poor growth).

Transfusion with HbA-containing erythrocytes may improve oxygen transport to the tissues in the sick preterm infant. However, this treatment has been reported also to increase the risk of ROP.

During the first weeks of life, the hematocrit and Hb levels decline steadily, in part because of a progressive increase in blood volume but also a result of suppression of erythropoiesis caused by improved tissue oxygenation. This physiologic anemia of infancy reaches a low point at 2–3 months of age, with Hb levels of 9–11 g/dl. At this time the HbF content of the blood has been largely replaced by HbA. As a result, oxygen delivery at the tissues is actually improved. Provided that nutrition is adequate, the Hb level now increases gradually over several weeks to 12–13 g/dl, which is maintained during early childhood.

The preterm infant demonstrates an earlier and greater fall in Hb content, reaching 7–8 g/dl in those weighing less than 1,500 g at birth. This finding is the result of a short erythrocyte life span, rapid growth, and low level of erythropoietin production. The early "physiologic" anemia of the preterm infant is often followed by a continuing "late" anemia, which is secondary to nutritional deficiencies. In the infant in the neonatal intensive care unit, this anemia is also commonly caused by repeated blood sampling. Iron therapy is not effective in correcting this situation and may even cause other problems (e.g., hemolysis, infection). Anemia of the preterm infant may lead to tachycardia, tachypnea, poor feeding and growth, diminished activity, and apnea. In severe states, congestive heart failure may occur.

Suggested Additional Reading

Alverson DC: The physiologic impact of anemia in the neonate. Clin Perinatol 22:609–625, 1995.

Anaemia in premature infants [Editorial]. Lancet 2:1371, 1987.

Burrows FA, Klinck JR, Rabinovitch M, and Bohn DJ: Pulmonary hypertension in children: perioperative management. Can Anaesth Soc J 33:606–628, 1986.

Delivoria-Papadopoulos M, Roncevic NP, and Oski FA: Post-natal changes in oxygen transport of term, premature and sick infants: the role of 2,3-diphosphoglycerate and adult hemoglobin. Pediatr Res 5:235, 1971.

Fisher DJ and Towbin J: Maturation of the heart. Clin Perinatol 15:421–446, 1988.

Friedman WF: The intrinsic properties of the developing heart. Prog Cardiovasc Dis 15:87, 1972.

Gregory GA: The baroresponses of preterm infants during halothane anaesthesia. Can Anaesth Soc J 29:105, 1982.

Holland BM, Jones JG, and Wardrup CAJ: Lessons from the anemia of prematurity. Hematol Oncol Clin North Am 1:355, 1987.

James LS and Rowe RD: The pattern of response of pulmonary and systemic arterial pressures in newborn and older infants to short periods of hypoxia. J Pediatr 51:5, 1957.

O'Brien RT and Pearson HA: Physiologic anemia of the newborn infant. J Pediatr 79:132, 1971.

Palmer RM, Ferrige AG, and Moncada S: Nitric oxide release accounts for the biologic activity of endothelium derived relaxing factor. Nature 327:524–526, 1987.

Rowe MI and Marchildon MB: Physiologic considerations in the newborn surgical patient. Surg Clin North Am 56:245, 1976.

Strauss RG: Red blood cell transfusion practices in the neonate. Clin Perinatol 22:641–655, 1955.

Swiet M, Fayers P, and Shinebourne EA: Systolic BP in a population of infants in the first year of life: the Brompton Study. Pediatrics 65:1028, 1980.

Wallgren G, Barr M, and Rudhe U: Hemodynamic studies of induced acute hypo- and hypervolemia in the newborn infant. Acta Paediatr Scand 53:1, 1964.

Wallgren G, Hansen JS, and Lind J: Quantitative studies of the human neonatal circulation: III. Observations on the newborn infant's central circulatory responses to moderate hypovolemia. Acta Paediatr Scand Suppl 179:43, 1967.

Walsh SZ, Meyer WW, and Lind J: The Human Fetal and Neonatal Circulation: Function and Structure. Charles C Thomas, Springfield, IL, 1974.

METABOLISM: FLUID AND ELECTROLYTE BALANCE

Glucose Metabolism

At term the neonate has stores of glycogen that are located mainly in the liver and myocardium. These are used during the first few hours of life until gluconeogenesis becomes established. Small-for-gestational-age and preterm infants may have inadequate glycogen stores and may fail to establish adequate gluconeogenesis.

Hypoglycemia is common in the stressed neonate (Table 2–6). Blood glucose levels should be measured frequently in sick neonates, and levels lower than 40 mg/100 ml or 2.2 mmol/L should be corrected by continuous infusion of 10% dextrose (5–8 mg/kg/min). Symptoms of hypoglycemia (jitteriness, convulsions, apnea) should be treated immediately by slow injection of 10% dextrose (1–2 ml/kg). Neurologic damage occurs in up to 50% of infants with symptomatic hypoglycemia. Infants of diabetic mothers and those with Beckwith-Wiedemann syndrome must be treated with particular care, because a therapeutic dose of intravenous glucose may precipitate hyperinsulinemia and serious rebound hypogly-

Table 2–6. Factors Associated with Hypoglycemia in Neonates

Prematurity
Perinatal stress
Sepsis
Small for gestational age
Polycythemia
Hypoxia
Excess insulin
    Infant of diabetic mother
    Beckwith-Wiedemann syndrome

cemia. A slow infusion of glucose (4–8 mg/kg/min) is recommended for these infants.

Older infants and young children rarely become hypoglycemic during an excessively long preoperative fasting period. Late trends are away from long periods of preoperative fasting (*see* page 70).

Hyperglycemia is a common iatrogenic problem of small infants receiving intravenous therapy, probably as a result of inadequate insulin release and continued hepatic glucose production. The effects of hyperglycemia can be serious. Osmotically induced cerebral fluid shifts may lead to cerebral hemorrhage, and glycosuria may cause diuresis resulting in water and electrolyte depletion. Some evidence suggests that hyperglycemia may also increase the extent of neurologic damage during a cerebral hypoxic-ischemic event. It is essential that glucose therapy be carefully controlled to avoid hyperglycemia.

Calcium Metabolism

Calcium is actively transported across the placenta to meet the needs of the fetus. This transport accelerates near term and may cause a decline in maternal calcium levels. After birth, the infant must depend on its own calcium reserves. However, parathyroid function is not fully established, and vitamin D stores may be inadequate. As a result, hypocalcemia must be anticipated—especially in the preterm infant—after birth trauma, neonatal asphyxia, any severe neonatal illness, or blood transfusion. Correction of metabolic acidosis in the neonate by administration of sodium bicarbonate may also precipitate hypocalcemia.

Symptoms of hypocalcemia include twitching, increased muscle tone, and convulsions. (Obviously, hypocalcemia is not always easily distinguished from hypoglycemia.) The Chvostek sign may be present, but confirmation depends on laboratory test results (total serum calcium, less than 7 mg/dl or 1.75 mmol/L; ionized calcium, less than 4 mg/dl or 1.0 mmol/L) or on the response to therapy. The infant prone to hypocalcemia is treated with continuous calcium chloride infusion at a rate of 5 mg/kg/hr. Symptomatic hypocalcemia requires infusion of 10% calcium gluconate (100–200 mg/kg), with continuous electrocardiographic monitoring. Note that calcium-containing solutions may cause severe skin damage, leading to slough if they leak from the intravenous line into the tissues. They should preferably be given through a central line.

Magnesium Metabolism

Magnesium and calcium metabolism are closely related: an imbalance in one may affect the other. Magnesium levels affect parathyroid hormone secretion, and the renal excretion of calcium and that of magnesium are interrelated. Chronic hypomagnesemia is commonly accompanied by hypocalcemia secondary to the effect on parathyroid function.

Hypomagnesemia is more common in preterm infants, small-for-gestational-age infants, infants of diabetic mothers, and infants with intestinal disease. It may also complicate massive blood transfusion. Hypomagnesemia results in abnormal muscle activity, tremors, seizures, and cardiac arrhythmias.

Hypermagnesemia may complicate renal failure, or, in the neonate, it may be a consequence of the administration of magnesium sulfate to the mother. It may result in depression of the central nervous and respiratory systems, hyporeflexia, and hypotension.

Bilirubin Metabolism

In the full-term infant, unconjugated hyperbilirubinemia during the first week of life (physiologic jaundice) occurs secondary to an increased bilirubin load, limited hepatic cell uptake of bilirubin, and deficient hepatic conjugation to the water-soluble glucuronide. Serum bilirubin levels seldom exceed 7 mg/dl or 103 µmol/L. In preterm infants, higher levels (10–15 mg/dl or 170–255 µmol/L) are commonly reached. These persist for a longer period, owing to a higher bilirubin load and delayed maturation of the hepatic conjugation pathway. The preterm infant may sustain neurologic damage at lower serum bilirubin levels (6–9 mg/dl) than does the full-term infant (20 mg/dl). This predisposition is a result of the infant's less effective blood-brain barrier and may be exacerbated by hypoxia, acidosis, or hypothermia, or a low level of serum albumin and hence decreased binding sites. The preterm infant must be carefully monitored for increased serum bilirubin levels, and specific treatment should be administered as required. Treatment includes phototherapy and possibly exchange transfusion. Some drugs (e.g., diazepam, sulfonamides, furosemide) displace protein-bound bilirubin and therefore increase the danger of neurologic damage. There are no reports of anesthetic drugs (except benzodiazepines) producing adverse changes in bilirubin levels, but hypoxia, acidosis, hypothermia, and hypoalbuminemia may all increase the danger.

Suggested Additional Reading

Hall SC, Przybylo HJ, and Roth AG: 5% and 10% dextrose intravenous solutions during neonatal surgery. Anesthesiology 69:A738, 1988.

Kliegman RM: Problems in metabolic adaptation: glucose, calcium, and magnesium. In Klaus MH and Fanaroff AA (eds.): Care of the High Risk Neonate, 4th ed. WB Saunders, Philadelphia, 1993, pp 282–301.

Kwang-Sun L, Gartner LM, Eidelman AI, and Ezhuthachan S: Unconjugated hyperbilirubinemia in very low birth weight infants. Clin Perinatol 4:305, 1977.

Long TMW: An unusual case of symptomatic hypoglycaemia in a child. Anaesthesia 44:765–766, 1989.

Poland RL and Ostrea EM: Neonatal hyperbilirubinemia. In Klaus MH and Fanaroff AA (eds.): Care of the High Risk Neonate, 4th ed. WB Saunders, Philadelphia, 1993, pp 302–322.

Sieber FE, Smith DS, Traystman RJ, and Wollman H: Glucose: a re-evaluation of its intraoperative use. Anesthesiology 67:72–81, 1987.

Steward DJ: Hyperglycemia: something else to worry about. Paediatr Anaesth 2:81–83, 1992.

COMPOSITION AND REGULATION OF BODY FLUIDS

The management of fluid and electrolyte treatment demands knowledge of the maturation of renal function in the infant and the differences in the volumes of the fluid compartments and fluid turnover.

Body Water

The amount of total body water is relatively greater in neonates and infants than in adults. Its distribution also differs, the proportion of extracellular fluid (ECF) being greater in neonates and young children. In the preterm infant the ECF exceeds the intracellular fluid (ICF), whereas in the older child and adult the ECF is only half the volume of the ICF (Table 2–7). Normal levels of serum electrolytes in the newborn are listed in Table 2–8.

Neonatal Renal Function and Water Balance

In the neonate, renal function is determined by a high renal vascular resistance—which results in low renal blood flow and a low glomerular filtration rate (GFR)—and by a limited tubular function. The preterm infant has an even lower GFR, and it increases less rapidly over the first weeks of life than it does in the full-term infant. The GFR of the neonate increases with fluid loading, but only to a limited capacity. Consequently, the infant cannot readily handle an excessive water load and may be unable to excrete excess electrolytes or other substances dependent

Table 2–7. Extracellular and Intracellular Fluid Compartments (% of Body Weight)

Fluid	Preterm Neonate	Full-term Neonate	Infant (7–8 Mo)	Adult
ECF	50	35–40	30	20
ICF	30	35	35	45

Table 2–8. Normal Blood Chemistry

Parameter	Preterm Neonate	Full-term Neonate	2 Yr to Adult
Serum chloride (mEq/L)	100–117	90–114	98–106
Serum potassium (mEq/L)	4.6–6.7	4.3–7.6	3.5–5.6
Serum sodium (mEq/L)	133–146	136–148	142
Blood glucose (mg/dl)	40–60	40–80	70–110
Total protein (g/dl)	3.9–4.7	4.6–7.7	5.5–7.8
$PaCO_2$ (mmHg)	30–35	33–35	35–40

on glomerular filtration. The GFR is further decreased by hypoxia, hypothermia, or congestive cardiac failure.

The limited tubular function impairs the infant's ability to modify the glomerular filtrate for conservation or excretion. For this reason sodium losses may be large, especially in the preterm infant, and must be balanced by intake. These losses are further increased if the GFR is increased by a high fluid intake; hence, the tendency of the neonate to hyponatremia. Glucose reabsorption is also limited in the preterm infant, and glycosuria may occur. In the patient with marked hyperglycemia, the resultant osmotic diuresis may lead to severe dehydration. The ability of the tubule to excrete acid is reduced in the preterm infant, thus impairing renal compensation in acidosis. The capacity to excrete H^+ increases with gestational age. Newborn infants have a lower renal threshold for bicarbonate than adults, and this leads to lower serum bicarbonate levels. The limitations of renal function summarized above necessitate careful fluid and electrolyte replacement therapy planned to match losses. Renal vascular resistance declines and renal function matures rapidly over the first few weeks of life in the full-term infant. Preterm infants show less rapid changes in renal function.

Fluid loss and hence the replacement requirement is related to insensible fluid losses, urine output, and metabolic rate. Insensible fluid losses are relatively high during infancy, major factors being the high level of alveolar ventilation and the thin skin of low-birth-weight infants. Fluid losses are markedly increased by the use of radiant heat and/or phototherapy. Because of the infant's proportionally higher water turnover and the limited ability to concentrate urine and conserve water, dehydration develops rapidly when intake is restricted or losses occur.

Maintenance Requirements

Although maintenance requirements are directly related to $\dot{V}O_2$ and caloric expenditure and are more accurately expressed in milliliters per square meter of surface area, it is most convenient to relate them to body weight. Fluid requirements for full-term neonates are reduced (40–60 ml/kg per 24 hours) during the first few days of life as excess fluid present at birth is being excreted. By 1 week of age, the requirements are increased. Table 2–9 shows the volumes of fluid required during the period of high metabolic activity in infants weighing 4–20 kg.

Fluid, Na^+, and K^+ requirements can be met by the intravenous infusion of appropriate volumes of a solution of two-thirds 5% glucose and one-third N saline, containing 20 mEq of K^+ per liter.

Suggested Additional Reading

Arant BS: Fluid therapy in the neonate-concepts in transition. J Pediatr 101:387, 1982.

Guignard JP: Renal function in the newborn infant. Pediatr Clin North Am 29:777, 1982.

Jones DP and Chesney RW: Development of tubular function. Clin Perinatol 19:33–57, 1992.

Leighton Hill L: Body composition, normal electrolyte concentrations, and the maintenance of normal volume, tonicity, and acid-base metabolism. Pediatr Clin North Am 37:241–256, 1990.

Long TMW: An unusual case of symptomatic hypoglycemia in a child. Anaesthesia 44:765–766, 1989.

Marks KH, Gunther RC, Rossi JA, and Maisels J: Oxygen consumption and insensible water loss in premature infants under radiant heaters. Pediatrics 66:228–232, 1980.

Rice HE, Caty MG, and Glick PL: Fluid therapy for the pediatric surgical patient. Pediatr Clin North Am 45:719–727, 1998.

Seikaly MG and Arant BS: Development of renal hemodynamics: glomerular filtration and renal blood flow. Clin Perinatol 19:1–13, 1992.

PHYSIOLOGY OF TEMPERATURE HOMEOSTASIS

Because of their large surface area relative to body weight and their lack of heat-insulating subcutaneous fat, infants tend to lose heat rapidly

Table 2–9. Daily Maintenance Requirements for Fluid, Electrolytes, and Carbohydrates in Relation to Weight

Weight	H_2O (ml/kg)	Na^+ (mEq/kg)	K^+ (mEq/kg)	Carbohydrate (g/kg)
Newborn*				
1,000 g	≤200	3.0	2.0–2.5	≤10
1,000–1,499 g	≤100	2.5	2.0–2.5	
1,500–2,500 g	≤160	2.0	1.5–2.0	≤8
2,500 g	≤150	1.5–2.0	2.0	≤5
4–10 kg	100–120	2.0–2.5	2.0–2.5	5–6
10–20 kg	80–100	1.6–2.0	1.6–2.0	4–5
20–40 kg	60–80	1.2–1.6	1.2–1.6	3–4
Adult	2,500–3,000 ml total	50 mEq total	50 mEq total	100–150 g total

*Adjust according to postnatal age, exposure to phototherapy, reduced insensible losses with assisted ventilation, etc.

(From The Hospital for Sick Children: Residents' Handbook of Pediatrics, 6th ed. Toronto, Canada, 1979, with permission.)

when placed in a cool environment. This heat is lost by radiation, conduction, and convection. Further heat is lost by evaporation of water in the respiratory tract and through the skin. Evaporative heat loss via the skin is a significant factor in the preterm infant and is related to increased skin permeability. Heat loss from the body surface by radiation is related to the temperature of surrounding objects (e.g., the wall of the incubator) and not to the surrounding air temperature. A single-walled incubator does not prevent radiant heat loss if the wall temperature is below that of the infant.

When heat loss occurs, heat production within the body must be increased to maintain a normal core temperature. In adults and older children, this heat production is principally a function of involuntary muscular activity (shivering) accompanied by increased $\dot{V}O_2$, both of which can be prevented by the administration of a neuromuscular blocking drug. Infants rely primarily on nonshivering thermogenesis to generate heat. This mechanism, which also results in increased $\dot{V}O_2$, occurs mainly in the brown adipose tissue, which makes up 2%–6% of the full-term infant's body weight (less in the preterm infant) and is located around the scapulae, in the mediastinum, and surrounding the kidneys and adrenal glands. The cells of this "brown fat" have many mitochondria and fat vacuoles, and the tissue has a rich blood and autonomic nerve supply. Increased metabolic activity in brown fat is initiated by norepinephrine released at the sympathetic nerve endings. Hydrolysis of triglyceride to fatty acids and glycerol occurs with associated increased $\dot{V}O_2$ and heat production. Brown fat deposits decline during the first weeks of extrauterine life.

Exposure to a cool environment together with a decline in central temperature normally triggers thermoregulatory vasoconstriction in unanesthetized infants and children. This vasoconstriction tends to limit further heat loss from the body surface. It is now recognized that the mechanisms for controlling body temperature are well developed in the full-term newborn. However, a decline in core temperature results when compensatory increases in heat production cannot match heat losses. On exposure to a cool environment, increased metabolic activity is initiated in the brown fat so as to maintain the core temperature. This is accompanied by a progressively increased $\dot{V}O_2$ as the temperature gradient between the skin and the environment widens. Oxygen consumption is minimal when this gradient is less than 2°C. Exposure to a cool environment also leads to increased glucose use and acid metabolite formation.

The physiologic responses to cooling lead to increased oxygen and glucose use and result in acidosis, all of which may compromise the sick infant. The infant with chronic hypoxemia (e.g., cyanotic congenital heart disease) is unable to compensate if exposed to a low ambient temperature and cools rapidly. To eliminate the need for compensatory responses, sick neonates should be maintained in a neutral thermal environment—that is, in an ambient temperature that minimizes $\dot{V}O_2$ (Table 2–10).

During anesthesia the normal thermoregulatory response of the infant to cold stress is lost and no increase in oxygen consumption is

Table 2-10. Neutral Thermal Environment Temperatures (°C)

Age	1,200 g	Weight 1,200–1,500 g	1,500–2,500 g	2,500 g
0–6 hr	34–35.4	33.9–34.4	32.8–33.8	32.0–33.8
6–12 hr	34–35.4	33.5–34.4	32.2–33.8	31.4–33.8
12–24 hr	34–35.4	33.3–34.3	31.8–33.8	31.0–33.7
24–36 hr	34–35	33.1–34.2	31.6–33.6	30.7–33.5
36–48 hr	34–35	33.0–34.1	31.4–33.5	30.5–33.3
48–72 hr	34–35	33.0–34.0	31.2–33.4	30.1–33.2
72–96 hr	34–35	33.0–34.0	31.1–33.2	29.8–32.8
4–12 days	—	33–34*	31–33.2	29.5–31.4
2–3 wk	—	32.2–34*	30.5–33.0	—
3–4 wk	—	31.6–33.6*	30.0–32.7	—

*1,500 g.

observed in response to a cool environment. In addition, normal thermoregulatory skin vasoconstriction is inhibited. Anesthetized infants and children tend to have increased heat loss and a drop in body temperature. There is also a redistribution of body heat away from the central core to the periphery. Measures to minimize heat loss and avoid cold stress are important during anesthesia and are outlined on page 109.

Suggested Additional Reading

Adamsons K Jr, Gandy GM, and James LS: The influence of thermal factors upon oxygen consumption of the newborn human infant. J Pediatr 66:495, 1965.

Bennett EF, Patel KP, and Grundy EM: Neonatal temperature and surgery. Anesthesiology 46:303, 1977.

Bissonette B: Body temperature and anesthesia. Anesthesiol Clin North Am 9:849–864, 1991.

Bissonette B and Sessler DI: The thermoregulatory threshold in infants and children anesthetized with isoflurane and caudal bupivacaine. Anesthesiology 73:1114–1118, 1990.

Heiser MS and Downes JJ: Temperature regulation in the pediatric patient. Semin Anesthesiol 3:37–42, 1984.

Hey EN and Katz G: The optimum thermal environment for naked babies. Arch Dis Child 45:328, 1970.

Kennaird DL: Oxygen consumption and evaporative heat loss in infants with congenital heart disease. Arch Dis Child 51:34–41, 1976.

Lindahl SGE, Grigsby EJ, Meyer DM, and Beynen FMK: Oxygen uptake, body, skin and room temperatures in anesthetized infants and children. Anesthesiology 69:A765, 1988.

Plattner O, Semsroth M, Sessler DI, et al.: Lack of non-shivering thermogenesis in infants anesthetized with fentanyl and propofol. Anesthesiology 86:772–777, 1997.

Silverman WA and Sinclair JC: Temperature regulation in the newborn infant. N Engl J Med 274:92–146, 1966.

Chapter 3

Pharmacology of Pediatric Anesthesia

ROUTES OF ADMINISTRATION

Intravenous. The intravenous route is the most certain route to deliver drugs to the bloodstream under all conditions and should be the principal route for all anesthetic drugs given parenterally. Be very careful to check all drugs and doses before administration. In the case of less commonly used drugs (e.g., antibiotics), ensure that the manufacturer's directions as to speed of injection, dilution, and so forth, are carefully followed. Rapid injection of some drugs (e.g., vancomycin) may cause severe physiologic effects (e.g., cardiac arrest).

N.B. Drugs preferably should not be injected into central hyperalimentation lines, because infection or thrombosis of the line might result. Be very careful that all intravenous tubing is flushed after drugs are administered to ensure that no drugs remain in the tubing!

Intramuscular. Drugs administered intramuscularly are rapidly absorbed *(absorption is more rapid from the arm (deltoid) muscle than from the leg muscle)*, especially in small children. However, this route is much less *reliable* in patients with shock or hypovolemia, and there is a danger that repeated doses may have a cumulative effect when muscle tissue perfusion improves. Intramuscular injections are painful and should be avoided in conscious children.

Intralingual. Injections into the tongue have been suggested for use in an emergency (e.g., succinylcholine). *We have never found a use for this technique and do not recommend it.*

Intratracheal. Drugs sprayed into the trachea are rapidly absorbed, and this may be a useful emergency route if an intravenous route is not available (e.g., to administer atropine or epinephrine during cardiopulmonary resuscitation).

Rectal. Use of suppositories (acetaminophen) or rectal administration of drugs (e.g., pentobarbital, methohexital) are usually well accepted by young children (3 years and younger). Absorption is less certain than with other routes, possibly in part because of the first-pass effect of the liver and the variable volume and pH of the rectal contents. Unanesthetized children older than 3 years of age may be upset by use of the rectal route.

Oral. Preoperative medication and postoperative analgesics may be given to selected patients by this route, which is readily accepted by children, but drug absorption is somewhat unpredictable. The oral route cannot be used if vomiting or other gastrointestinal dysfunction exists. Many drugs are very rapidly and predictably absorbed across the oral mucous membrane (e.g., fentanyl, midazolam) if administered as a lozenge or if placed under the tongue. The oral transmucosal route is a potentially very useful route for drug therapy in children.

Intranasal. Some drugs are well absorbed across the nasal mucous membrane and are rapidly effective by this route (e.g., sufentanil, midazolam). However, children are usually upset at having nose drops instilled, and this route has not gained wide acceptance. There is also a concern that some drugs (e.g., midazolam) might be neurotoxic if absorbed via the olfactory area.

DISTRIBUTION OF ADMINISTERED DRUGS

In infants and young children, the relative sizes of the body fluid compartments differ from those in the adult. The extracellular fluid compartment is large; hence, drugs that are distributed throughout this space (e.g., succinylcholine) are required in larger doses.

Protein binding is less in neonates because of lower total serum protein levels and lower levels of specific proteins (e.g., α_1-acid glycoprotein). More of the administered drug is free in the plasma to exert a clinical effect. For this reason, lower doses of such drugs as barbiturates are indicated.

The composition of the body also has an influence on drug distribution; neonates have little fat or muscle tissue. Drugs normally distributed to these tissues will have a longer half-life.

METABOLISM AND ELIMINATION OF DRUGS

The half-lives of drugs that are metabolized in the liver in the neonate and small infant are generally longer than those in the adult (e.g., opioid analgesics). Hepatic blood flow and hepatocellular enzymatic activity are the primary determinants of the rate of metabolism of a drug by the liver. Hepatic blood flow may be reduced in the small infant because of increased intra-abdominal pressure, congestive cardiac failure, and, in the first few postnatal days, patent ductus venosus. The conjugation pathways for drug metabolism are immature in small infants and are not fully active until 2–3 months of age. Hence, drugs such as morphine have a considerably longer half-life. In addition, alternative pathways for drug metabolism may result in the accumulation of metabolites, some of which may be pharmacologically active.

Older infants and young children demonstrate a rapid elimination of some drugs, reflecting the high hepatic blood flow and enhanced metabolic activity in the child's liver.

Drugs excreted via the kidney (e.g., pancuronium) are dependent on the glomerular filtration rate or tubular secretion capacity, both of which are reduced during the first few weeks of life.

DRUGS USED IN ANESTHESIA
Agents for General Anesthesia
Inhalation Agents

Inhaled anesthetic drugs increase in concentration in the alveoli more rapidly in children than in adults. Alveolar levels approach inspired levels most rapidly in infants. This is a result of the high level of alveolar ventilation in relation to functional residual capacity, the higher proportion of vessel-rich tissues that rapidly equilibrate with blood levels, and the lower blood-gas partition coefficients (PCs) of volatile anesthetics in infants. Therefore, induction of anesthesia is more rapid in infants and small children. The rapid increase in alveolar, blood, and tissue concentrations of potent inhalation agents may account in part for the precipitous decreases in blood pressure that occur when higher concentrations of these agents are given, especially during controlled ventilation.

Excretion of inhaled anesthetic agents, and therefore recovery, is also more rapid in infants and small children, provided that ventilation is not depressed. The alveolar level of nitrous oxide (N_2O) decreases to 10% within 2 minutes after discontinuation of 70% N_2O, a level not reached until 10 minutes in adults.

The minimal alveolar concentration (MAC) for all anesthetic agents is greater in infants than in older children and adults but is less in full-term neonates and especially in preterm neonates (Table 3–1). The reasons for this are unknown.

Nitrous Oxide

N_2O is commonly used in pediatric anesthesia to speed and facilitate induction and to provide analgesia/amnesia during maintenance. It may also be administered to sedate and to provide analgesia before intravenous induction of anesthesia. N_2O is odorless and insoluble (PC, 0.47), and in high concentrations it enhances the rate of uptake of the volatile agents into the alveoli, accelerating the induction of anesthesia. The analgesic effects of N_2O may be useful to complement the anesthesia regimen during maintenance. The effects of N_2O on ventilation appear to equal those of equipotent concentrations of halothane. N_2O mildly depresses cardiac output and systemic blood pressure in infants, but it has little effect on pulmonary artery pressure or pulmonary vascular resistance, even in those with pulmonary vascular disease. In infants and small children, the cardiovascular effects of N_2O + either halothane or isoflurane to 1.5 MAC are similar to those of equipotent (1.5 MAC) concentrations of either halothane or isoflurane in oxygen. N_2O rapidly diffuses into any gas-containing space within the body; this contraindicates its use in those patients with lung cysts, pneumothorax, lobar emphysema, necrotizing enterocolitis, bowel obstruction, and so forth. N_2O also diffuses into the middle ear and may displace the graft during tympanoplasty. In some patients with a normal ear and an intact eardrum, postoperative absorption of N_2O from the middle ear results in atelectasis of the drum and a later complaint of earache. A relationship between N_2O and postoperative vomiting has not been established in pediatric studies.

Halothane

Halothane is an almost ideal anesthetic agent for children, although its popularity in pediatric anesthesia has waned since the introduction of sevoflurane into clinical practice. Halothane is moderately soluble in blood (PC, 2.3) and its washin is slow compared with other anesthetics. Halothane provides a smooth inhalation induction with minimal irritant effects on the respiratory system. The level of anesthesia is easily controlled and can be changed rapidly. The MAC in children with mental handicaps may be 25% less than in children without handicaps.

Table 3–1. Minimal Alveolar Concentration (MAC%) of Volatile Agents

Age	Halothane	Isoflurane	Sevoflurane	Desflurane
Preterm neonate	0.55	1.3–1.4	Not available	Not available
Full-term neonate	0.87	1.6	3.2	9.1
Infant	1.2	1.8	3.2	9.4
Child	0.95	1.6	2.5	8.5

During halothane anesthesia, a dose-dependent depression of spontaneous ventilation occurs; there is usually an increase in respiratory rate, but tidal volume and minute ventilation decrease considerably. This results in an increase in end-tidal carbon dioxide. The level of ventilation returns toward normal during surgical stimulation and is quite variable throughout anesthesia. Halothane inhibits intercostal muscle activity. Diaphragmatic ventilation predominates, and paradoxic movement of the chest wall may occur. Even very low blood levels of halothane cause severe depression of the ventilatory response to hypoxia in young volunteers. It is likely that this effect occurs in all pediatric patients. Severe laryngeal spasm may occur during light planes of halothane anesthesia, especially on extubation of the trachea. This effect can be avoided by extubating the trachea while the child is still deeply anesthetized or completely awake. Alternatively, lidocaine (1–2 mg/kg IV) given slowly before extubation may prevent laryngospasm. Halothane is a potent bronchodilator and is very useful in children with asthma.

Halothane depresses myocardial contractility, especially in small infants. It also produces bradycardia and thus causes a fall in cardiac output. Atropine prevents bradycardia and therefore tends to maintain cardiac output, but it cannot reverse the reduced myocardial contractility caused by halothane. Neonates are especially sensitive to the myocardial depressant effects of halothane (*see* page 28). Severe hypotension may ensue if high concentrations of halothane are administered to infants and children, particularly when ventilation is controlled. This is a result of myocardial depression and subsequent decreased cardiac output as the concentration of halothane rapidly increases in the child's myocardium.

The infant's blood pressure is very sensitive to changes in cardiac output. Vasoconstriction is less effective than in the adult. Halothane also depresses reflex baroresponses. Inspired halothane concentrations should be limited to 0.5%–1% during controlled ventilation, and the blood pressure should be carefully monitored. In children with cardiac failure, the myocardial depressant effects of halothane are prominent, and severe hypotension may occur.

Arrhythmias also occur during halothane anesthesia. Ventricular premature beats are common, especially during spontaneous ventilation with halothane. If they occur, ventilation should be assisted or controlled; and if they persist, another volatile agent (e.g., isoflurane) should be substituted for halothane. Junctional rhythm and wandering pacemaker may also be seen during halothane anesthesia. This is usually of little consequence but might compromise the patient who has other disease of the heart. Halothane sensitizes the myocardium to exogenous catecholamines, and arrhythmias may occur when these compounds are injected (e.g., to infiltrate the skin). Studies indicate that children tolerate higher levels of injected epinephrine than adults do. Epinephrine in doses up to a maximum of 10 μg/kg mixed with lidocaine and injected into the tissues of healthy children appears to be safe. Serious arrhythmias may occur if halothane is administered to children who have been receiving theophylline medication chronically; other agents should be used. Halothane and other volatile agents inhibit hypoxic pulmonary vasoconstriction and thereby disrupt the mechanism that normally redistributes perfusion away from underventilated alveoli. This increased shunt may result in a clinically significant decrease in arterial oxygen saturation, especially in infants with lung disease (e.g., bronchopulmonary dysplasia).

Shivering and muscle rigidity are common during emergence from halothane anesthesia. These effects may be of concern after orthopaedic surgery and for patients in whom the additional oxygen demands of shivering might be detrimental. In such cases, an alternative anesthetic technique may be more appropriate.

Halothane is metabolized 15%–20% in adults in vivo, but the extent of metabolism is less in infants and small children than in adults. Halothane is occasionally a cause of hepatic failure in adults, but very few well-documented cases of liver dysfunction have been reported in children, despite its wide and often repeated use in this age group. The evidence suggests that halothane hepatitis does rarely occur in children, supported by the fact that halothane-related antibodies can be detected. Significant episodes are extremely rare, however, and it would appear that the disease runs a less fulminant course in children than in adults. The reason for the reduced susceptibility of prepubertal children to halothane hepatitis is not known. Contraindications to halothane include a history of unexplained posthalothane jaundice.

Halothane, like most other potent inhalational anesthetic agents, increases cerebral blood flow and therefore may increase intracranial pressure (ICP). At low concentrations, this effect is minimal, however; if hyperventilation is employed, the ICP does not increase significantly even in those with intracranial space-occupying lesions. In fact, halothane has been widely used for pediatric neurosurgery and has proved most useful. Complications after halothane are infrequent. After a brief halothane anesthesia for minor surgery, most children recover to full activity very soon.

Enflurane

This inhaled agent has several disadvantages compared with other agents and, as a result, is not commonly administered to children in North America.

Isoflurane

Isoflurane, a stereoisomer of enflurane, is a polyhalogenated methyl ethyl ether. Its relatively low solubility in blood (PC, 1.43) facilitates a more rapid washin to the alveoli, compared with halothane. Isoflurane is a stable compound that is metabolized less than 0.2% in vivo. It is eliminated almost completely unchanged via the lungs; therefore, recovery should be very complete.

Despite its low solubility, isoflurane is not suited to inhalational induction because its pungent odor irritates airway reflexes (coughing, laryngospasm, breath-holding, and decreased arterial oxygen saturation) and delays induction compared with halothane (± 7 versus ± 4 minutes, respectively). However, isoflurane can be successfully introduced, especially after an intravenous induction, provided that the concentration is increased slowly. Recovery after isoflurane anesthesia is quite rapid and not measurably different from halothane. The incidence of laryngospasm during extubation and emergence is similar to that with halothane, and extubation should be carefully managed. Isoflurane has slightly greater depressant effects on the respiratory system than halothane, because the respiratory rate tends to decrease more. For this reason, controlled ventilation is required.

The cardiovascular effects of isoflurane differ from those of halothane. At equipotent concentrations, isoflurane and halothane decrease blood pressure in children to similar extents, although heart rate is better maintained with isoflurane. The effect of isoflurane on cardiac output may be less with isoflurane. Vasodilatation during isoflurane anesthesia explains the greater decrease in blood pressure compared with halothane. Isoflurane may be useful to control blood pressure, for example during induced hypotension. Whether isoflurane has a lesser myocardial depressant effect than halothane has been a matter of some controversy. It had been suggested that isoflurane causes less myocardial depression, but late studies indicate that its effect on cardiac contractility is very similar to that of halothane. Isoflurane does depress the reflex baroresponses in the neonate. This impairs the ability to compensate for changes in arterial blood pressure and to respond to hypovolemia. Isoflurane does not sensitize the myocardium to the effects of catecholamines or theophylline.

Isoflurane potentiates nondepolarizing neuromuscular blocking drugs to a greater extent than halothane. This effect allows reduced doses of relaxant drugs to be used, and it is reversible when isoflurane is withdrawn. Isoflurane, like enflurane and desflurane, reacts with desiccated soda lime and Baralyme to release carbon monoxide into the breathing circuit *(see below)*.

Desflurane

Desflurane is a fluorinated ether with a boiling point of 23°C and a very low solubility in blood (PC, 0.42). It is a very stable compound, and less than 0.02% is metabolized in vivo. The effects of desflurane on the cardiovascular system at 1 MAC anesthesia are similar to those with other ether inhalational anesthetics, although bradycardia is rare. In adults, when desflurane is the sole anesthetic agent, sudden increases in the inspired concentration can lead to profound central sympathetic discharge, resulting in sudden increases in blood pressure and heart rate. Similar responses have not been reported in children.

Desflurane is very pungent and irritant to the airway; breath-holding and laryngospasm are very common. Similar to isoflurane, it is not suited for inhalational inductions in children. It can, however, be used for maintenance after induction with halothane, sevoflurane, or intravenous drugs. Emergence from desflurane anesthesia is very rapid, but this may result in delirium, particularly if pain is present. The incidence of emergence delirium after desflurane anesthesia is greater than after other agents. Desflurane is less convenient to use than other agents, because its low boiling point demands special consideration in vaporizer design. A higher concentration is required to maintain anesthesia, and it will prove expensive unless low, fresh gas flows are used.

Desflurane may be given with carbon dioxide absorbents in closed circuits or low flow conditions to contain costs. However, desflurane interacts with desiccated soda lime or Baralyme and may produce potentially toxic concentrations of carbon monoxide. Amsorb, a new calcium-based carbon dioxide absorbent that is free of sodium and potassium hydroxide, does not interact to produce carbon monoxide.

Sevoflurane

Sevoflurane, a fluorinated methyl isopropyl ether, has a low solubility in blood (PC, 0.63) and is not irritating to the airway. Sevoflurane is the first ether anesthetic that does not irritate the airway in children; its effects on airway reflexes are comparable to those of halothane. It is an ideal agent for inhalation induction, and this can most rapidly be accomplished by administering a high concentration of the drug together with N_2O. It is not necessary to slowly introduce sevoflurane into the gas mixture. A single breath taken from functional residual capacity and inspiring 8% sevoflurane can induce anesthesia rapidly and smoothly in children older than 6 years of age. The other respiratory and circulatory effects of sevoflurane do not differ markedly from those of isoflurane.

Sevoflurane is metabolized (5%) in vivo with the release of inorganic fluoride; maximum levels occur within 2 hours after termination of the anesthetic. However, the blood levels produced are lower than the threshold for fluoride-induced nephrotoxicity, and the levels rapidly fall in children. Sevoflurane is also hydrolyzed in the presence of soda lime or Baralyme (but not Amsorb) to five compounds, compound A (which is potentially nephrotoxic) being the most common. However, evidence from nonhuman primates suggests that sevoflurane may be administered in a closed circuit for up to 25 MAC-hours before nephrotoxicity is a serious risk.

Emergence from sevoflurane anesthesia is smooth and rapid, although care must be taken to ensure adequate analgesia at this time (e.g., regional block, opioid analgesics) to decrease the risk of emergence delirium. There is some evidence that recovery of fine coordination over the first few hours after anesthesia is more complete than after halothane.

Summary

1. The MAC of anesthetic drugs is greater in infants and children than in neonates or adults (e.g., the MAC of halothane is greater than 1% in children but only about 0.8% in adults).
2. The smaller the child, the more rapid the uptake of anesthetics into the alveoli.
3. High concentrations of potent inhalation agents can cause serious hypotension in infants and young children, particularly when

ventilation is controlled. *Beware: overdose of volatile agents is a leading cause of serious complications.*

4. Halothane-induced hepatic failure is rare in children younger than 14 years of age.

5. Although halothane remains an agent for general use in pediatric patients, sevoflurane has challenged its widespread use and may replace it in the near future.

6. *MAC is as follows: intubation, halothane (1.3) or sevoflurane (2.7); extubation, halothane (1.4) or sevoflurane (2.3); and LMA insertion, halothane (1.5) or sevoflurane (2.0).*

Suggested Additional Reading

Agnor RC, Sikich N, and Lerman J: Single breath vital capacity rapid inhalation induction in children: 8% sevoflurane versus 5% halothane. Anesthesiology 89:379–384, 1998.

Aono J, Ueda W, Mamiya K, et al.: Greater incidence of delirium during recovery from sevoflurane anesthesia in preschool boys. Anesthesiology 87:1298–1300, 1997.

Brandom BW, Brandom RB, and Cook DR: Uptake and distribution of halothane in infants: in vivo measurements and computer simulations. Anesth Analg 62:404, 1983.

Cameron CB, Robinson S, and Gregory GA: The minimum anesthetic concentration of isoflurane in children. Anesth Analg 63:418–420, 1984.

Davis PJ, Cohen IT, McGowan FX, and Latta K: Recovery characteristics of desflurane versus halothane for maintenance of anesthesia in pediatric ambulatory patients. Anesthesiology 80:298–302, 1994.

Dubois MC, Piat V, Constant I, et al.: Comparison of three techniques for induction of anaesthesia with sevoflurane in children. Paediatr Anaesth 9:19–23, 1999.

Frei FJ, Haemmerle MH, Brunner R, and Kern C: Minimum alveolar concentration for halothane in children with cerebral palsy and severe mental retardation. Anaesthesia 52:1056–1060, 1997.

Friesen RH and Lichtor JL: Cardiovascular effects of inhalation induction with isoflurane in infants. Anesth Analg 62:411, 1983.

Kenna JG, Neuberger J, Mieli-Vergani G, et al.: Halothane hepatitis in children. Br Med J 294:1209–1211, 1987.

Lerman J, Robinson S, Willis MM, and Gregory GA: Anesthetic requirements for halothane in young children 0–1 month and 1–6 months of age. Anesthesiology 59:421–424, 1983.

Lerman J, Sikich N, Kleinman S, and Yentis S: The pharmacology of sevoflurane in infants and children. Anesthesiology 80:814–824, 1994.

Lindahl SGE, Hulse MG, and Hatch DJ: Ventilation and gas exchange during anaesthesia and surgery in spontaneously breathing infants and children. Br J Anaesth 56:121–129, 1984.

Lindahl SGE, Yates AP, and Hatch DJ: Respiratory depression in children at different end tidal halothane concentrations. Anaesthesia 42:1267–1275, 1987.

Murat I, Lapeyre G, and Saint-Maurice C: Isoflurane attenuates baroreflex control of heart rate in human neonates. Anesthesiology 70:395–400, 1989.

Murray DJ, Forbes R, Murphy K, and Mahoney L: Nitrous oxide: cardiovascular effects in infants and small children during halothane and isoflurane anesthesia. Anesth Analg 67:1059–1064, 1988.

Murray DJ, Vanderwalker G, Matherne P, and Mahoney L: Cardiovascular effects of halothane and isoflurane in infants and small children using pulsed Doppler echocardiography. Anesthesiology 67:211–217, 1987.

Phillips AJ, Brimacombe JR, and Simpson RL: Anaesthetic induction with isoflurane or halothane: oxygen saturation during induction with isoflurane or halothane. Anaesthesia 43:927–929, 1988.

Renfrew CW, Murray JM, and Fee JPH: A new approach to carbon dioxide absorbents. Acta Scand Anaesth 41(Suppl 12):58–60, 1998.

Salintre E and Rackow H: The pulmonary exchange of nitrous oxide and halothane in infants and children. Anesthesiology 30:388, 1969.

Taylor RH and Lerman J: Minimum alveolar concentration of desflurane and hemodynamic responses in neonates, infants, and children. Anesthesiology 75:975–979, 1991.

Taylor RH and Lerman J: Induction and maintenance characteristics of anaesthesia with desflurane in infants and children. Can J Anaesth 39:6–13, 1992.

Walton B: Halothane hepatitis in children. Anaesthesia 41:575–578, 1986.

Watcha MF, Forestner JE, Connor MT, et al.: Minimum alveolar concentration of halothane for tracheal intubation in children. Anesthesiology 69:412–416, 1988.

Wolf WJ, Neal MB, and Peterson MD: The hemodynamic and cardiovascular effects of isoflurane and halothane anesthesia in children. Anesthesiology 64:328–333, 1986.

Intravenous Agents

The intravenous route is widely used for both induction and maintenance of anesthesia in children. It has been reported that skillful, painless intravenous induction may cause fewer psychological sequelae than inhalation induction. The anesthesiologist should be skilled in painless venipuncture, and the assistance of an experienced nurse should be available. Needles and syringes should be kept out of the child's sight at all times, and the word *needle* specifically should be avoided. Music, pictures, television, or bubble blowing help to distract the child during venipuncture. A disposable 26- or 27-gauge "butterfly" needle is easy to conceal during insertion and to leave in place for short procedures. Use of topical EMLA cream (a eutectic mixture of lidocaine and prilocaine) or Ametop (amethocaine) facilitates painless venipuncture; apply 90 minutes (EMLA cream) or 30 minutes (Ametop) before the procedure. Alternatively, N_2O (inspired concentration, 50%–70%) may be given by mask to sedate the child and provide analgesia for venous cannulation.

If the patient arrives in the operating room with a peripheral intravenous infusion running, this can be used as a route to administer induction drugs. If at all possible, injections should not be made into central or intravenous hyperalimentation lines.

Thiopental

Thiopental is still the most commonly used intravenous induction agent for infants and children of all ages. Onset of anesthesia is rapid but smooth, usually accompanied by a very brief period of apnea. Cardiovascular changes are minimal in the healthy child. Neonates are especially sensitive to barbiturates. This finding is related to the reduced protein binding of the drug in the serum of the neonate. However, older infants may require larger than usual doses to induce anesthesia (Table 3–2). Contraindications to thiopental are similar to those in adults. Intravenous induction should not be used when there is a possible airway problem, and barbiturates should not be used for children with porphyria. As in adults, barbiturates should be administered with extreme care in patients

Table 3–2. Effect of Age on Effective Dose of Thiopental	
Age	**Effective Dose (mg/kg)**
Neonate	3–4
Infant	6–7
Child	5–6

who may be hypovolemic and in those with limited cardiac reserve. Thiopental reduces intraocular and cerebrospinal fluid pressure and hence may be especially useful for induction of patients having neurosurgical or ocular procedures.

Methohexital

Methohexital is sometimes provided as an alternative to thiopental. In children, the induction dose is approximately 1.5 mg/kg. Although some authors have reported that recovery after methohexital is faster than after thiopental, careful testing of coordination has shown little difference between the two drugs. Methohexital often causes muscle twitching or hiccups—effects that can be minimized by avoiding large doses. Intravenous injection of 1% methohexital commonly causes pain along the injected vein; this can be minimized by adding a small amount of plain lidocaine (e.g., 1 mg lidocaine per milliliter of solution).

Propofol

Propofol (2,6-diisopropylphenol) is a short-acting hypnotic that is associated with a very rapid and pleasant recovery. Propofol has rapidly replaced thiopental as the induction agent of choice in ambulatory surgery. Propofol is hydrophobic and therefore is prepared in Intralipid, an emulsion in soybean oil that supports bacterial growth. Extreme caution regarding asepsis is required, and all unused solutions should be discarded in accordance with the manufacturer's instructions. There are now two preparations available, one containing ethylenediamine tetraacetic acid (EDTA) and the other sodium metabisulfite. The latter may trigger bronchospasm in asthmatic children. Anaphylactoid reactions have been reported after the use of both formulations. The dose required for induction of anesthesia ranges from 2.5 to 5 mg/kg; larger doses may be required for younger infants and unpremedicated patients. The respiratory and cardiovascular effects of a sleep dose (2.5–3.5 mg/kg) are similar to those of thiopentone; a short period of apnea may occur, and there is a slight decline in blood pressure.

Airway reflexes are depressed by propofol; this is useful for cases involving airway instrumentation (e.g., laryngeal mask insertion) and generally results in a good airway during emergence. The hypertensive response to endotracheal intubation is less after an induction sequence with propofol plus a relaxant than after thiopental plus a relaxant. Extraneous (frequently choreiform) movements are common on induction, especially if lower doses are provided.

Pain is common at the site of injection but is less severe if the drug is given into a free-flowing infusion or into a large antecubital vein, both of which are unlikely in the small child at induction. The addition of 1% lidocaine (1 mg/ml) to the propofol emulsion is the most effective means to minimize pain on injection, probably because of its action in altering the pH of the solution. Recovery is more rapid after short procedures if propofol rather than thiopental is used for induction. However, propofol has little advantage over thiopental if the operation lasts longer than 1 hour.

Propofol may be infused continuously for maintenance of anesthesia in children to provide a form of total intravenous anesthesia. This approach may offer the advantage of rapid recovery with minimal sequelae and may also facilitate anesthesia in special locations where space is limited.

The infusion rates required by pediatric patients vary depending on other concurrent medications, but they tend to be greater than those needed in adults. When infusions are used to maintain anesthesia, the administration rate should be adjusted to match the predicted elimination of the drug (to maintain a constant blood level) and to prevent the signs of light anesthesia. The infusion may be adjusted manually or controlled by a computer. In either case, the rate should be dictated by the pharmacokinetic parameters for the child's age group. Although these parameters vary considerably more in children than in adults, clinically useful dosage schedules for children have been developed (Table 3–3). For brief or minor surgeries, we have found intermittent intravenous boluses of propofol to be both effective and efficient.

Experience with propofol in pediatric hospitals suggests that its most useful applications may lie outside the operating room—in magnetic resonance imaging and other imaging studies, radiotherapy, and invasive procedures that include medical procedures, burn dressing changes, and endoscopies. Propofol has a potent antiemetic effect, and postoperative nausea is rare.

Table 3–3. Infusion Regimen for Propofol in Children

No other opioid or anesthetic agents used.

Loading sleep dose: 2.5–5 mg/kg

Initial infusion rate (first 10 min): 200–300 μg/kg/min or 12–18 mg/kg/hr

Subsequent infusion rate (next 10 min): 200 μg/kg/min or 12 mg/kg/hr

Final infusion rate: 150 μg/kg/min or 9 mg/kg/hr

These rates must be adjusted or supplemental doses administered if signs of light anesthesia appear.

If an opioid is used, these infusion rates may be reduced by 25%.

Propofol has been used for prolonged sedation in pediatric intensive care units. However, this practice is no longer recommended because myocardial failure and postinfusion neurologic dysfunction have been reported in children after prolonged infusions, particularly in septic children.

Midazolam

Midazolam is a water-soluble benzodiazepine that has been used for premedication, for sedation during endoscopic procedures (in a dose of 0.2–0.3 mg/kg IV), and for amnestic supplementation to general anesthesia. Ventilation and cardiovascular homeostasis are maintained. Midazolam has also been found satisfactory for producing sedation in children in pediatric intensive care units; a loading dose of 0.2 mg/kg has been used, after which an infusion at a rate of 2–6 mg/kg/min is required. It is not an effective agent for induction of anesthesia because of the large doses required and the variability in response. Midazolam is most widely given as an oral premedication (*see* page 79).

Ketamine Hydrochloride

Ketamine, a phencyclidine derivative for general anesthesia, came into clinical use in 1964. It has been utilized extensively in pediatric anesthesia for a wide variety of situations, but with the introduction of propofol it has limited appeal today.

Ketamine's effects on the central nervous system are unlike those of any other anesthetic agent in common use. It produces profound analgesia, unconsciousness, cataleptic state, and amnesia. Ketamine increases cerebral blood flow, ICP, and cerebral metabolic rate. The airway is usually well maintained, but airway obstruction or laryngospasm may occur. Some degree of respiratory depression with brief periods of apnea may occur after induction. Because the protective laryngeal reflexes are depressed, gastric contents may be regurgitated and aspirated. Ketamine increases both the heart rate and the mean arterial pressure, although its direct effect on the isolated heart is a depressant one. In healthy subjects, cardiac output is increased and peripheral vascular resistance is little changed. These indirect cardiovascular responses are mediated by adrenergic pathways.

Ketamine has minimal gastrointestinal effects, although nausea and vomiting may occur. There have been no reports of hepatic or renal damage after its administration. Its most serious disadvantage is a very high incidence of emergence phenomena, ranging from hallucinations and bad dreams to frank psychosis. These phenomena can be significantly reduced by adequate premedication with a benzodiazepine and by providing the patient's recovery in a quiet area. Although such effects may seem less common in children, the high incidence of these phenomena and others has limited ketamine's use. The effects on ICP and cerebral blood flow have led most centers to abandon this drug during neuroradiologic or similar procedures. Some still use it for cardiac catheterization. Ketamine has no effect on visceral pain and therefore is unsatisfactory for abdominal surgery.

Ketamine has been widely used for children with burns that require skin grafting procedures. In such cases, the advantage of an early return to normal nutrition outweighs any of the drug's disadvantages. It is also useful for minor superficial procedures in infants. Ketamine may also be valuable for anesthesia in children with right-to-left intracardiac shunt, epidermolysis bullosa, or Stevens-Johnson syndrome; for induction of anesthesia in severely shocked patients; for general anesthesia when facilities are limited as in some underdeveloped countries; and in large-scale disasters.

Summary

Of the intravenous agents available, thiopental remains the most popular and widely administered for induction in children, although propofol is rapidly gaining in popularity. All of the newer agents have problems relating to administration, making it unlikely that they will supplant thiopental. Ketamine may still have advantages in a few selected cases. Maintenance of a state of deep sedation/general anesthesia using a propofol infusion is a helpful technique for many procedures.

Rectal Methohexital

Methohexital is effective by the rectal route: 15 mg/kg of a 1% solution usually induces sleep in 6–8 minutes. Rarely, ventilatory obstruction or depression may occur; therefore, the child must be observed closely until he falls asleep. The anesthesiologist should be in attendance with equipment to establish an airway discretely at hand. Once the child is anesthetized, the induction may be continued with a volatile agent; gently assisted ventilation may be needed at this stage. This is a pleasant method of induction, and it is especially suitable for apprehensive patients younger than 3 years of age, who may remain in their mother's arms until they fall asleep.

Methohexital should be administered from a syringe, using a well-lubricated #10 catheter, which should be inserted 3–4 cm. A small volume of air in the syringe enables the total dose to be flushed into the rectum. A diaper should be placed under the child, because soiling sometimes occurs.

Opioid Drugs

Morphine, meperidine, and fentanyl have been administered extensively as part of balanced anesthesia in children. The newer agents alfentanil, sufentanil, and remifentanil have also been used in pediatric patients. Administration by infusion after loading doses is optimal, although bolus doses are often used intraoperatively. In addition to providing analgesia, fentanyl and sufentanil, when given in adequate dosage, may block neuroendocrine and pulmonary vascular responses to stress.

Morphine

Morphine provides excellent analgesia and sedation and remains a most satisfactory agent for postoperative systemic analgesia. Neonates have been considered more sensitive to the ventilatory depressant effects of morphine than to those of meperidine (pethidine). Various factors have been postulated to account for this sensitivity, including differences in permeability of the blood-brain barrier. Probably the most important factor is the relatively slower, less predictable clearance of the drug in the neonate, which tends to result in higher blood levels. The decline in the blood level after discontinuation of a morphine infusion may also be delayed in small infants. Indeed, sometimes a transient increase may be observed, possibly as a result of enterohepatic recirculation of the drug. Provided that careful monitoring and suitably low infusion rates are used, morphine can be safely administered by continuous infusion even in the neonate. The patient should be monitored for 24 hours after discontinuation of a morphine infusion.

Fentanyl

Fentanyl is potent but short-acting. Its metabolism in infants is dependent on age: neonates, and especially preterm infants, metabolize fentanyl more slowly than older infants do. Increased intra-abdominal pressure (e.g., repaired omphalocele, intestinal obstruction) further slows the clearance of fentanyl by reducing hepatic blood flow. As a sole analgesic agent during anesthesia, 12–15 μg/kg is required to prevent cardiovascular responses to surgery. Supplemental fentanyl may not be required for 60–90 minutes. If it is planned to extubate the trachea after surgery, an infusion of 2–4 μg/kg/hr may be used to supplement N_2O during balanced anesthesia. Larger doses should not be given to small infants unless they are ventilated or closely monitored postoperatively. Rebound of fentanyl blood levels may occur and may cause depression of ventilation; therefore, if large doses have been given, the patient must be carefully watched. Infants older than 3 months of age may be less sensitive to fentanyl-induced ventilatory depression and have been demonstrated to metabolize the drug more rapidly. Bradycardia may occur after use of fentanyl unless it is preceded by a vagal blocking drug (e.g., atropine, pancuronium). Muscle rigidity may occur with the potent analgesics but is rare in infants and children.

Infants who receive large doses of fentanyl over a prolonged period may develop tolerance to the drug, and a significant number may also show signs of dependence. This effect is common in infants who have been treated with a fentanyl infusion while receiving extracorporeal membrane oxygenation for a period of days. Such infants subsequently require very large doses to prevent response to a surgical stimulus. It may then be appropriate to use other anesthetic or analgesic drugs if necessary. Neonatal abstinence syndrome may occur when fentanyl is withdrawn after continued use; it is characterized by crying, hyperactivity, fever, tremors, poor feeding and sleeping, and—in the extreme case—vomiting and convulsions. These sequelae can be avoided by careful tapering of the narcotic dosage.

Alfentanil

Alfentanil has a more rapid onset and a shorter duration of action than fentanyl. It is less lipid soluble than fentanyl and is highly protein bound. Most of the drug is metabolized in the liver. Less than 1% is excreted via the kidney unchanged. Clearance of the drug is slower and more variable in young infants, especially preterm infants. Otherwise, in older infants and children, the pharmacokinetics are similar to those in adults. The drug has minimal cardiovascular effects. Alfentanil, 35 μg/kg as a bolus followed by intermittent doses of 10 μg/kg every 10–15 minutes, has been suggested as suitable for children. A continuous infusion may be preferred. Recovery after alfentanil is reported to be very rapid and complete. However, this is a very potent drug and all children should be closely observed for signs of residual or recurring respiratory depression. Because vomiting after alfentanil is common, a prophylactic antiemetic should be considered.

Sufentanil

Sufentanil is 10 times as potent as fentanyl and has a shorter elimination half-life. The clearance rate is slower in infants younger than 1 month of age. Sufentanil has been administered in high doses for cardiac surgery in infants, producing good cardiovascular stability with minimal depression of ventricular function. Sufentanil in large doses may favorably influence the metabolic and neuroendocrine response to major cardiovascular surgery in infants.

Remifentanil

Remifentanil, an ultra-short-acting synthetic opioid, represents a new class of opioids that must be administered as a continuous intravenous infusion. It is available as a lyophilized powder and requires reconstitution. The intravenous loading dose is 0.5–2.0 μg/kg, and the maintenance dose is 0.05–2.0 μg/kg/min. The maintenance dose may be reduced by half if a potent inhaled agent is coadministered. The kinetics of remifentanil are unique: its elimination half-life, which is 3–10 minutes, is independent of both the dose and the duration of administration of the infusion. Its action is terminated by hydrolysis of an ester bond by ubiquitous tissue esterase enzymes. As an analgesic, the potency of remifentanil is similar to that of fentanyl but 20- to 30-fold greater than that of alfentanil. The side effects of remifentanil are similar to those of other opioids and include bradycardia, apnea, chest wall rigidity, and vomiting.

Nonsteroidal Anti-inflammatory Drugs

Acetaminophen

Acetaminophen is an analgesic and antipyretic drug without anti-inflammatory actions. It is metabolized well by infants and children of all ages. It is useful as an analgesic for mild pain and is also useful as an opioid-sparing adjunct for more severe pain. It is usually given in doses of 10–15 mg/kg PO or up to 20 mg/kg PR. However, there is evidence to suggest that larger doses may be more effective. Doses of 25–30 mg/kg PO or 40 mg/kg PR are found to achieve more effective blood levels. The total dose should not exceed 90 mg/kg per 24 hours. *Beware: hepatic failure may occur with overdose and is a particular risk in the seriously ill child.*

Indomethacin and Ibuprofen

Indomethacin and ibuprofen were demonstrated to reduce postoperative morphine requirements and to improve pain relief in a series of children. Ibuprofen has fewer side effects and is a safer drug to use in children.

Ketorolac

Ketorolac is a nonsteroidal analgesic that is available for parenteral use either intramuscularly or intravenously. It is considered to be a moderately potent analgesic that is devoid of respiratory depression, vomiting, sedation, and urinary retention effects. In clinical trials ketorolac has been shown to be effective and is opioid-sparing. The dose is usually 1.0 mg/kg IV, repeated every 6 hours up to a maximum 24-hour dose of 90 mg. The elimination half-life of ketorolac in children is similar to that in adults: 5 hours.

It is recommended that the drug be used for short periods (i.e., several days) only, because of the risk of nephrotoxicity. Ketorolac should be administered with caution to patients with impaired renal or hepatic function. Like most nonsteroidal anti-inflammatory drugs (NSAIDs), ketorolac reversibly inhibits platelet function and may result in increased bleeding, especially if it is administered before or early in the surgical procedure. Postoperatively, ketorolac does not appear to lead to increased bleeding, although most clinicians avoid it for surgeries where bleeding may be problematic (adenotonsillectomy, cleft palate, and so forth).

Neuroleptics

Droperidol is a powerful tranquilizer that potentiates sedatives and hypnotics. It has a potent antiemetic effect but sedates children postoperatively, thus limiting it for ambulatory surgery. Droperidol and fentanyl have been given together to produce tranquility and analgesia during procedures performed using local analgesia (neuroleptanalgesia) or to supplement N_2O (neuroleptanesthesia).

Neuroleptanalgesia is most useful when the patient's cooperation is required during major surgery. The patient should be monitored very closely afterward, because droperidol potentiates all other depressant drugs and its effects may continue for some hours.

Opioid Antagonists

There may rarely be a need for an antagonist after the administration of narcotics as adjuncts to general anesthesia.

Naloxone Hydrochloride

Naloxone hydrochloride (Narcan), an *N*-allyl derivative of oxymorphone HCl, antagonizes narcotics, but unlike previous agents it has no narcotic effects. In addition (unlike *N*-allyl-normorphine or levallorphan), it is also an antagonist to the opioid effects of pentazocine. Naloxone does not decrease barbiturate-induced respiratory depression and therefore is useful when it is unknown which drugs are contributing to the depression. Respiratory depression may be reversed with as little as 0.5–1.0 µg/kg, although larger doses (up to 100 µg/kg) may be required. Repeated small doses reverse the respiratory depression without reversing the analgesic effects. The same dose of naloxone that reverses the respiratory depression may be administered again, but intramuscularly, to ensure naloxone will antagonize the opioid effects for a prolonged period. The naloxone dosage should always be titrated slowly until the desired effect is achieved. Naloxone is contraindicated in patients who may be opioid dependent.

Suggested Additional Reading

Acetaminophen

Anderson BJ: What we don't know about paracetamol in children. Paediatr Anaesth 8:451–460, 1998.

Heubi JE, Barbacci MB, and Zimmerman HJ: Therapeutic misadventures with acetaminophen: hepatotoxicity after multiple doses in children. J Pediatr 132:22–27, 1998.

Romsing J, Hertel S, Harder A, and Rasmussen M: Examination of acetaminophen for outpatient management of postoperative pain in children. Paediatr Anaesth 8:235–239, 1998.

Thiopental

Jonmarker C, Westrin P, Larsson S, and Werner O: Thiopental requirements for induction of anesthesia in children. Anesthesiology 67:104–107, 1987.

Kingston HGG, Kendrick A, Sommer KM, et al.: Binding of thiopental in neonatal serum. Anesthesiology 72:428–431, 1990.

Sorbo S, Hudson RJ, and Loomis JC: The pharmacokinetics of thiopental in pediatric surgical patients. Anesthesiology 61:666–670, 1984.

Westrin P, Jonmarker C, and Werner O: Thiopental requirements for induction of anesthesia in neonates and in infants one to six months of age. Anesthesiology 71:344–346, 1989.

Propofol

Browne BL, Prys Roberts C, and Wolf AR: Propofol and alfentanil in children: infusion and dose requirements for total intravenous anaesthesia. Anaesthesia 69:570–576, 1992.

Jones RD, Chan K, and Andrew LJ: Pharmacokinetics of propofol in children. Br J Anaesth 65:661–667, 1990.

Marsh B, White M, Morton N, and Kenney GN: Pharmacokinetic model driven infusion of propofol in children. Br J Anaesth 67:41–48, 1991.

Martin TM, Nicholson SC, and Bargas MS: Propofol anesthesia reduces emesis and airway obstruction in pediatric outpatients. Anesth Analg 76:144–148, 1992.

McFarlan CS, Anderson BJ, and Short TG: The use of propofol infusions in paediatric anesthesia: a practical guide. Paediatr Anaesth 9:209–216, 1999.

Patel DK, Keeling PA, Newman GB, and Radford P: Induction dose of propofol in children. Anaesthesia 43:949–952, 1988.

Midazolam

Booker PD, Beechey A, and Lloyd-Thomas AR: Sedation of children requiring artificial ventilation using an infusion of midazolam. Br J Anaesth 58:1104–1108, 1986.

Cole WHJ: Midazolam in paediatric anaesthesia. Anaesth Intensive Care 10:36–39, 1982.

Silvasi DL, Rosen DA, and Rosen KR: Continuous intravenous midazolam infusion for sedation in the pediatric intensive care unit. Anesth Analg 67:286–288, 1988.

Ketamine

Hollister GR and Burn JMB: Side effects of ketamine in pediatric anesthesia. Anesth Analg 53:264, 1974.

Yeung ML and Lin RSH: Laryngeal reflexes in children under ketamine anaesthesia. Br J Anaesth 44:1089, 1972.

Rectal Methohexital

Forbes RB, Murray DJ, Dillman JB, et al.: Pharmacokinetics of 2% rectal methohexital in children. Anesthesiology 69:A757, 1988.

Goresky GV and Steward DJ: Rectal methohexitone for induction of anaesthesia in children. Can Anaesth Soc J 26:213, 1979.

Liu LMP, Gaudrealt P, Friedman PA, et al.: Pharmacodynamics of rectal methohexital in children. Anesthesiology 59:A450, 1983.

Opioid Drugs

Arnold JH, Truog RD, Orav EJ, et al.: Tolerance and dependence in neonates sedated with fentanyl during extracorporeal membrane oxygenation. Anesthesiology 73:1136–1140, 1990.

Davis PJ, Killian A, Stiller RL, et al.: Alfentanil pharmacodynamics in premature infants and older children. Anesthesiology 69:A758, 1988.

Davis PJ, Robinson KA, Stiller RL, and Cook DR: Sufentanil kinetics in infants and children. Anesthesiology 63:A472, 1985.

Goresky GV, Koren G, Sabourin MA, et al.: The pharmacokinetics of alfentanil in children. Anesthesiology 67:654–659, 1987.

Greeley WJ and deBruijn NP: Changes in sufentanil pharmacokinetics within the neonatal period. Anesth Analg 67:86–90, 1988.

Greeley WJ, deBruijn NP, and Davis DP: Pharmacokinetics of sufentanil in pediatric patients. Anesthesiology 65:A442, 1986.

Hertzka RE, Gauntlett IS, Fisher DM, and Spellman MJ: Fentanyl induced ventilatory depression: effects of age. Anesthesiology 70:213–218, 1989.

Johnson KL, Erickson JP, Holley FO, and Scott JC: Fentanyl pharmacokinetics in the pediatric population. Anesthesiology 61:A441, 1984.

Killian A, David PJ, Stiller RL, et al.: Influence of gestational age on pharmacokinetics of alfentanil in neonates. Dev Pharm Ther 15:83–85, 1990.

Koehntop DE, Rodman JH, and Brundage DM, et al.: Pharmacokinetics of fentanyl in neonates. Anesth Analg 65:227–232, 1986.

Purcell-Jones G, Dorman F, and Sumner E: The use of opioids in neonates: a retrospective study of 933 cases. Anaesthesia 42:1316–1320, 1987.

Singleton MA, Rosen JI, and Fisher DM: Pharmacokinetics of fentanyl for infants and adults. Anesthesiology 61:A440, 1984.

Way WL, Costley EC, and Way EL: Respiratory sensitivity of the newborn infant to meperidine and morphine. Clin Pharmacol Ther 6:454, 1965.

Yaster M: The dose response of fentanyl in neonatal anesthesia. Anesthesiology 66:433–435, 1987.

Youngberg JA, Subaiya C, Graybar GB, et al.: Alfentanil for day stay surgery in children: an evaluation. Anesth Analg 63:284, 1984.

Nonsteroidal Anti-inflammatory Drugs

Forrest JB, Heitlinger EL, and Revell S: Ketorolac for postoperative pain management in children. Drug Safety 16:309–329, 1997.

Maunuksela EL, Olkkola KT, and Korpela R: Does prophylactic intravenous infusion of indomethacin improve the management of postoperative pain in children. Can J Anaesth 35:123–127, 1988.

Romsing J, Ostergaard D, Walther-Larsen S, and Valentin N: Analgesic efficacy and safety of preoperative versus postoperative ketorolac in paediatric tonsillectomy. Acta Anaesth Scand 42:770–775, 1998.

Neuromuscular Blocking Drugs

Neuromuscular blocking drugs are often used in pediatric anesthesia to facilitate tracheal intubation and muscle relaxation for controlled ventilation and surgery. These drugs require special attention because their effects in infants may differ from those in adults. The neuromuscular junction in infancy has less reserve than that of the adult. Fade occurs at high rates of stimulation. This has led to the suggestion that infants show a myasthenic response and would be sensitive to nondepolarizing relaxants. In fact, to produce a similar degree of block, infants and adults require similar doses of relaxants on a milligram-per-kilogram basis. This may be attributed to the combined effects of a larger volume of distribution and a greater degree of block for a specific plasma concentration in the infant. It is important to note that although the average doses of nondepolarizing relaxants in infants are similar to those in adults, the variability in dose requirements is much greater. This may be related to the larger number of extrajunctional receptors in the skeletal muscles of infants. It is prudent to monitor the degree of neuromuscular block carefully as a guide to dosage.

Succinylcholine

Succinylcholine is the only depolarizing relaxant in clinical use. Its onset and offset of action are more rapid than those of any other relaxant. It may be administered by any one of three routes: intravenously, intramuscularly, or intralingually. Intravenous succinylcholine (2 mg/kg) has an onset of action of 20–30 seconds and reaches its maximum effect within 40 seconds. Intramuscular administration of succinylcholine (4 mg/kg) has a slightly slower onset of action compared with the intravenous route.

Intralingual succinylcholine is used only for emergencies when other routes are not accessible.

Infants require a relatively higher dose of succinylcholine than adults (2 versus 1 mg/kg, respectively), despite the lower plasma cholinesterase activity in infants younger than 6 months of age. The greater dose requirement results from distribution of the drug throughout the relatively large extracellular fluid compartment. Recovery is similar to that in the adult. The cholinesterase activity, although lower, is quite adequate to metabolize the drug.

Cardiac arrhythmias, in the form of bradycardia, occur commonly after a single dose of intravenous succinylcholine in children. Bradycardia can be prevented by preceding succinylcholine administration with a single intravenous dose of atropine (0.01–0.02 mg/kg). Intramuscular succinylcholine (4 mg/kg) changes the heart rate and rhythm minimally, even in unatropinized anesthetized children.

Although myoglobinemia and myoglobinuria occur more commonly after succinylcholine in children than in adults, especially if halothane precedes succinylcholine, the incidence of strong fasciculations and muscle pains is less. However, children who are ambulatory should be pretreated with a nondepolarizing relaxant to prevent postoperative muscle pains. Serious rhabdomyolysis, severe myoglobinuria, and cardiac arrest may occur in children with myopathies including Duchenne muscular dystrophy.

Masseter spasm is reported to occur in as many as 1 in 100 cases if intravenous succinylcholine is given after induction of anesthesia with halothane. The significance of masseter spasm and its relation, if any, to malignant hyperthermia are unclear. All reports indicate that the malignant hyperthermia trait is very much less common. Masseter spasm is extremely rare after induction of anesthesia with thiopental followed by succinylcholine (i.e., without simultaneous halothane administration). If it occurs in this situation, it must be considered a significant warning sign of possible malignant hyperthermia trait. The sequence of thiopental plus succinylcholine does not commonly result in masseter spasm and remains the most effective means of securing the airway rapidly.

Succinylcholine causes less increase in intragastric pressure in infants and young children than in older children and adults. Intraocular pressure increases transiently after succinylcholine administration because of greater tension in the extraocular muscles. Succinylcholine should be avoided if the injured eye has a large laceration, if intraocular pressure is to be measured (i.e., in glaucoma), or if forced duction testing is planned (i.e., in strabismus surgery).

Serum potassium levels increase after succinylcholine administration in children with burns more than 24 hours old, massive trauma, major neurologic disease, or renal failure compounded by neuropathy. It has been suggested that dreaming during anesthesia may be more common if repeated doses of succinylcholine are given.

d-Tubocurarine

d-Tubocurarine (3 mg/ml concentration in 5-ml ampule) was not available for a number of years owing to concerns about quality control at manufacturing facilities. It is currently available worldwide but is not often used. Curare is effective for relaxation during maintenance of anesthesia for surgery of intermediate duration (longer than 1 hour). It causes a release of histamine that is age dependent (i.e., less in the younger child). Volatile agents, especially isoflurane, potentiate the action of curare and reduce the requirements for this drug. Maintenance doses are 0.3–0.4 mg/kg when volatile agents are used and 0.4–0.5 mg/kg when they are not. The effects of curare on the cardiovascular system include hypotension, but they are less in infants and children than in adults. In children, even small doses of curare depress ventilation; therefore, ventilation must be controlled whenever curare is administered. Curare should not be given to asthmatic patients, in whom bronchospasm secondary to histamine release may occur.

Pancuronium

Pancuronium (1 or 2 mg/ml concentration in a 5-ml ampule) is five times as potent as *d*-tubocurarine, and the duration of its action is longer. Initial doses of 0.1 mg/kg permit intubation in about 2 minutes. Supplementary doses should be given carefully, using a nerve stimulator for guidance; each dose should be only 10%–20% of the initial paralyzing dose.

Pancuronium causes much less histamine release than does *d*-tubocurarine, and it is the preferred relaxant for surgery of longer duration in asthmatics. Pancuronium causes an increase in heart rate and blood pressure, particularly when given as a rapid intravenous bolus. These effects are more pronounced in younger patients. In preterm infants, pancuronium causes a sustained tachycardia and hypertension and increased plasma epinephrine level. Pancuronium is excreted principally via the kidney and should not be given to patients whose renal function is impaired, as prolonged neuromuscular block may occur.

Atracurium

Atracurium, a benzylisoquinolonium, is a nondepolarizing neuromuscular blocking agent with a brief duration of action (±30 minutes)—less than that of *d*-tubocurarine or pancuronium. It is a mixture of 10 stereoisomers that vary in potency and side effects. It is used infrequently now, having been replaced by *cis*-atracurium. Atracurium degrades at physiologic pH to inactive compounds (Hofmann elimination) and hence has a predictable rate of elimination even in the presence of severe hepatic or renal disease. Its shorter duration of action and constant rate of metabolism make this drug ideal for administration by continuous infusion. In children, an initial bolus of 0.3 mg/kg followed by an infusion of 6 μg/kg/hr results in satisfactory relaxation during halothane or isoflurane anesthesia. Slightly larger doses are required if opioids are substituted for volatile agents. Atracurium usually has little effect on the cardiovascular system. It does release histamine, especially if large doses are given rapidly, and should not be given to patients with asthma. Bronchospasm has been described after use of the drug in adults and children. A rash is common, but significant hypotension is rare. Rarely, precipitous and severe hypotension has occurred after the use of atracurium, especially when it has been given in a large dose (more than 0.4 mg/kg) and preceded by thiopental. Anaphylaxis was reported in an infant after induction with thiopental and paralysis with atracurium.

Cis-atracurium

Cis-atracurium is one of the 10 stereoisomers of atracurium besylate. It was isolated and purified because it conferred the most stable hemodynamics and least histamine release of the isomers. It has a relatively slow onset of action. The dose for tracheal intubation is 0.15–0.2 mg/kg, which yields an effective duration of action of approximately 35 minutes. *Cis*-atracurium may also be administered by infusion at a dose of 1.5 μg/kg/min. Termination of its action is similar to atracurium, via Hofmann elimination and ester hydrolysis. The duration of action of *cis*-atracurium is unaffected by renal or hepatic failure; therefore, it is a drug of choice in such situations.

Vecuronium

Vecuronium (lyophilized powder), a steroidal relaxant, is an intermediate-acting nondepolarizing neuromuscular blocking agent. Its duration of action is 35–45 minutes in children but may be longer (70 minutes or longer) in small infants. The effective dose in 95% of patients (ED_{95}) for vecuronium is greater in children 2–10 years old (81 mcg/kg) than in infants (47 mcg/kg) or adolescents (55 mcg/kg). It is a highly specific drug, devoid of cardiovascular effects and histamine release. The duration of action of vecuronium increases in the presence of some forms of liver disease or impaired renal function. Because vecuronium has no vagal blocking effect, bradycardia may occur if vagotonic drugs (e.g., fentanyl, halothane) are coadministered; atropine may be required. Vecuronium may be administered as an infusion. Infants require a considerably lower rate than older children (approximately 60 μg/kg/hr versus 150 mg/kg/hr, respectively).

Rocuronium

Rocuronium, a steroid-based relaxant, differs from vecuronium in its potency (one-sixth as potent as vecuronium) and in its availability in a solution that is stable at room temperature. The intubating dose is 0.7 mg/kg, with a dose of 1.0–1.2 mg/kg recommended for a rapid-sequence induction. It is devoid of cardiovascular and histamine effects, similar to vecuronium, although bradycardia may occur. Recovery after 1.2 mg/kg requires about 40 minutes, although this dose may be antagonized earlier. Elimination is unchanged in renal failure but may be prolonged by up to 100% in hepatic failure.

Mivacurium

Mivacurium is a synthetic nondepolarizing neuromuscular blocking agent with a short duration of action; it is hydrolyzed by plasma cholinesterase. A dose of 0.1–0.2 mg/kg produces a profound degree of blocking in less than 2 minutes, but the onset of blocking is not as rapid as with succinylcholine. The duration of action is approximately half of that of vecuronium. The cardiovascular effects of the drug are minimal. Its short duration of action suggests that it may prove useful for intubation for minor procedures and possibly for infusion, especially when the extent of neuromuscular block must be adjusted rapidly (e.g., when muscle power must be assessed or motor evoked potentials monitored). Because the recovery time is related to plasma cholinesterase activity, prolonged effects may be expected in those children with abnormality of the plasma cholinesterases.

Rapacuronium

Rapacuronium has a rapid onset and a short duration of action. A dose of 1.5 mg/kg usually produces good intubating conditions within 1 minute. The duration of effective clinical action of this dose is about 20 minutes. Repeat dosing is not recommended because a more potent metabolite is formed, which may lead to prolonged neuromuscular block. This is therefore a single-dose drug for short procedures. The drug has minimal cardiovascular effects.

Antagonism of Neuromuscular Block

Nondepolarizing neuromuscular blocking agents should always be antagonized unless it is very obvious that the patient has completely recovered normal neuromuscular function. Antagonism may not be fully effective in patients who are hypothermic (less than 35°C); therefore, controlled ventilation should be continued. Rarely, antibiotics potentiate the neuromuscular blocking drugs in infants or children to the extent that they cannot be antagonized. This possibility must be considered, especially in those receiving aminoglycoside derivatives (e.g., neomycin, gentamicin, tobramycin).

The adequacy of antagonism of relaxants may be difficult to judge, especially in infants. The train of four should demonstrate four equal contractions. Muscle tone can be examined and is often best judged by flexion of the elbows and hips. The ability to generate an inspiratory pressure of 25 cmH$_2$O has been suggested as a useful index. When any doubt whatsoever exists about the adequacy of the antagonism, controlled ventilation should continue and recovery of neuromuscular function should be reevaluated periodically.

Commonly used regimens to antagonize the nondepolarizing muscle relaxants in infants and children are as follows:

1. Neostigmine (0.05 mg/kg) mixed with atropine (0.02–0.025 mg/kg is effective and results in few and insignificant cardiac arrhythmias even in those with congenital heart disease. Glycopyrrolate does not have any advantage over atropine during antagonism and may not prevent neostigmine-induced bradycardia.
2. Edrophonium (1 mg/kg) after atropine (20 µg/kg) may be used.

Edrophonium has a more rapid onset of action than neostigmine, and its vagotonic action appears early. These findings have led to the practice of administering atropine before the edrophonium.

Suggested Additional Reading

Bennett EJ, Ramamurthy S, Dalal FY, and Salem ME: Pancuronium and the neonate. Br J Anaesth 47:75, 1975.

Brandom BW, Cook DR, Woelfel SK, et al.: Atracurium infusion requirements in children during halothane, isoflurane, and narcotic anesthesia. Anesth Analg 64:471–476, 1985.

Bryson HM and Faulds D: *Cis*-atracurium besylate. Drugs 53:848–866, 1997.

Bush GH and Stead AL: The use of *d*-tubocurarine in neonatal anaesthesia. Br J Anaesth 34:721, 1962.

Cook DR, Brandom BW, Stiller RL, et al.: Pharmacokinetics of atracurium in normal and liver failure patients. Anesthesiology 61:A433, 1984.

Cook DR and Fischer CG: Neuromuscular blocking effects of succinylcholine in infants and children. Anesthesiology 42:662, 1975.

Fisher DM, O'Keefe C, Stanski DR, et al.: Pharmacokinetics and dynamics of *d*-tubocurarine in infants, children, and adults. Anesthesiology 55:A391, 1981.

Goudsouzian NG: Maturation of neuromuscular transmission in the infant. Br J Anaesth 52:205–213, 1980.

Goudsouzian NG: The physiology and pharmacology of neuromuscular transmission in infants and children. In DJ Steward (ed.): Some Aspects of Paediatric Anaesthesia. Excerpta Medica, Amsterdam, 1982, pp 59–77.

Goudsouzian NG: Atracurium in infants and children. Br J Anaesth 58(Suppl 1):23S–28S, 1986.

Goudsouzian NG, Alifimoff JK, Eberl C, et al.: Neuromuscular and cardiovascular effects of mivacurium in children. Anesthesiology 70:237–242, 1989.

Goudsouzian NG, Donlon JV, Savarese JJ, and Ryan JF: Reevaluation of dosage and duration of action of *d*-tubocurarine in the pediatric age group. Anesthesiology 43:416, 1975.

Goudsouzian NG, Ryan JF, and Savarese JJ: The neuromuscular effects of pancuronium in infants and children. Anesthesiology 41:95, 1974.

Hobbs AJ, Bush GH, and Downham DY: Perioperative dreaming and awareness in children. Anaesthesia 43:560–562, 1988.

Kaplan RF, Fletcher JE, Hannallah RS, et al.: The potency (ED_{50}) and cardiovascular effects of rapacuronium (Org 9487) during narcotic-nitrous oxide-propofol anesthesia in neonates, infants and children. Anesth Analg 89:1172–1176, 1999.

Meretoja OA, Taivainen T, Erkola O, et al.: Dose-response and time-course of effect of rocuronium bromide in paediatric patients. Eur J Anaesthesiol Suppl 11:19–22, 1995.

Meretoja OA, Taivainen T, and Wirtavuori K: *Cis*-atracurium during halothane and balanced anaesthesia in children. Paediatr Anaesth 6:373–378, 1996.

Meretoja OA, Wirtavuori K, and Neuvonen PJ: Age dependence of the dose-response curve of vecuronium in pediatric patients during balanced anesthesia. Anesth Analg 67:21–26, 1988.

Montgomery CJ and Steward DJ: A comparative study of intubating doses of atracurium, *d*-tubocurarine, pancuronium, and vecuronium in children. Can J Anaesth 35:31–35, 1988.

Nightingale DA: Use of atracurium in neonatal anaesthesia. Br J Anaesth 58(Suppl 1):32S–36S, 1986.

Nightingale DA and Bush GH: A clinical comparison between tubocurarine and pancuronium in children. Br J Anaesth 45:63, 1973.

Salem MR, Toyama T, Wong AY, et al.: Haemodynamic responses to antagonism of tubocurarine block with atropine-neostigmine mixture in children. Br J Anaesth 49:901, 1977.

Woolf RL, Crawford MW, and Choo SM: Dose response of rocuronium bromide in children anesthetized with propofol. Anesthesiology 87:1368–1372, 1997.

Zsigmond ED and Downs JR: Plasma cholinesterase activity in newborns and infants. Can Anaesth Soc J 18:278, 1971.

Reversal of Muscle Relaxants

Fisher DM, Cronnelly R, Miller RD, and Sharma M: The neuromuscular pharmacology of neostigmine in infants and children. Anesthesiology 59:220–225, 1983.

Fisher DM, Cronnelly R, Sharma M, and Miller RD: Clinical pharmacology of edrophonium in infants and children. Anesthesiology 61:428–433, 1984.

Mason LJ and Betts EK: Leg lift and maximum inspiratory force clinical signs of neuromuscular blockade reversal in neonates and infants. Anesthesiology 52:441–442, 1980.

Salem MR, Ylagan LB, and Angel JJ: Reversal of curarization with atropine-neostigmine mixture in patients with congenital heart disease. Br J Anaesth 42:991–998, 1970.

Wong AY, Salem MR, and Mani M, et al.: Glycopyrrolate as a substitute for atropine in the reversal of curarization in pediatric cardiac patients. Anesth Analg 53:412–418, 1974.

LOCAL ANALGESIC DRUGS

Local analgesic drugs are now very widely used in pediatric patients, particularly in the management of postoperative pain (Table 3–4).

Pharmacology

The pharmacokinetics are different in infants and small children, compared with older children and adults:

1. Absorption of the drugs is rapid, the cardiac output and regional tissue blood flows are higher, and the epidural space contains less fat

Table 3–4. Maximum Doses of Commonly Used Local Analgesics for Pediatric Patients*

Agent	Dose (mg/kg)
Lidocaine	
Plain	5
With epinephrine	10
Bupivacaine	3
Tetracaine	2
Procaine	15
Chloroprocaine	15

*Doses may vary according to the site of injection.

tissue to buffer uptake. Drugs sprayed into the airway are very rapidly absorbed.

2. The volume of distribution of the drug is larger. Plasma levels of bupivacaine after administration of a standard 3 mg/kg dose into the epidural space are therefore significantly lower in infants than in young children and adults. This greater volume of distribution also extends the elimination half-life.

3. The extent of protein binding is less; serum albumin and α_1-acid glycoprotein levels are low in the neonate. Bilirubin may further reduce the potential for protein binding. Caution is advised when local analgesia is being considered in the jaundiced neonate.

4. The rate of metabolism of local analgesic drugs is reduced in very young infants:

   a. Plasma cholinesterase activity is reduced, which may prolong the metabolism of the ester-type drugs. For example, the plasma half-life of procaine or chloroprocaine is extended in the neonate.

   b. The hepatic pathways for conjugation of the amide local analgesics are immature. The neonate has a reduced capacity to metabolize mepivacaine and bupivacaine; however, by 1–6 months of age, the latter is cleared as rapidly as in adults. Older infants and children metabolize drugs much more rapidly because of their relatively large liver size.

5. The metabolism of prilocaine may result in methemoglobinemia. This may be more significant in infants, who have lower levels of the enzyme methemoglobin reductase.

Other Effects

Epinephrine

Epinephrine is added to local anesthetic drugs to extend their action. It also acts as a marker for intravascular injection, although tachycardia may be more difficult to assess in children. Epinephrine may interact with halothane and precipitate arrhythmias, but doses up to 10 μg/kg by infiltration are considered safe in children. Epinephrine extends the duration of action of bupivacaine to a greater extent in infants and young children than in older patients.

Toxicity

Compared with adults, neonates may exhibit signs of central nervous system toxicity at lower blood levels of a drug. Local analgesic blocks in pediatric patients are commonly performed during general anesthesia. This practice tends to mask any signs of neurologic toxicity. Because potent volatile anesthetic agents (e.g., halothane) may augment the cardiac effects of the local anesthetic drugs, caution is advised.

Intravenous lidocaine in normal doses may produce toxic effects in children with right-to-left cardiac shunting, because the normal first-pass

absorption within the pulmonary circulation is bypassed. The dose
should be reduced by at least 50% in such cases.

Suggested Additional Reading

Bokesch PM, Castenada AR, Ziemer G, and Wilson JM: The influence of a right
to left shunt on lidocaine pharmacokinetics. Anesthesiology 67:739–744, 1987.

Eyres RL, Hastings C, Brown TCK, and Oppenheim RC: Plasma bupivacaine
concentrations following lumbar epidural anaesthetic in children. Anaesth Intensive Care 14:131–135, 1986.

Karl HW, Swedlow DB, Lee KW, and Downes JJ: Epinephrine-halothane interactions in children. Anesthesiology 58:142–145, 1983.

Lerman J, Strong HA, Ledez KM, et al.: Effects of age on the serum concentration of alpha 1 acid glycoprotein and the binding of lidocaine in pediatric
patients. Clin Pharm Ther 46:219–225, 1989.

Mazoit JX and Dubousset AM: Pharmacology and pharmacokinetics. In Saint-
Maurice CS and Schulte Steinberg O (eds.): Regional Anaesthesia in Children.
Appleton & Lange, Norwalk, CT, 1990, pp 39–59.

Warner MA, Kundel SE, Offord KO, et al.: The effects of age, epinephrine,
and operative site on duration of caudal analgesia in pediatric patients. Anesth
Analg 66:995–998, 1987.

Chapter 4

Techniques and Procedures of Pediatric Anesthesia

ROUTINE PREPARATION FOR SURGERY

Preoperative Assessment

A careful assessment of the patient must be made at the time of the preoperative visit. Although many children are healthy, some have diseases with significant implications for the anesthesiologists. A thorough review of the history is the first essential; this must usually be obtained from the patient's chart and from the parents. Review the systems and look particularly for special problems that may complicate anesthesia (Table 4–1). When a significant history is obtained, it is important to establish the exact current status of the disease; this may require consultation with the pediatrician and other physicians. Although many children are not taking any regular medications, some may be receiving treatment that has implications for management during the perioperative period. Always ask about medications and drug allergies. Some important pediatric medications and their significance are detailed in Table 4–2. Throughout the preoperative interview, strive to gain the confidence of the patient and the parents. In establishing rapport, always invite questions.

Preoperative Feeding Orders

Infants and children must not be subjected to unnecessarily prolonged preoperative fasting. The higher rate of fluid turnover in young patients dictates that fluid restriction leads quite rapidly to dehydration and hypovolemia. In addition, excessive fasting may precipitate hypoglycemia and/or metabolic acidosis. Studies have clearly shown that healthy children may safely be given clear fluids up to 2 hours before induction of general anesthesia. The volume and acidity of the gastric contents are not increased when this regimen is used. Indeed, it has been reported that a small drink of apple juice 2 hours before anesthesia may reduce gastric contents at induction, possibly by stimulating gastric emptying. In addition, it reduces hunger and thirst.

Breast milk remains in the stomach for a longer period than clear fluids; infants who are breast-fed should be fasted for at least 4 hours. Infant formula remains in the stomach even longer than breast milk; formula-fed infants should be fasted 6 hours. Solids and semisolids remain in the stomach longer than fluids do. Regular formula feedings may be given up to 6 hours preoperatively to children younger than 2 years of age; clear fluids may then be given up to 2 hours preoperatively.

Children older than 2 years of age should have no solid food on the day of surgery but may be offered drinks of clear fluids (water, ginger ale, apple juice, and so on are considered clear fluids; milk and orange juice are *not*) up to 2 hours preoperatively. Those children who are scheduled for afternoon surgery may be given a soft breakfast early in the morning. These rules must, of course, be modified in special cases (e.g., for diabetic patients).

All patients having emergency surgery, those with gastrointestinal disease, and any others at increased risk for vomiting during induction must be treated differently. They should have nothing by mouth, intravenous fluids as indicated, and rapid sequence induction of anesthesia. Patients for whom any period of fluid deprivation might pose a risk (e.g., those with polycythemia associated with congenital heart disease) should have an intravenous infusion established at the commencement of any prolonged period of restricted oral intake.

Prophylaxis Against Hemorrhage

Ensure that the newborn infant undergoing surgery has been given vitamin K_1 to prevent hemorrhage due to lack of vitamin K–dependent factors. Aqueous vitamin K_1 (1 mg IM or IV) corrects such deficiency within a few hours and therefore should be given as early as possible.

Basic Laboratory Tests

Routine laboratory tests are now considered unnecessary for most children who require anesthesia; however, in some regions, they are a legislated preoperative requirement. Preoperative urinalysis has not been found useful in detecting significant diseases or in routine screening in the pediatric population. Hemoglobin (Hb) determination is likewise of little value in otherwise healthy children. Mild degrees of anemia have not been shown to increase the risk of anesthesia and do not alter the anesthesia technique selected. Most authorities now recommend that these tests may be omitted for healthy patients undergoing minor sur-

Text continued on page 77

Table 4–1. Review of the Medical History—Possible Implications for Anesthesia

Systems	History	Concerns for the Anesthesiologist
Central nervous system	Seizures	Adequacy of seizure medication, recent control of convulsions. Phenytoin increases nondepolarizing relaxant and fentanyl requirements, produces gingival hyperplasia and bleeding, and may cause hepatic dysfunction. Ketamine, enflurane, and methohexital are relatively contraindicated.
	Hydrocephalus	Possible raised intracranial pressure. Repeated anesthesias. Possible need for prophylactic antibiotics to prevent shunt infection.
	Head injury	Possible raised intracranial pressure. Current status. Possible danger of hyperkalemia with succinylcholine.
	Cerebral tumor	Possible raised intracranial pressure, vomiting, change in electrolyte status. Chemotherapeutic agents and possible drug interactions.
	Cerebral palsy	Nutritional status, presence of chronic infections. Possible history of chronic aspiration and difficulties with positioning. Intelligence may be normal—careful psychological preparation needed.
	Down syndrome	Optimal cooperation at induction may be a problem. (Possibly get help from parent.) Airway (large tongue, subglottic stenosis). Heart disease. Evidence of joint hypermobility and indications of atlantoaxial instability.
	Neuromuscular disease	Hyperkalemia with succinylcholine. Altered response to nondepolarizing relaxants. Ventilatory reserve. Cardiac involvement.
	Meningomyelocele	Associated hydrocephalus. History suggesting latex allergy. Renal infections. Impaired renal function. Difficulty positioning. Repeated surgery—careful psychological preparation needed.
Cardiovascular system	Heart murmur	Innocent murmur vs. significant lesion. Need for prophylactic antibiotics. Risk of paradoxic embolism.
	Cyanosis	Hemoconcentration—avoid fluid restriction; risk of hyperviscosity. Coagulopathy secondary to hyperviscosity; check coagulogram. Reduced response to hypoxemia—caution with premedication. Risk of air embolism via intravenous routes.

System	Condition	Considerations
	Dyspnea, tachypnea	Evidence of congestive cardiac failure. History of medication with digoxin.
	Sweating	Digoxin level. History of diuretic therapy. Electrolyte levels.
	Previous heart surgery	Need for prophylactic antibiotics. Cardiac conduction defects. Pacemaker. History of arrhythmias.
Respiratory system	Hypertension	Renal disease, coarctation of the aorta, endocrine disease.
	Prematurity	Risk of perioperative apnea.
	Respiratory distress syndrome	Present postconceptual age, gestational age at birth. Anemia. History of apnea, residual chronic respiratory disease, impaired gas exchange. History of prolonged ventilation, residual subglottic stenosis.
	Recent upper respiratory tract infection	Evidence of acute infection. Pyrexia. Lower respiratory tract infection. Reactive airways prone to secondary infection.
	Bronchiolitis	Reactive airways, evidence of bronchospasm.
	Croup	Possible subglottic stenosis. ?Avoid intubation, use LMA.
	Asthma	Reactive airways. Current status. Theophylline therapy (blood level). β-Agonist drug therapy, history of corticosteroid therapy (prescription supplements). Develop a plan to ensure optimal status preoperatively.
	Cystic fibrosis	Present pulmonary function. Any acute infection? Can condition be improved? Can regional analgesia be used? Present drug therapy. Nutritional status. Emotional status.
Gastrointestinal system	Gastroesophageal reflux	Evidence of aspiration pneumonia. Reactive airways and bronchospasm. Recent food intake, risk of regurgitation, and need for antacid and H_2 blockers. Evidence predicting difficult intubation.
	Vomiting	Nutritional and hydration status. Electrolyte values. Urine output. Immediate full stomach danger.
	Diarrhea	Nutritional, fluid, and electrolyte status.
	Liver disease	Risk of hypoglycemia. Drug metabolism. Increased requirements for nondepolarizing relaxants.

Table continued on following page

Table 4-1. Review of the Medical History—Possible Implications for Anesthesia *Continued*

Systems	History	Concerns for the Anesthesiologist
Genitourinary system	Renal failure	Anemia and coagulopathy, electrolyte abnormality, volume status. Acid-base status. Hypertension and incipient congestive cardiac failure. History of infection? Impaired immunity? Psychological status.
	Bladder surgery	Is history suggestive of latex allergy?
	Extrophy	Is history suggestive of latex allergy?
Endocrine system	Diabetes mellitus	Current status and therapy. Plans for perioperative management. Need for planning with surgeon and endocrinologist.
	Thyroid disease	Current status and medication? Euthyroid? Enlarged thyroid effect on the airway.
	Pituitary disease	Intracranial pressure? Adrenal insufficiency? Thyroid function? Diabetes insipidus?
	Adrenal disease	Need for corticosteroid therapy? Volume and electrolyte status.
Hematopoietic system	Anemia	What is cause? Possible medical therapy. Urgency of surgery. Will anemia affect the course of anesthesia? Is transfusion indicated?
	Bruising or bleeding	Is coagulopathy present? Are further tests required? Preoperative therapy? Order products.
	Sickle cell disease	Trait or disease? Are other abnormal hemoglobins present (Hb electrophoresis results)? Is preoperative preparation required?
Muscular system	Muscular dystrophy	Risk of hyperkalemia with succinylcholine. Avoid nondepolarizing relaxants if possible. Ventilatory reserve? Cardiac function? Will postoperative ICU admission be necessary?

(Modified from Cote CJ, Todres ID, and Ryan JF. Preoperative evaluation of pediatric patients. In Ryan JF, Todres ID, Cote CJ, and Goudsouzian NG (eds.): A Practice of Anesthesia for Infants and Children. Grune & Stratton, Orlando, FL, 1986, p 27, with permission.)

Table 4–2. Concurrent Medication—Possible Implications for Anesthesia

Drug	Implications for Anesthesia
Analgesic, anti-inflammatory	
Acetylsalicylic acid (ASA, aspirin)	Prolonged bleeding time due to platelet inactivation; check bleeding time if ASA given within 10 days.
Nonsteroidal anti-inflammatory drugs (NSAIDs; e.g., ibuprofen, ketorolac)	Affect platelet aggregation and prolong bleeding time. Effect of antihypertensive agents may be decreased. Ketorolac decreases diuretic effect of furosemide.
Antibiotics	Many of the "mycins" may potentiate neuromuscular blockade. Monitor neuromuscular block, check reversal carefully.
Aminoglycosides	May potentiate succinylcholine and nondepolarizing relaxant drugs. Renal toxicity.
Clindamycin	Cardiac depression when given rapidly. May potentiate nondepolarizing relaxant drugs.
Erythromycin	May prolong the effect of alfentanil. Decreases theophylline clearance rates. Potentiates anticoagulant effect of wafarin.
Gentamicin	May prolong the effect of succinylcholine. Potentiates nondepolarizing relaxant drugs.
Vancomycin	Potentiates nondepolarizing relaxant drugs. Rapid administration (<1 hr) may cause "red man syndrome" with severe cardiovascular collapse.
Anticancer agents	All may cause blood dyscrasia, coagulopathy, anorexia, nausea, stomatitis, and reduced resistance to infection.
Doxorubicin (Adriamycin)	Cardiotoxic, may cause arrhythmias.
Daunorubicin (Cerubidine)	Severe cardiac depression with halothane, especially likely when cumulative dose exceeds 250 mg/m² (or 150 mg/m² plus radiation).
Bleomycin	Pulmonary fibrosis—may be exacerbated by excess oxygen. Limit carefully.
Busulfan	Inhibits plasma cholinesterases. May prolong the effect of succinylcholine.
Cyclophosphamide	Inhibit plasma cholinesterases; prolonged effect of succinylcholine or mivacurium.

Table continued on following page

Table 4–2. Concurrent Medication—Possible Implications for Anesthesia
Continued

Drug	Implications for Anesthesia
Anticonvulsants	
Phenytoin	May cause blood dyscrasia, hypotension, bradycardia, arrhythmia.
Mephenytoin	May increase requirements for nondepolarizing relaxants and may cause peripheral neuropathy.
Valproic acid	May cause hypotonia. Hepatotoxic.
Antihypertensive drugs	Severe hypotension may occur with potent anesthetics, especially if patient is dehydrated.
Captopril	Hyperkalemia with potassium-sparing diuretics (spironolactone). Indomethacin reduces antihypertensive effect.
Clonidine	Must not be abruptly withdrawn—severe hypertension may result. Interaction with β-blockers—bradycardia, hypotension.
Hydralazine (Apresoline)	May cause systemic lupus erythematosus (SLE)-type syndrome. Decreases tachycardia with atropine.
Labetalol	May prolong spinal analgesia with tetracaine. Cimetidine may potentiate labetalol action.
Prazosin (Minipress)	May potentiate effects of ketamine. Diuretics potentiate antihypertensive effect.
Antiviral agent	
Acyclovir	Nephrotoxic, bone marrow depression.
β-Agonist agents (e.g., albuterol, Alupent)	May cause tachycardia, hypertension, arrhythmia. Albuterol has increased effect with tricyclic antidepressants or monoamine oxidase inhibitors. Blocked by β-blocking drugs.
β-Blocking drugs	May cause bronchospasm, block effects of albuterol. Potentiate cardiac depression caused by halothane. May cause bradycardia with anticholinesterase drugs (e.g., neostigmine).
Calcium channel blockers	Potentiate nondepolarizing relaxant drugs. Severe bradycardia or heart block with β-blocking drugs.
Verapamil, nifedipine	May interact with β-blockers to cause severe cardiac depression.

Table 4–2. Concurrent Medication—Possible Implications for Anesthesia *Continued*

Drug	Implications for Anesthesia
Corticosteroid preparations	Chronic therapy may lead to depression of the hypothalamic pituitary axis; severe collapse may occur perioperatively. Supplemental steroid therapy should be ordered preoperatively.
Digoxin	May potentiate bupivacaine toxicity. Hypokalemia, if induced (e.g., by hyperventilation), predisposes to arrhythmias.
Diuretics	All may result in electrolyte disturbances.
Acetazolamide (Diamox)	Produces hyperchloremic metabolic acidosis.
Furosemide	May prolong effect of d-tubocurarine. Hypokalemia, if present, may prolong action and delay reversal of relaxant drugs.
Ophthalmic topical drugs	
Echothiopate (anticholinesterase)	Inhibits plasma cholinesterases. Prolonged apnea with succinylcholine and mivacurium.
Phenylephrine	May cause tachycardia and hypertension.
Timolol (β-blocker)	May exacerbate asthma.
Theophylline	Severe arrhythmias may occur with halothane; check blood level.

gery. All small infants, especially those who were born preterm, should have an Hb determination to exclude anemia, which is more common in infants and may increase the risk of complications. Older children with systemic diseases and those with a history of anemia, and those who may lose significant amounts of blood intraoperatively, should also have a preoperative Hb determination. A sickle cell test is necessary for all patients at risk. If the result is positive, an Hb electrophoresis should be ordered.

Premedication

Drugs may be given preoperatively to block unwanted autonomic reflex (vagal) responses, produce preoperative sedation and tranquility, facilitate separation from parents if necessary, and smooth the induction of anesthesia.

Vagal Blocking Drugs

Vagal blocking drugs (atropine, hyoscine, glycopyrrolate) are no longer routinely given to children preoperatively. Brisk vagal responses may occur during anesthesia in infants and children. In every case atropine should immediately be available for use if it becomes necessary.

Serious bradycardia may occur in young patients and may lead to significant hypotension or more dangerous arrhythmias. This can result from instrumentation of the airway, manipulation of the eye, traction of the peritoneum, or administration of cholinergic drugs (halothane, succinylcholine). The heart rate should be continuously monitored during anesthesia. If bradycardia occurs, it should be treated promptly, either by withdrawal of the precipitating stimulus or by intravenous atropine.

Atropine is the preferred anticholinergic in children. It is more effective in blocking the cardiac vagus nerve and causes less drying of secretions than hyoscine or glycopyrrolate. Respiratory tract secretions, in fact, are not a serious problem with current potent agents (e.g., halothane, isoflurane, sevoflurane). What is needed is an effective block of the cardiac vagus nerve.

Children require larger doses of atropine than adults to achieve the same effect on the heart rate. If indicated, atropine (0.02 mg/kg; maximum, 0.6 mg) may be given intravenously at induction; if thiopental is used, it may be mixed with this drug. This is the preferred method; it ensures effective drug action and spares the child a painful intramuscular injection and subsequent dry mouth. If successful venipuncture is in doubt, the same dose of atropine should be given orally 90 minutes or intramuscularly 30 minutes preoperatively to ensure a peak effect at the time of induction. Atropine may also be given per rectum if a rectal barbiturate is used for induction of anesthesia. In an emergency, the usual dose of atropine diluted in 2 ml of saline is rapidly effective by the intratracheal route.

Infants with established bradycardia have a longer onset time for the chronotropic effect of intravenous atropine, because of their reduced cardiac output. Therefore, if bradycardia is thought to be caused by excessive vagal action, atropine should be given as early as possible. *The most common cause for intraoperative bradycardia in infants or children is hypoxia, so the first treatment for any unexpected bradycardia is ventilation with oxygen.*

Contraindications to the use of atropine are few in the pediatric age group; patients with heart disease who might tolerate tachycardia poorly (i.e., aortic stenosis) deserve special attention.

It had been suggested that children with Down syndrome are sensitive to atropine; however, careful studies failed to confirm this hypothesis, and such children should be given the usual doses.

True allergy to atropine is extremely rare (if it exists), but it is not uncommon for parents to state that their child is "allergic" to atropine. This claim has usually been prompted by the appearance of a rash after a previous atropine administration. This erythematous rash commonly involves the upper part of the body and is thought to be caused by histamine release.

Sedatives and Tranquilizers

There is a voluminous literature and many widely divergent opinions concerning sedative premedication for children. Until recently, there was no really effective drug for this purpose. Sedatives, narcotics, or hypnotics may not ensure calm cooperation at the time of induction, but they may significantly increase the likelihood of postoperative depression, delirium, or vomiting.

The oral route has become most popular for premedication of healthy children. The introduction of midazolam has provided us with a drug that may be taken orally and can be effective in calming the child, easing separation from the parents, and smoothing induction of anesthesia; it is not surprising that midazolam has become the most widely preferred pediatric sedative premedicant.

Midazolam

Midazolam is a water-soluble benzodiazepine with a more rapid onset and shorter duration of action than diazepam. The drug may be given orally, nasally, rectally, or intravenously. For healthy infants and children, the oral route is preferred; a dose of 0.5–0.75 mg/kg of the cherry-flavored solution produces sedation and tranquility in most patients within 10–20 minutes, after which time its effects start to wane. In infants the drug may be placed under the tongue with a medicine dropper; this technique ensures rapid oral transmucosal absorption. Higher doses (up to 1 mg/kg) may be used if the child is very upset, but such doses can cause respiratory depression, so the child should be closely monitored.

Midazolam (0.2 mg/kg) via the intranasal route is effective but usually upsets the child, so this route is not recommended. Rectal midazolam (0.3 mg/kg) may be useful for small infants who cannot take the drug orally, but the onset of sedation is less predictable. Children with an intravenous infusion running may be given midazolam 0.1 mg/kg IV immediately before coming to the operating room (OR).

Oral midazolam produces sedation and tranquility with some antegrade amnesia, does not significantly affect the volume or acidity of gastric contents, but does improve cooperation on separation from parents and during induction. Recovery is not delayed after a 1-hour operation, but after a brief procedure (10 minutes) early recovery may be delayed. Some children given midazolam are more restless during emergence after a brief procedure.

There is some evidence that effective midazolam premedication reduces the incidence of adverse behavioral outcomes after hospitalization for surgical procedures; however, it is also suggested that some children have an increased incidence of bad dreams if this drug is used.

Lorazepam

Lorazepam has been used successfully for premedication of adult patients and is also very useful for adolescents. In a dose of 1–2 mg it produces good anxiolysis with a significant degree of amnesia. However, doses that produce sedation and amnesia in younger children also result in an unacceptable incidence of unpleasant side effects.

Ketamine

Ketamine may be given orally in doses of up to 6 mg/kg but must be accompanied by oral atropine if excessive secretions are to be avoided. The combination of oral midazolam (0.3–0.5 mg/kg) and oral ketamine (3–5 mg/kg) produces very effective sedation for the more disturbed child. If this combination is used, the child should be closely observed as the drugs become effective. The combination should not be used when heavy sedation might be dangerous (e.g., in the child who possibly has a difficult airway). Immediate postoperative emergence delirium was reported in a 12-year-old given 6 mg/kg ketamine; the authors recommended that oral ketamine not be used for operations lasting less than 1 hour.

Opioids

Opioids are rarely indicated as premedication agents for healthy children, unless pain is present. Opioids have traditionally been given via intramuscular injection, which children find unpleasant. Dizziness, nausea, and vomiting are common after their use. Meperidine is a poor sedative and can cause vomiting; therefore, its use as a premedicant in pediatric patients makes little sense.

Fentanyl in the form of an Oralet (lozenge) is available as a premedicant in the United States. This formulation takes full advantage of the rapid effect that may be obtained by oral transmucosal absorption of the drug. The fentanyl Oralet produces good sedation together with analgesia that complements the anesthesia regimen and may extend into the postoperative period. Provided the total dose administered is less than 15 μg/kg, significant respiratory depression is unlikely, but the patient should be continuously monitored with pulse oximetry. As with all opioids, fentanyl may increase the incidence of postoperative nausea and/or vomiting.

Special Considerations

1. Neurosurgical patients who may have increased intracranial pressure should not receive any sedative premedication.
2. Atropine should not be given intramuscularly to children with pyrexia, because it may exacerbate the fever by abolishing sweating. If needed, it may be given intravenously at the time of induction.
3. Some patients undergoing correction of strabismus are assessed by the ophthalmologist immediately before the operation and should not be heavily sedated. They may receive atropine (0.02 mg/kg intravenously) at induction to block the oculocardiac reflex.

Suggested Additional Reading

Black AE: Medical assessment of the paediatric patient. Br J Anaesth 83:3–15, 1999.

Cote CJ: Preoperative preparation and premedication. Br J Anaesth 83:16–28, 1999.

Feld LH, Champeau MW, van Steenis CA, and Scott JC: Preanesthetic medication in children: a comparison of oral transmucosal fentanyl citrate versus placebo. Anesthesiology 71:374–377, 1989.

Feld LH, Negus JB, and White PF: Oral midazolam preanesthetic medication in pediatric outpatients. Anesthesiology 73:831–834, 1990.

Henderson JM, Brodsky DA, Fisher DM, et al.: Preinduction of anesthesia in pediatric patients with nasally administered sufentanil. Anesthesiology 67:A495, 1987.

Kain ZN, Mayes LC, Wang SM, and Hofstadter MB: Postoperative behavioral outcomes in children: effects of sedative premedication. Anesthesiology 90:758–765, 1999.

Kallar SK and Everett LL: Potential risks and preventive measures for pulmonary aspiration: new concepts in preoperative fasting guidelines. Anesth Analg 77:171–182, 1993.

Karl HW, Rosenberger JL, Larach MG, and Ruffle JM: Transmucosal administration of midazolam for premedication of pediatric patients: comparison of nasal and sublingual routes. Anesthesiology 78:885–891, 1993.

McGraw T and Kendrick A: Oral midazolam and postoperative behaviour in children. Paediatr Anaesth 8:117–121, 1998.

Peters CG and Brunton JT: Comparative study of lorazepam and trimeprazine for oral premedication in paediatric anaesthesia. Br J Anaesth 54:623, 1982.

Riva J, Lejbusiewicz G, Papa M, et al.: Oral premedication with midazolam in paediatric anaesthesia: effects on sedation and gastric contents. Paediatr Anaesth 7:191–196, 1997.

Saint-Maurice C, Meistelman C, Rey E, et al.: The pharmacokinetics of rectal midazolam for premedication in children. Anesthesiology 65:536–538, 1986.

Splinter WM and Schreiner MS: Preoperative fasting in children. Anesth Analg 89:80–89, 1999.

Splinter WM, Stewart JA, and Muir JG: The effect of preoperative apple juice on gastric contents, thirst, and hunger in children. Can J Anaesth 36:55–58, 1989.

Steward DJ: Psychological preparation and premedication. In Gregory GA (ed.): Pediatric Anesthesia, 4th ed. Churchill Livingstone, New York, 1994.

Zimmerman G and Steward DJ: Bradycardia delays the onset of intravenous atropine in infants. Anesthesiology 65:320–322, 1986.

MANAGEMENT OF THE AIRWAY

Mask Anesthesia

1. During mask anesthesia, always have equipment for endotracheal intubation immediately at hand.
   a. A selection of suitably sized tubes with connectors in place (Table 4–3)
   b. A laryngoscope with suitable blades
   c. A syringe that contains atropine and one that contains succinylcholine
2. Select a mask that fits the contours of the face and minimizes the dead space if possible; the Rendell Baker mask is ideal for infants

Table 4–3. Approximate Size and Length of Pediatric Endotracheal Tubes[a]

Approximate Age of Patient (yr)	Internal Diameter (ID) (mm)[b]	Length (cm) Oral	Nasal
Premature	2.5 (for infants <1,500 g) to 3.0 (for infants >1,500 g)	11	13.5
Newborn	3.5	12	14
1	4.0	13	15
2	4.5	14	16
4	5.0	15	17
6	5.5	17	19
8	6.0	19	21
10	6.5	20	22
12	7.0	21	22
14	7.5	22	23
16	8.0	23	24

[a]Thin-walled, uncuffed tubes of clear PVC.
[b]Formula: (age of patient in years ÷ 4) + 4.0 = size of tube ID in millimeters. The tube diameters listed are given only as a guide. Always prepare a selection of tubes, and use the one with the best fit (*see* text).

and small children; however, the anesthesiologist may occasionally find it easier to achieve a good seal with a cushion-type mask. Certainly the latter type is more suitable for resuscitation carts, because nurses find them easier to use.
3. The relatively large tongue in infants and adenoid hypertrophy in older children may cause obstruction. If this occurs, insert an oropharyngeal airway of suitable size.
4. Infants have soft laryngeal cartilages and tracheal rings. Therefore, the anesthesiologist's finger may compress the airway during mask anesthesia. Monitor breath sounds, end-tidal carbon dioxide ($EtCO_2$), and the movement of the reservoir bag continuously.

Endotracheal Intubation

Laryngoscopy

1. Ensure that the head is correctly positioned and supported.
   a. For infants and young children (younger than 6 years of age), the head should be on the level of the table and supported in a low head ring. At this age the larynx is high in the neck and there is no advantage to flexing the neck to bring the head into a "sniffing position." Pressure applied to the cricoid cartilage region of the anterior aspect of the neck (applied in a posterior and cephalad direction) may be used, if required, to view the glottis.
   b. For older children and adolescents, place a small pillow under

the head to slightly flex the cervical spine and improve the intubation angle and the view of the glottis.

c. Beware of conditions that may be associated with an unstable cervical spine (e.g., Down syndrome, Marfan syndrome). In such cases, extreme care should be taken to limit head movement.

2. Examine the teeth carefully; many children have loose deciduous teeth. The teeth must be kept in view throughout laryngoscopy: retract the lip with your thumb and exert no pressure on the teeth during intubation. If a very loose tooth is present, this fact should be noted preoperatively and the parents should be informed that it may be safer to remove it once the child is asleep. If the tooth is removed, it should be retained and given to the parents after the operation.

3. In infants and children, the anesthesiologist's view of the glottis may be obscured by the epiglottis unless it is elevated with the tip of the blade. If a straight blade is used, this is easily accomplished. In small infants it is sometimes a problem to lift the epiglottis without its slipping off the laryngoscope blade. If this happens, advance the blade into the hypopharynx and slowly withdraw it until the glottis slips off the blade and the base of the epiglottis is firmly held.

4. Insufflation of oxygen into the pharynx during laryngoscopy (especially in infants or those with a difficult airway) improves oxygenation during attempts at intubation. Specially designed blades with an oxygen port are available (Oxyscope*), or a suction catheter may be taped to any blade and supplied with 4 L/min of oxygen.

Intubation

1. The optimal size of the tube is the largest one that passes easily through the glottis and subglottic regions without incurring resistance. The presence of a leak around an uncuffed tube at 20 cmH$_2$O positive pressure depends on a number of factors (including head position and muscle relaxation). In deciding that the tube size is appropriate, many clinicians depend more on the absence of any resistance when the tube passes through the cricoid region than on the need to hear an audible leak. In fact, there is increasing use of cuffed tracheal tubes in children in the OR *(see below)*.

2. Clear, thin-walled polyvinyl chloride (PVC) tubes (Z79-approved) are preferred. The "Murphy eye" type of tube is not recommended, because the additional side hole encourages accumulation of secretions and accelerates tube blockage.

3. Cuffed tubes may be preferred for major surgery, for patients who may be difficult to ventilate, and for those at high risk for regurgitation of stomach contents. Even in infants and young children, the use of a cuff does not increase postoperative morbidity. The use of a cuffed tube reduces the need to change tubes, reduces OR pollution, and may reduce the risk of aspiration. It also obviates the need to have a close fit in the subglottic region to ensure

---

*Anesthesia Medical Specialties, Santa Fe Springs, CA.

effective ventilation. For this reason it may be preferable, in patients with a known tendency to subglottic stenosis (e.g., Down syndrome), to use a tube of smaller diameter together with a cuff to seal the airway. Small-sized cuffed tubes are now available with a wall thickness similar to that of uncuffed tubes.

4. Endotracheal connectors must have a lumen at least equal to the internal diameter (ID) of the tube and must be firmly inserted.
5. The correct placement of the tube should immediately be confirmed by observation of the capnograph trace. Ventilation should then be checked in all areas of both lungs. The trachea of the infant and young child is short; it is only 5 cm long in the neonate. The tip must be accurately placed at midtracheal level to minimize the risk of an endobronchial intubation or accidental extubation. Note carefully the length of tube that is passed through the cords, and check the tube length marking at the teeth. This confirms the approximate position of the tip (Fig. 4–1). Tubes must be firmly taped in place, preferably near the middle of the mouth, where they are less likely to kink.
6. Pressure by anesthetic hoses and other equipment on the patient's face or head must be prevented by the use of suitable padding (e.g., Dalzofoam).
7. The anesthesia circuit and tube must be carefully positioned and supported to prevent any traction on the tube that might cause it to kink. *Pediatric endotracheal tubes kink very easily, and this is still a potential cause of disastrous accidents.*

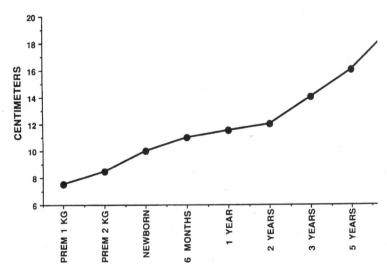

Figure 4–1. Correct distance from teeth to midtrachea for endotracheal intubation.

8. Remember that extension of the neck withdraws the tip of the tube proximally in the trachea and flexion advances the tube; 1–3 cm of movement may occur between full flexion and full extension in infants. Position the tube carefully and consider the effects of changing the head position. Always recheck the ventilation to all areas after repositioning the patient.

9. Some neonates and infants have a congenitally short trachea, which increases the danger of endobronchial intubation. This condition is often associated with DiGeorge syndrome but may occur in association with other syndromes.

A Note on Awake Intubation of the Neonate. It was common practice to intubate the newborn awake; however, it is now usual to induce anesthesia first. Intubation is more likely to be successful and less desaturation occurs if the infant is first anesthetized. Awake intubation has been demonstrated to cause rises in blood pressure and intracranial pressure that are similar to those that have been measured during crying and coughing. There is a concern that the risk of intraventricular hemorrhage may be increased in preterm infants who are intubated awake, although this risk has never been established. If awake intubation is deemed necessary, a local anesthetic solution should be applied to the mouth and palate to reduce the infant's distress and struggling. The use of a laryngeal mask airway (LMA) to establish the airway should be considered *(see below)*.

Suggested Additional Reading

Bosman YK and Foster PA: Endotracheal intubation and the head posture in infants. S Afr Med J 59:71, 1977.

Charlton AJ and Greenhough SG: Blood pressure response of neonates to tracheal intubation. Anaesthesia 43:744–746, 1988.

Cook-Sather SD, Tulloch HV, Cubina ML, et al.: A comparison of awake versus paralyzed tracheal intubation in infants for pyloromyotomy. Anesthesiology 83:A1151, 1995.

Eckenhoff JE: Some anatomic considerations of the infant larynx influencing endotracheal intubation. Anesthesiology 12:401, 1951.

Khine HH, Corddry DH, Kettrick RG, et al.: Comparison of cuffed and uncuffed endotracheal tubes in young children during general anesthesia. Anesthesiology 86:627–631, 1997.

Koka BV, Jeon IS, Andre JM, et al.: Postintubation croup in children. Anesth Analg 56:501, 1977.

Lane GA, Pashly NRT, and Fishman RA: Tracheal and cricoid diameters in the preterm infant. Anesthesiology 53:S326, 1980.

Ledbetter JL, Rasch DK, Pollard TG, et al.: Reducing the risks of laryngoscopy in anaesthetised infants. Anaesthesia 43:151–153, 1988.

Morgan GAR and Steward DJ: Linear airway dimensions in children: including those with cleft palate. Can Anaesth Soc J 29:1, 1982.

Ring WH, Adair JC, and Elwyn RA: A new endotracheal tube. Anesth Analg 54:273, 1975.

Wells AL, Wells TR, Landing BH, et al.: Short trachea, a hazard in tracheal intubation of neonates and infants: syndromal associations. Anesthesiology 71:367–373, 1989.

Westhorpe RN: The position of the larynx in children and its relationship to the ease of intubation. Anesth Intensive Care 15:384–388, 1987.

The Laryngeal Mask Airway

The LMA is an oropharyngeal tube provided with an anatomically conforming elliptical inflated rim designed to encircle the laryngeal inlet. If correctly inserted, the mask tip lies against the upper esophageal sphincter, the sides against the pyriform fossa, and the upper border against the base of the tongue. It was primarily designed as a substitute for mask anesthesia in spontaneously ventilating patients, but more recently its use has been extended to some patients with controlled ventilation. In children, controlled ventilation without distention of the stomach may be possible if peak airway pressures are maintained at less than 20 cmH_2O. The LMA does not protect the airway should vomiting or regurgitation occur. Seven sizes are available in the standard model.*

Size 1:   For neonates and infants up to 5 kg (cuff volume, 2–4 ml)
Size 1.5: For infants of 5–10 kg (cuff volume, 4–6 ml)
Size 2:   For infants and children 10–20 kg (cuff volume, 10 ml)
Size 2.5: For children 20–30 kg (cuff volume, up to 14 ml)
Size 3:   For children, adolescents, and small adults (cuff volume, 25 ml)
Size 4:   For normal adults (cuff volume, 35 ml)
Size 5:   For large adults (cuff volume, 40 ml)

Insertion of the mask is performed after induction of adequate anesthesia by inhalation or by an intravenous injection of propofol. The cuff should be checked before it is inserted. After the cuff has been completely deflated and the mask well lubricated, it is inserted blindly along the curve of the palate and down into the pharynx, with the aperture positioned anteriorly, until a resistance is felt. The cuff is then inflated and ventilation is checked. An alternative method of insertion in children has also been suggested: with the cuff partly inflated, the LMA is inserted upside down and then rotated 180° as it enters the pharynx. In either case a black guideline on the proximal visible tube should lie centrally against the upper incisors when the tube is in place and correctly oriented. Coughing and laryngospasm may occur if insertion is attempted at too light a level of anesthesia; such complications may be more common in infants and small children than in adults.

Studies have shown that, when the LMA is in position, the tip of the tube lies in the hypopharynx but the relationship of the cuff to the epiglottis and laryngeal aperture may vary somewhat despite an apparently good airway.

Some difficulty with insertion may be encountered in up to 25% of patients; this is more likely in the smaller patients having a size 1 or size 1.5 LMA inserted. In a very small percentage of patients, it may be impossible to place the LMA correctly.

When correctly positioned, the LMA provides a good airway with less

---

*Sizes 2 and up are also available with a flexible reinforced tube. In some cases, when weight and age do not relate normally, the optimal size varies.

resistance than an endotracheal tube. It avoids instrumentation through the glottis and frees the anesthesiologist from holding the mask. It may find applications during imaging procedures and radiotherapy and for other short procedures where mask anesthesia with spontaneous ventilation might be used. Somewhat surprisingly, some have found the LMA to be useful during adenotonsillectomy, and it has been suggested that less aspiration of blood occurs with the LMA than with an uncuffed endotracheal tube.

Some special applications of the LMA include the child with a difficult airway, in whom it may be used as a prelude to fiberoptic endoscopy and intubation. The LMA can be inserted in awake infants (e.g., those with Pierre Robin syndrome) and used to provide an airway to induce and deepen anesthesia before endotracheal intubation. The LMA also may be advantageous in infants with tracheal stenosis, in whom passage of an endotracheal tube would severely reduce an already compromised airway diameter. It must be remembered that the LMA does not guarantee the airway as does an endotracheal tube, and it does not protect against aspiration.

At the end of the procedure, the LMA may be left in place until protective reflexes have returned, or it may be removed while the patient is still deeply anesthetized. Removal while the patient is anesthetized results in fewer airway complications and less desaturation, but a face mask should be applied until the patient is able to maintain a safe airway. The incidence of postoperative sore throat is similar whether an LMA or an endotracheal tube is used.

Suggested Additional Reading

Asai T, Fujise K, and Achida M: Use of the laryngeal mask airway in a child with tracheal stenosis. Anesthesiology 75:903–904, 1991.

Boehringer LA and Bennie RE: Laryngeal mask airway and the pediatric patient. Int Anesthesiol Clin 36:45–60, 1998.

Dubreuil M, Laffon M, Plaud B, et al.: Complications and fiberoptic assessment of size 1 laryngeal mask airway. Anesth Analg 76:527–529, 1993.

Grebenik CR, Ferguson C, and White A: The laryngeal mask airway in pediatric radiotherapy. Anesthesiology 72:474–477, 1990.

Haynes SR and Morton NS: The laryngeal mask airway: a review of its use in paediatric anesthesia. Paediatr Anaesth 3:65–67, 1993.

Heath MI and Williams PJ: The reinforced laryngeal mask airway for adenotonsillectomy. Br J Anaesth 72:726–735, 1994.

Laffon M, Plaud P, Dubousset AM, et al.: Removal of the laryngeal mask airway: airway complications in children, anaesthetized versus awake. Paediatr Anaesth 4:35–37, 1994.

Lopez-Gil M, Brimacombe J, and Alvarez M: Safety and efficacy of the laryngeal mask airway: a prospective study of 1400 children. Anaesthesia 51:969–972, 1996.

Markakis DA, Sayson SC, and Schreiner MS: Insertion of the laryngeal mask airway in awake infants with the Robin sequence. Anesth Analg 75:822–824, 1992.

Selby IR and Morris P: Intermittent positive pressure ventilation through a laryngeal mask in children: does it cause gastric dilation? Paediatr Anaesth 7:305–308, 1997.

Splinter WM, Smallman B, Rhine EJ, and Komocar L: Postoperative sore throat in children and the laryngeal mask airway. Can J Anaesth 41:1081–1083, 1994.

"Difficult Intubation"

Preoperative Assessment of the Airway

It is most important that the anesthesiologist carefully assess the airway before administration of anesthesia to determine the likelihood of obstruction during anesthesia induction and to judge the likely ease of endotracheal intubation.

Beware of any child who does not look quite normal or who has any syndrome or association of defects. Always anticipate the possibility of an abnormal airway. When there is any doubt, assume the airway will be difficult and be prepared. Review the history and examine the child carefully. Always examine any previous anesthesia records—but do not be lulled into a false sense of security by a previous uneventful anesthesia. First, not all anesthetic difficulties are detailed in the record or patient chart. But even if they were, the ease of intubation may change as the child grows. In some cases, intubation becomes easier, as in the child with a cleft palate and Pierre Robin syndrome. In others, it becomes more difficult, as in the child with Treacher Collins or Klippel-Feil syndrome.

The examination of the patient may provide clues as to the likely ease of intubation:

1. Check to assess the extent of mouth opening.
2. Check the extent of neck extension.
3. Check the shape and size of the mandible and maxilla.
4. Examine the mouth and tongue.

Limited mouth opening, restricted neck extension, a large tongue, or a "short" ramus of the mandible predicts difficulty with laryngoscopy and intubation. Inability to fully visualize the fauces and uvula suggests difficult intubation, but the Mallampati scoring system may be less reliable in the child and may fail to predict a difficult laryngoscopy. Successful laryngoscopy depends on the ability to displace the soft tissues of the oropharynx into the mandibular space. Any deformity that limits this space (short or shallow mandible) or increases oropharyngeal tissue (large tongue) can be expected to compromise efforts to see the glottis.

Management of the Difficult Pediatric Airway

It is most important to be prepared for every option. Make sure that all the equipment you may require is readily available. It is essential to keep all the "Difficult Pediatric Airway" supplies on a special cart that is located centrally and can be wheeled into any room where it is required. It is always advantageous to have expert assistance on hand. If there are other members of the department with special skills, do not hesitate to enlist their aid, even if their initial role is simply to stand by and provide moral support.

Preoperative administration of an anticholinergic drug may be advantageous to decrease secretions in the mouth and pharynx and minimize the possibility of laryngeal spasm. No heavy sedation should be administered; small doses of anxiolytics might be administered when necessary, using suitable caution and appropriate monitoring. Patients who cannot be fasted and require emergency surgery should be prepared with the use of histamine$_2$-blocking drugs and intravenous metoclopramide.

A recommended sequence to follow is outlined in the Pediatric Difficult Airway Algorithm summarized here.

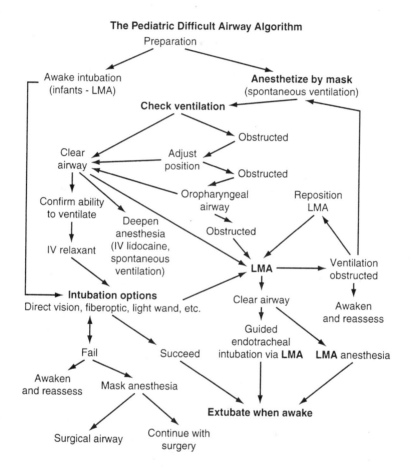

The Pediatric Difficult Airway Algorithm

The choice of anesthetized versus awake intubation is quite simple: pediatric patients, unlike adults, almost always require general anesthesia. Children are very easily upset and will not cooperate during attempts at awake intubation. Small infants may be severely stressed by attempts at awake intubation and are more easily and rapidly intubated when they are anesthetized. The exception is certain small infants (e.g., those with

Pierre Robin syndrome), in whom intubation may be managed by topical anesthesia of the mouth and insertion of a well-lubricated LMA while the patient is awake. The LMA can then be used as a route to induce anesthesia and, if necessary, to complete endotracheal intubation.

Standard Management

The classic traditional approach to the management of the difficult pediatric airway is by inhalational induction, deep volatile anesthesia, continued spontaneous ventilation, and direct laryngoscopy. This method is advantageous in that it does not require complex equipment and does immediately determine the status of the airway and the degree of difficulty of direct laryngoscopy. These details, along with the type of laryngoscope blade used and other data, can then be clearly recorded in the anesthesia record. *Although this procedure is still recommended as a standard basic management plan, some patients may be more effectively managed by early insertion of the LMA (see Alternative Methods).*

Induction of anesthesia should be performed by inhalation; intravenous hypnotic or relaxant drugs are contraindicated. Sevoflurane is preferred for a smooth, rapid induction, but once induction is complete it is advantageous to convert to halothane in oxygen. Emergence from halothane is less rapid and allows more time for endoscopy and attempts at intubation. As anesthesia is induced, the muscles of the tongue and pharynx relax. At this time obstruction may occur, and immediate measures may be required to reestablish a clear airway.

1. Adjust the position of the head with increased jaw thrust to lift the tongue from the posterior pharyngeal wall and open up the airway. A two-handed method is preferred, with one digit behind the most cephalad tip of the ascending ramus on each side of the mandible. The finger is wedged in the triangle formed at the base of the skull between the ascending ramus of the mandible anteriorly and the mastoid process posteriorly, immediately under the tragus. These two digits pull the mandible in an anterior and cephalad direction. This maneuver serves to sublux the mandible anteriorly as well as rotate the temporomandibular joint, thereby opening the mouth. Two thumbs hold the mask on the face.
2. Insert an oropharyngeal airway; but be aware that if the patient is too lightly anesthetized this procedure may result in coughing and laryngospasm. Make sure that the airway is appropriately sized for the patient; measure it against the outside of the face (the tip should extend just to the angle of the mandible).

When an airway is established, anesthesia is deepened with the use of halothane in oxygen. Three minutes before the first attempts at laryngoscopy and intubation, 1.5 mg/kg of intravenous lidocaine is administered slowly to reduce the likelihood of breath-holding or coughing during instrumentation. During laryngoscopy, oxygen may be insufflated into the pharynx via a catheter or by the use of a special laryngoscope blade. If an adequate view of the glottis is obtained, intubation can be performed; if not, other manipulations are required:

1. With the laryngoscope in place, apply posterior and cephalad pressure on the cricoid region of the neck to bring the larynx into view.
2. In some cases, a two-person approach to intubation is preferable. One person holds the laryngoscope with one hand and applies pressure (as just described) to align the axes of the larynx and oropharynx. Then the head is tilted to the left to enable the second person to see the larynx and insert the tube.
3. Inserting the straight blade at the extreme right side of the mouth behind the last molar tooth while rotating the head to the left and pushing the larynx to the right may permit visualization of the glottis even in patients with severe retrognathia.

An alternative procedure after induction of anesthesia, and after confirming the ability to ventilate the patient with bag and mask, is to administer a short-acting muscle relaxant. Laryngoscopy can then be attempted during apnea with complete muscular relaxation. This may make laryngoscopy and intubation slightly easier, but it does limit the time available for each intubation attempt. Infants and small children desaturate more rapidly during apnea than do older children or adults.

If laryngoscopy proves impossible by direct vision, the mask should be reapplied, deep anesthesia continued, and other options considered. It is wise not to persist with prolonged attempts at direct laryngoscopy, because these may become traumatic and result in bleeding, thus compromising the chances of success with other methods or by other persons.

Alternative Methods

Laryngeal Mask Airway. The introduction of the LMA has made possible many new approaches to management of the difficult airway, provided the mouth and pharynx are of adequate size. If intubation under direct vision is impossible, the LMA may be inserted without delay. Insertion of an LMA at any stage is usually successful in establishing a patent upper airway, but laryngeal spasm may occur if the patient is inadequately anesthetized. Once in place, the LMA can be used as a route for ventilation and oxygenation, to continue anesthesia, or as a conduit for flexible bronchoscopes, endotracheal tubes, airway catheters, light wands, or other equipment needed to complete intubation (Table 4–4).

Flexible Bronchoscope. In some patients it is impossible to insert an LMA (e.g., very small or scarred mouth) and it may be necessary to perform flexible bronchoscopy via the mouth or nose. The use of fiberoptic laryngobronchoscopes in pediatric patients has been facilitated by the development of small-diameter scopes that accommodate small endotracheal tubes. The Olympus* LF-P model has a diameter of only 2.2 mm but no suction channel; the Pentax† FI-10P has a diameter of

---

*America, Inc., Melville, N.Y.
†Pentax, Orangeburg, N.Y.

Table 4-4. Features of the LMA and Diameters of Endotracheal Tubes and Bronchoscopes That Can Be Passed

LMA Size	Patient Weight (kg)	LMA ID (mm)	Cuff Volume (mL)	Largest ETT (ID, mm) Inside LMA	Largest FOB Inside ETT (mm)	Type of FOB That Can Be Passed Through ETT
1	<6.5	5.25	2–5	3.5	2.7	Olympus PF27M, LF-P, ENF-P2, BF-N20, Pentax FB 10H, F1-10P
2	6.5–20	7.0	7–10	4.5	3.5	Olympus ENF-P3, BF-3C20 Pentax FNL-15S
2.5	20–30	8.4	14	5.0	4.0	Olympus LF1, LF2
3.0	30–70	10	15–20	6 cuffed	5.0	Olympus BF2TR, BF-P20D
4	>70	10	25–30	6 cuffed	5.0	Pentax FB-19H, FB-19H3

ETT, endotracheal tube; FOB, fiberoptic bronchoscope; ID, internal diameter.

3.5 mm with a built-in suction channel. A suction channel on the scope is a very desirable feature, because secretions frequently obscure the view.

If the nasal route is chosen, the patient should be prepared as outlined earlier, and vasoconstrictor nose drops should be administered. Anesthesia should be cautiously induced, as previously described, maintaining spontaneous ventilation. When the patient is adequately anesthetized, a well-lubricated endotracheal tube with a prewarmed tip should be passed through the nose and advanced to a level just above the vocal cords. Monitoring of the movement of the reservoir bag aids in this placement of the tube tip. The flexible bronchoscope can then be passed through an adaptor into the lumen of the endotracheal tube and advanced to the tip. At this point the glottis should immediately appear, and the scope can then be passed into the trachea.

Practice at flexible bronchoscopy on normal routine patients is essential if the anesthesiologist is to become adept at intubation of the difficult airway. When a very small endoscope is not available, alternative methods for pediatric patients have been suggested, such as visualizing the glottis with a larger scope and with direct vision to pass a stylet into the trachea, over which the endotracheal tube can subsequently be threaded.

Bullard Laryngoscope. The Bullard laryngoscope and other similar devices are designed to indirectly view the glottis and thereby make it possible to direct an endotracheal tube. All of these devices require practice, especially in the manipulation of the tube once the glottis is visualized. Initial experience should be gained with children who have a normal airway. The success rate for the experienced operator is reported to be high.

Light Wand Intubation. The use of a malleable lighted stylet, passed blindly into the trachea, makes it possible, with practice, to rapidly secure the airway. The stylet should be curved to suit the predicted shape of the patient's airway, and a suitable endotracheal tube is mounted on it. Always check that the lamp is screwed firmly in place. As the light passes into the trachea, the anterior neck can be seen to transilluminate. This is more easily seen with the room lights dimmed. The endotracheal tube can then be advanced over the stylet into the trachea. The method requires practice but may be successful in many patients with a difficult airway. It is limited by the size of tube that can be passed over the stylet (5.0–5.5 mm with the Flexi-Lum*; the Trachlight† can accommodate tubes as small as 3.5 mm ID). This technique can be used with general anesthesia, appropriate sedation, and regional or topical analgesia. The use of a light wand via the LMA has also been described.

Blind Nasotracheal Intubation

This is a technique that requires much practice. It is an art that few acquire in an era when advances in technology offer so many alternative methods. Blind nasoendotracheal intubation may still be necessary if all

---

*Concept Inc., Clearwater, FL.
†Trachlight, Laerdal Inc., Long Beach, CA.

else fails, or when equipment fails, and the patient's glottis cannot be visualized (*see* **N.B.** after item 7 below). The following are some hints:

1. Inspect the nares for size and patency; use the larger one. The success rate increases if the left nostril is used, because the bevel of most tubes is on the left. (Special tubes are made with the bevel on the right for use in the right nostril.)
2. Prepare and lubricate suitable tubes (ID 0.5 mm smaller than for oral intubation).
3. Use an inhalation induction (e.g., N_2O + O_2 + halothane); 5% CO_2 may be added to increase the tidal volume before intubation attempts. *Do not use intravenous induction agents or muscle relaxants.*
4. When the patient is deeply anesthetized, position the head slightly extended, as in the sniffing position.
5. Insert the tube through the nostril and advance it. It goes in one of five directions:
   a. Larynx—desired location.
   b. Right of larynx—withdraw the tube slightly; turn it to the left and turn the patient's head to the right.
   c. Left of larynx—withdraw the tube slightly; turn it to the right and turn the patient's head to the left.
   d. Esophagus—withdraw the tube slightly and extend the head maximally before advancing the tube again.
   e. Anterior to epiglottis—withdraw the tube slightly and flex the head.
6. If unsuccessful, repeat, using the other nostril.
7. Other useful maneuvers include
   a. Listening at the end of the tube for maximal gas exchange.
   b. Passage of a second tube through the other nostril to block the esophagus.
   c. External pressure to the neck, which may direct the glottis toward the tip of the tube.
   d. An angled stylet passed through the tube to direct the tip toward the glottic aperture.
   e. Use of a smaller-size tube for initial intubation; the tube can then be changed up in size by passing an airway exchange catheter and leaving it in place to guide the larger tube.

N.B. The technique of blind intubation requires considerable skill, which can be acquired only by extensive practice. It is a method that cannot be learned in the lecture hall but must be mastered by repeated practice. If the anesthesiologist is not sufficiently experienced and has no such skilled assistance at hand, some other technique may be preferable.

As a means to simpler blind intubation, an endotracheal tube or an airway exchange catheter passed blindly through an LMA frequently passes into the trachea.

Retrograde Intubation

This technique depends on threading a wire proximally through the vocal cords into the pharynx via a needle passed percutaneously into the trachea. This wire is then retrieved in the mouth and used to "railroad" a tube into the trachea. In infants and small children, the trachea is soft and can be difficult to locate, significantly reducing the chances of success. A modification of this technique passes the retrieved wire retrograde up the suction port of a bronchoscope. The scope is then guided into the trachea by the wire and can be used to position the tube.

Failed Intubation

If intubation options are failing, consider the following:

Should we awaken the patient and plan for another day?
Can this case be done with mask anesthesia?
Can this case be done with an LMA for airway support?
Do we need a surgical airway?

Extubation of the Trachea

1. Children are prone to laryngeal spasm on extubation, especially after halothane or isoflurane and if extubated during a light plane of anesthesia. Therefore,
   a. Before extubation, ensure that all facilities are available to ventilate with oxygen and to reintubate if necessary.
   b. Extubate when the child is fully awake (or, if indicated, deeply anesthetized).
   c. Extubation when the child is lightly anesthetized, coughing, or straining on the tube must be avoided.
   d. When judging whether the child is "awake" enough for extubation, wait until the eyes and mouth open spontaneously, all limbs are moving, and the child resumes regular spontaneous ventilation after coughing.
   e. Do not disturb the child unnecessarily during the awaking stage, so as to minimize coughing and bucking on the tube before the child is fully awake.
   f. All monitors should be left in place until successful extubation is complete.
2. Severe laryngospasm on extubation may be followed by pulmonary edema as the laryngospasm is relieved. If this occurs, it should be treated by continued positive pressure ventilation.
3. The following patients should be fully awake before extubation:
   a. All those in whom intubation was difficult.
   b. All those having emergency surgery; these patients may vomit gastric contents during emergence from anesthesia.
   c. All infants.
4. Some patients should not be allowed to cough and strain on the endotracheal tube during emergence (e.g., those having neurosurgery or intraocular surgery). This may be achieved with a planned "deep" extubation, preceded by careful suctioning of the stomach and pharynx. Lidocaine, 1–2 mg/kg IV administered slowly before extubation, also decreases the risk of coughing and breath-

holding. After the tube is removed, a face mask should be applied, the airway maintained, and oxygen administered until the child is awake. Studies suggest that oxygen saturation (SaO_2) levels are better maintained if extubation is performed while the child is still anesthetized and oxygen is then given by mask until the child is fully awake.
5. Patients who have had a mouth gag with tongue blade inserted by the surgeon (e.g., for cleft palate repair) are at risk for postoperative swelling of the tongue; always inspect the mouth before extubation.

Extubation of the Difficult Pediatric Airway. Extubation should be performed as a well-planned exercise, with the necessary equipment and personnel to reintubate the patient readily available. In selected patients trial extubation, leaving an airway exchange catheter in situ, may be indicated.

All patients with difficult airways should be extubated or have the LMA removed only after they have fully regained consciousness and when all danger of swelling in the region of the airway has passed. Corticosteroids (Decadron) have been used before extubation to decrease the likelihood of stridor, and all patients should be given humidified oxygen after the tube is removed.

The golden rule: If there is any doubt leave the trachea intubated!

Suggested Additional Reading

Baraka A: Intravenous lidocaine controls extubation laryngospasm in children. Anesth Analg 57:506–507, 1978.

Berry FA: Anesthesia for the child with a difficult airway. In Berry FA (ed.): Anesthetic Management of Difficult and Routine Pediatric Patients, 2nd ed. Churchill Livingstone, New York, 1990, p 173.

Borland LM and Casselbrant M: The Bullard laryngoscope: a new indirect oral laryngoscope (pediatric version). Anesth Analg 70:107–108, 1990.

Borland LM, Swan DM, and Leff S: Difficult pediatric endotracheal intubation: a new approach to the retrograde technique. Anesthesiology 55:577–578, 1981.

Cook-Sather SD, Tulloch HV, Cubina ML, et al.: A comparison of awake versus paralysed tracheal intubation in infants for pyloromyotomy. Anesthesiology 83:A1151, 1995.

Frei FJ and Ummenhofer W: Difficult intubation in paediatrics. Paediatr Anaesth 6:251–263, 1996.

Gunawardana RH: Difficult laryngoscopy in cleft lip and palate surgery. Br J Anaesth 76:757–759, 1996.

Harness SR and Morton NS: The laryngeal mask airway: a review of its use in paediatric anesthesia. Paediatr Anaesth 3:65–67, 1993.

Holzman RS, Nargozian CD, and Florence FB: Lightwand intubation in children with abnormal upper airways. Anesthesiology 69:784–787, 1988.

Kopp VJ, Bailey A, Valley RD, et al.: Utility of the Mallampati classification for predicting difficult intubation in pediatric patients. Anesthesiology 83:A1147, 1995.

Markakis DA, Sayson SC, and Schreiner MS: Insertion of the laryngeal mask airway in awake infants with the Robin sequence. Anesth Analg 75:822–824, 1992.

Patel RI, Hannalah RS, and Norden J: Emergence airway complications in children: a comparison of tracheal extubation in awake and deeply anesthetised patients. Anesth Analg 72:266–270, 1991.

Pounder DR, Blackstock D, and Steward DJ: Tracheal extubation in children: halothane vs isoflurane, anesthetised vs awake. Anesthesiology 74:653–655, 1991.

Roy WL and Lerman J: Laryngospasm in paediatric anaesthesia. Can J Anaesth 35:93–98, 1988.

White AP and Billingham IM: Laryngeal mask guided tracheal intubation in paediatric anaesthesia. Paediatr Anaesth 2:265–267, 1992.

PEDIATRIC ANESTHETIC CIRCUITS

The ideal pediatric anesthetic circuit should be lightweight; with low resistance and dead space; with low compliance; adaptable to spontaneous, assisted, or controlled ventilation; and readily humidified and scavenged. These conditions are most nearly met by the T-piece systems; however, modified circle systems are also extensively used for pediatric patients.

The T-Piece and Its Variants

The T-piece, originally described by Ayre in 1937, was modified by Jackson Rees to provide for artificial ventilation. The T-piece relies on continuous flow from the fresh gas limb to flush expired gases from the expiratory limb. The performance of the T-piece therefore depends on the rate of fresh gas flow and the ventilation of the patient.

Before capnography became standard practice, fresh gas flows were selected using formulas developed to prevent rebreathing of exhaled gases or to achieve a specific $EtCO_2$ tension. However, these formulas proved to be unreliable. In fact, small fresh gas flows that permit some rebreathing are well tolerated by patients, provided a capnograph is used to maintain the $EtCO_2$ tension within acceptable limits. Indeed, it has become environmentally, economically, and physiologically rational to decrease the fresh gas flow and permit rebreathing with these circuits. Physiologically, exhaled gases contain anesthetics, humidity, heat, and carbon dioxide, all of which are desirable constituents of the inspired gases in a spontaneously breathing child. However, if capnography is not available, then minimum fresh gas formulas should be used to reduce the risk of rebreathing exhaled gases. These are shown in Table 4–5.

Because the T-piece has no valves, it cannot malfunction and has a very low resistance. However, kinking or obstruction of the expiratory limb can lead to high pressure within the circuit and might cause barotrauma. Because it is also lightweight and convenient and has minimal dead space, it is considered by many to be the ideal circuit for infants and young children, especially during spontaneous ventilation. However, the relatively high fresh gas flow required is a potential source of atmospheric pollution. (Whenever a T-piece is used, an exhaust system should—and can easily—be added to the expiratory limb or ventilator to remove waste anesthetic gases and vapors.)

The Bain coaxial system is a modification of the T-piece. It has essentially the same characteristics and requires the same fresh gas flows.

Table 4–5. Fresh Gas Flow Rates Required to Prevent Rebreathing[a] in a T-Piece System (Including Coaxial Circuits)

| Patient Weight (kg) | Flow Rate (L/min)[b] | |
	Mask Anesthesia	Endotracheal Anesthesia
5	8	6.0
10	8	6.0
15	10	7.5
20	12	9.0

[a]*Important.* The flow rates cited are those required to prevent rebreathing in the T-piece. Lower fresh gas flow rates, as recommended by some authors, result in a degree of rebreathing; this can be compensated for only if the patient can increase ventilation. We believe that during spontaneous ventilation the safest course is to eliminate rebreathing completely.

[b]These flow rates should be used during spontaneous ventilation. They are calculated from the following formulas, which were derived by Rose et al. as an extension of theoretical work by Seeley et al. Patients under 30 kg: Mask anesthesia: FGF = 4 × [1,000 + (100 × kg body wt)]. Intubated patients: FGF = 3 × [1,000 + (100 × kg body wt)]. Patients over 30 kg: Mask anesthesia: FGF = 4 × [2,000 + (50 × kg body wt)]. Intubated patients: FGF = 3 × [2,000 + (50 × kg body wt)]. The safety of these flow rates has been confirmed clinically.

Circle Absorber Semiclosed System

The adult circle absorber semiclosed system can be modified for use in pediatric patients by incorporating smaller-diameter breathing tubes. Pediatric circle systems are available and are routinely used in some centers. The circle system is more economical and provides limited humidification of inspired gases, but the higher circuit resistance and the possibility of valve malfunction lead some to prefer the T-piece system for infants and small children, especially during spontaneous ventilation. The circle system facilitates $EtCO_2$ monitoring, because there is less mixing of expired and inspired gases than occurs in the T-piece system. The integrity of the circle system and the presence and correct functioning of the valves must be carefully checked before each use.

Suggested Additional Reading

Ayre P: Anaesthesia for intracranial operation: new technique. Lancet 1:561, 1937.

Ayre P: Endotracheal anesthesia for babies, with special reference to hare-lip and cleft-palate operations. Anesth Analg 16:330, 1937.

Brown ES and Hustead RF: Resistance of pediatric breathing systems. Anesth Analg 48:842, 1969.

Harrison GA: Ayre's T-piece: a review of its modifications. Br J Anaesth 36:115, 1964.

Harrison GA: The effect of the respiratory flow pattern on rebreathing in a T-piece system. Br J Anaesth 36:206, 1964.

Rose DK, Byrick RJ, and Froese AB: Carbon dioxide elimination during spontaneous ventilation with a modified Mapleson D system: studies in a lung model. Can Anaesth Soc J 25:353, 1978.

Seeley HF, Barnes PK, Conway CM: Controlled ventilation with the Mapleson D system: a theoretical and experimental study. Br J Anaesth 49:107, 1977.

HUMIDIFICATION OF ANESTHETIC GASES

Humidification of inspired gases during anesthesia is recommended (1) to prevent damage to the respiratory tract by dry gases and (2) to minimize heat loss via the respiratory tract and thereby assist in maintaining normothermia.

Dry gases inhibit ciliary activity and lead to the accumulation of inspissated secretions, which may, in the extreme, progress to obstruct the endotracheal tube. Degenerative changes in cells exfoliated from the trachea after exposure to dry gas have been described, but an increased incidence of postoperative morbidity from pulmonary complications remains unproved.

Humidified anesthetic gases significantly reduce heat loss during the operation. This is valuable in newborn infants, especially those who are preterm or small for gestational age. The use of a heated humidifier with a heated fresh gas delivery tube* is preferred for small infants. The temperature of inspired gases should be maintained at 35°–36°C and must be monitored by a thermistor probe at the patient end of the fresh gas line. When a heated humidifier is being used, extreme care should be taken to ensure that it does not run dry. When using humidifiers with a heated wire breathing circuit, be aware that they may overheat if used improperly; always check to see that correct gas flows are maintained, and do not cover the circuit or rest it on the patient's body.

An alternative means of humidification for older children is the use of a heat and moisture exchanger (HME) at the point of connection of the endotracheal tube to the circuit. The HME conserves approximately 50% of the water normally lost via the respiratory tract and thus prevents a corresponding heat loss. The HME is most efficient with smaller tidal volumes and higher respiratory frequency, so it is quite useful in pediatric cases. Studies have demonstrated that the inspired gases entering the trachea have a water content of approximately 24 mg/L when an HME is used. Disposable HMEs with a paper insert (Humid-vent†) are available and are easily attached to the breathing circuit. A miniature version (Mini-Humid-vent†) is also available for use with small tubes and infants weighing less than 10 kg. The use of a Mini-Humid-vent with tubes of 5 mm ID or larger significantly increases airway resistance. Always monitor ventilation carefully when an HME is used.

The circle system provides some humidification of inspired gases, but if a dry fresh gas is delivered into the inspiratory limb, the actual humidity is dictated by the ratio of fresh gas flow to minute ventilation. The temperature of the gases delivered via the inspiratory limb does not usually exceed room temperature, and this also limits the water content of the inspired gases. Therefore, the circle system is less effective than the other methods described.

In brief, a heated humidifier that delivers heated humidified gases via a heated inspiratory breathing tube delivers the most moisture to the

---

*Fisher & Paykell Healthcare, New Zealand.
†Gibeck-Dryden Corp., Indianapolis, IN.

lungs and is the most effective means of maintaining normothermia in small infants. The HME is less effective but is simple to use and is certainly much better than nothing, even when the circle system is in use.

Suggested Additional Reading

Bissonnette B, Sessler DI, and LaFlamme P: Passive and active inspired gas humidification in infants and children. Anesthesiology 71:350–354, 1989.

Jones BR, Ozaki GT, Benumof JL, and Saidman LJ: Airway resistance caused by a pediatric heat and moisture exchanger. Anesthesiology 69:A786, 1988.

MacKuanying N and Chalon J: Humidification of anaesthetic gases for children. Anesth Analg 53:387, 1974.

Rashad KF and Benson DW: Role of humidity in prevention of hypothermia in infants and children. Anesth Analg 46:712, 1967.

CONTROLLED VENTILATION DURING ANESTHESIA

During anesthesia, ventilation may be controlled by manual or mechanical ventilation.

Manual Ventilation. This is used at times, especially during induction and when there is any doubt about the adequacy of ventilation. It has been claimed that manual ventilation enables the anesthesiologist to monitor compliance continuously and to compensate rapidly for changes. There is some question about the ability of individual anesthesiologists to detect even complete airway obstruction just by the feel of the bag. However, if there is any doubt about the adequacy of ventilation or in the event of sudden deterioration in the patient's vital signs, it is wise to switch to manual ventilation. Then the adequacy of ventilation should be confirmed by auscultation of the lungs, observation of chest movement, and the $EtCO_2$ concentration.

Rapid ventilation with small tidal volumes provides optimal results in the newborn, because this pattern of ventilation tends to maintain the functional residual capacity and prevent airway closure. $EtCO_2$ levels should be monitored continuously, because the appropriate respiratory rate is frequently overestimated in newborns when ventilation is controlled. In this way, hyperventilation (and consequent respiratory alkalosis) can be avoided.

Mechanical Ventilation. Mechanical ventilators are widely used and have the advantage of maintaining a relatively constant level of ventilation while freeing the anesthesiologist to perform many other functions. Remember that in small patients the compression volume of the anesthesia circuit is likely to exceed the tidal volume that is delivered to the patient. Therefore, the readings of volume observed on a ventilator bag are meaningless. The adequacy of ventilation must be judged by auscultation of the chest and observation of chest movement, along with $EtCO_2$ or arterial carbon dioxide levels.

A mechanical ventilator can be used in conjunction with the T-piece; connection of the ventilator to the expiratory limb of the T-piece produces intermittent inflation of the lungs. Most standard types of adult ventilators can be used for this purpose, but low inspiratory flow rates must be set on the ventilator controls (the gas flow from the ventilator is complemented by the fresh gas flow into the T-piece during inspiration). Set flow and pressure at their lower limits; then, when the ventilator is attached to the patient circuit, gradually increase these settings to produce a satisfactory pattern of ventilation as judged by auscultation of the lungs and observation of expansion of the thorax. During major surgery, the level of ventilation should be confirmed by blood gas analysis and/or measurement of $EtCO_2$ levels. When using a mechanical ventilator with the T-piece:

1. Incorporate a pressure-relief valve (set to release at 40 cmH_2O) into the anesthetic circuit to prevent barotrauma to the lungs if the equipment malfunctions.
2. Attach a low-pressure alarm to warn of accidental disconnection of the ventilator.

During controlled ventilation, avoid excessive hyperventilation and maintain the arterial carbon dioxide concentration ($PaCO_2$) at near-physiologic levels. When the T-piece is used, it is possible to regulate the $PaCO_2$ quite accurately by limiting the fresh gas flow while slightly hyperventilating the patient. This introduces a controlled degree of rebreathing to compensate for the hyperventilation. Because of the interindividual variability in fresh gas flow requirements, the fresh gas flow for any child should be adjusted until an acceptable $EtCO_2$ tension is achieved with a given level of rebreathing.

The following fresh gas flow rates* result in a $PaCO_2$ of 35–40 mmHg:

Patients weighing 10–30 kg: 1,000 cc + 100 cc/kg
Patients weighing more than 30 kg: 2,000 cc + 50 cc/kg
Minute ventilation should be set at double the rate of fresh gas flow.

Suggested Additional Reading

Ramanthan S, Chalon J, and Turndorf H: A safety valve for the pediatric Rees system. Anesth Analg 55:741, 1967.

Rose DK and Froese AB: The regulation of $PaCO_2$ during controlled ventilation of children with a T-piece. Can Anaesth Soc J 26:104–113, 1979.

Seeley HF, Barnes PK, and Conway CM: Controlled ventilation with the Mapleson D system: a theoretical and experimental study. Br J Anaesth 49:107, 1977.

Spears RS, Yeh A, Fisher DM, and Zwass MS: The "educated hand": can anesthesiologists assess changes in neonatal pulmonary compliance manually? Anesthesiology 75:693–696, 1991.

Steward DJ: The "not so educated hand" of the pediatric anesthesiologist. Anesthesiology 75:555–556, 1991.

---

*Higher rates of fresh gas flow are required if there is a large leak around the endotracheal tube. Flowmeters are accurate only to ±10%; therefore, the end-tidal or $PaCO_2$ must be checked for all major procedures.

MONITORING DURING ANESTHESIA

Routine Monitoring Methods

Monitoring during anesthesia must always include the following:

1. **Pulse oximeter:** apply before induction and leave in place until the patient arrives in the recovery room; it may give useful information during transport and during the recovery room stay. The light source and sensor must be positioned to transilluminate part of the body (earlobe, finger, toe, palm of hand, or sole of foot, depending on the size of the patient). Placement on the earlobe or buccal angle rather than the finger may result in a slightly faster initial response time during acute desaturation. The sensor should be protected to prevent outside light or pressure from interfering with the reading. Pulse oximetry has proved most effective in providing an early warning of developing hypoxemia. Failure of the pulse oximeter to detect and record a pulsatile flow may provide useful warning information about the patient's circulatory status. If the pulse oximeter fails, check the patient first—then, if necessary, troubleshoot the equipment!

   Pulse oximetry is accurate throughout a wide variation in hematocrit, but severe degrees of anemia or hemoconcentration may compromise this accuracy. In patients with cyanotic congenital heart disease the oximeter tends to overestimate saturation at lower readings.

   The presence of fetal hemoglobin (HbF) in young infants has no clinically significant effect on the detection of hypoxemia by the pulse oximeter. Hyperbilirubinemia does not affect the oximetry measurements.

   Nail polish or disease of the nails may affect the performance of the monitor, but accurate readings of saturation can be made though pigmented skin. Methemoglobin (MetHb) or carboxyhemoglobin (CoHb), if present, affect the accuracy of readings. MetHb has a nonlinear effect, causing underestimation or overestimation of saturation; CoHb causes an overestimation of saturation.

   An arterial saturation of 80%–95% has been demonstrated to indicate a PaO_2 of 40–80 mmHg in most patients—a safe range for the preterm infant. But, because of the slope of the Hb/O_2 association curve, pulse oximetry is less precise in the assessment of hyperoxia than it is in hypoxia. If considered necessary, an arterial sample can be obtained to confirm which level of saturation is appropriate in terms of PaO_2 for each patient. This level of saturation can then be maintained by varying the fraction of inspired oxygen (FiO_2).

   The complications of pulse oximetry are few, but severe burns have occurred when an incorrect sensor from a different manufacturer has been substituted. Burns may also occur when pulse oximetry is incorrectly used in the magnetic resonance imaging suite.

2. **Stethoscope, precordial or esophageal:** there must be provision to monitor heart and breath sounds throughout anesthesia.

3. **Blood pressure (BP) cuff** of suitable width: the cuff should occupy two-thirds of the upper arm. If the cuff is too narrow, the BP readings are falsely high; if it is too wide, they are falsely low. A width of 4 cm is recommended for full-term neonates. An automatic BP cuff (e.g., Dinamap) may be used, but ensure that it is set to provide frequent readings.

4. **Electrocardiogram.**

5. **Thermistor probe** (axillary, esophageal, or rectal) (*see* Management of Body Temperature, *below*).

6. **End-tidal carbon dioxide:** This measurement provides a useful, noninvasive means to measure the adequacy of ventilation and pulmonary perfusion. It also provides a most reliable indicator of successful endotracheal intubation and should be used whenever intubation is performed. Two types of monitors are available, measuring carbon dioxide "in-line" at the connector or by sidestream sampling from the circuit. The latter method is more commonly used. However, it is not as easy to apply in infants and small children owing to the small size of the ventilatory volumes. When a partial rebreathing circuit is used (e.g., a T-piece plus ventilator), end-tidal sampling must be obtained from within the lumen of the endotracheal tube for all small patients (i.e., those weighing less than 12 kg) if useful numbers are to be obtained. If a nonrebreathing circuit is used (e.g., circle, Siemens ventilator, or Sechrist infant ventilator), proximal sampling at the endotracheal connector gives valid results even for small patients. The presence of a leak around the endotracheal tube may also affect end-tidal sampling, especially when positive end-expiratory pressure is applied; in these circumstances the $EtCO_2$ waveform may disappear completely.

   $EtCO_2$ measurements underestimate the $PaCO_2$ in children who have congenital heart disease with a right-to-left shunt or mixing lesion; the lower the saturation, the greater the $PaCO_2$-$EtCO_2$ gradient. In those with left-to-right shunting, the accuracy of $EtCO_2$ readings is unaffected.

7. **Peripheral nerve stimulator** should be used whenever relaxant drugs are administered.

8. **An arterial line** should be inserted for direct measurement of BP and to provide for intermittent blood gas analysis when required. The radial or femoral artery is usually cannulated (*see below*); rarely, the axillary artery may be used. Do not use the brachial artery, which has poor collateral vessels. (*See* Precautions with Arterial Lines, *below.*)

9. **Urine output:** record for all patients undergoing major surgery and all who have hypovolemic shock or whose renal function may be impaired.

10. **Central venous pressure (CVP):** record from a catheter inserted

centrally via the internal or external jugular vein *(see below)*. The external jugular is a less reliable route for CVP monitoring but is often useful for fluid replacement and drug infusions. The CVP should always be monitored in patients in whom major blood loss and/or impaired cardiac performance is anticipated.

Cannulation Techniques

Radial Artery Cannulation

The left radial artery is often preferred for arterial puncture.

1. Locate the artery by palpation; if this is difficult, use the Doppler flowmeter—or, in small infants, transilluminate the wrist with a bright cold light.
2. Use careful aseptic technique and prepare the skin with povidone-iodine (Betadine). (Your finger, which is used to palpate the artery, should be prepared also. Use a glove only on the hand that holds the needle.)
3. Make a small skin incision over the artery with an 18-gauge needle. This prevents damage to the tip of the cannula during skin puncture.
4. Perform arterial puncture; as soon as blood issues into the hub of the needle, turn the needle so that the bevel faces down.
5. Advance the cannula gently into the artery (Fig. 4–2).
6. If it will not advance, withdraw until blood flows freely and carefully insert a fine guidewire,* then advance the cannula over the wire.
7. If you fail to enter the artery at all, remove the needle and palpate the artery again, critically evaluating its alignment with the skin puncture. Then try again!
8. Apply antibiotic spray or ointment to the skin puncture site and cover with a sterile dressing (e.g., Tegaderm†).
9. Secure cannula carefully with adhesive tape. All connections should be Luer-Lok or similar to prevent accidental bleeding.

Femoral Artery Cannulation

In some patients the radial artery cannot be cannulated or is inappropriate (e.g., after surgery of the aortic arch). In such cases the femoral artery may be used.

1. Place a low pad under the patient to elevate the pelvis.
2. Palpate the femoral artery below the inguinal ligament.
3. Apply skin preparation and drapes; use sterile gloves.
4. Puncture the artery below the inguinal ligament using a 20-gauge needle. Punctures superior to the inguinal ligament introduce the risk of a retroperitoneal bleed.

---

*0.45 mm × 25 cm spring wire guide (Ref # AW-04018), Arrow International Inc., Reading, PA.

†3M Health Care Inc.

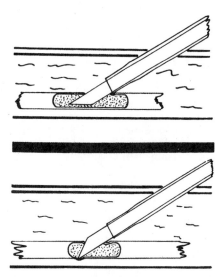

Figure 4–2. Advantage of turning the needle bevel down when inserting an intravenous cannula into a small vein or artery. (From Filston HC and Johnson DG: Percutaneous venous cannulation in neonates and infants: a method for catheter insertion without cutdown. Pediatrics 48:896–901, 1971, with permission of the American Academy of Pediatrics.)

5. Avoid needling the head of the femur; aseptic necrosis may result in infants and young children.
6. When the artery is entered, insert a guidewire and use it to introduce a 3F catheter or similar. Secure the catheter carefully in place and cover it with a clear plastic dressing.

If the artery is difficult to palpate the use of a Doppler flowmeter or a Doppler tipped-needle (Smart Needle) may facilitate arterial puncture.*

Precautions with Arterial Lines

Regarding any arterial cannulation:

1. Insert the cannula with meticulous asepsis.
2. Secure all connections, using Luer-Lok fittings, to exclude the danger of accidental disconnection and hemorrhage. Plug sampling taps when not in use. Tape stopcocks in the "line-open" position if they will be hidden under the drapes and inaccessible.
3. For radial lines, immobilize the forearm and wrist on a padded splint to prevent accidental decannulation.
4. Use a continuous flush device, but beware of accidental fluid overload. Use 1 N or 0.5 N saline with heparin (1,000 IU/500 ml).

---

*Peripheral Systems Group, Mountainview, CA.

Do not use dextrose, because of increased risk of infection of the line.
5. Beware of embolization.
   a. Do not reinfuse blood removed during sampling.
   b. Do not use high pressure to attempt to clear a blocked cannula.
   c. Infuse only small volumes of flush fluid after sampling. In small infants, volumes of only 0.5–1.0 ml injected into the radial artery may flow retrograde into the cerebral vessels.
6. Remove the arterial line as soon as it has served its purpose. Complications (especially arterial thrombosis and sepsis) increase with the duration of cannulation of the vessel.

Internal Jugular Vein Cannulation

The use of an ultrasound probe (Site Rite*) improves the success rate and decreases the incidence of complications.

1. Position the patient—head to left, 20° Trendelenburg, with a rolled towel under the shoulders to reduce concavity of the neck.
2. If available, use the Site Rite or other ultrasound probe to locate and mark the position of the internal jugular vein (IJV) at the level of the cricoid cartilage. It is helpful to also note the relation of the IJV to the carotid artery at this level.
3. Prepare and drape, and glove.
4. Insert the needle through the skin at 45° over the marked course of the IJV until the vein is punctured: a flow of venous blood is usually obtained as the needle is being slowly withdrawn.
5. Hold the needle very still, pass the guidewire, and complete the cannulation.

If ultrasound is not available, cannulation must be performed using anatomic landmarks:

1. Palpate the carotid pulse medial to the sternocleidomastoid and pick this muscle up to identify its bulk at the level of the thyroid cartilage prominence.
2. Make a skin stab (#11 blade) at the anterior border of the sternomastoid at the level of the thyroid prominence (if the patient weighs less than 15 kg) or at the level of the cricothyroid membrane (if more than 15 kg), taking care to avoid the external jugular vein.
3. Use a 22-gauge plastic cannula (e.g., Angiocath†). Advance this through the skin stab medial to the sternomastoid at an angle of 30° to skin toward the ipsilateral axilla. Aspirate intermittently to identify venous blood. If the vein is not entered, withdraw very slowly, aspirating continuously. The vein is more often successfully located on withdrawal. If unsuccessful, repeat the needle insertion in a more medial direction toward the ipsilateral nipple. Throughout this procedure, use care to avoid the carotid pulsation.

---

*Dymax Corp., Pittsburgh, PA.
†Becton Dickinson Infusion Therapy Systems Inc., Sandy, UT.

4. When the vein is found, advance the cannula and verify easy aspiration of blood.
5. Insert a guidewire and complete cannulation by the Seldinger technique.

N.B. In cyanotic patients, it is advisable to attach the needle or a cannula to a transducer and confirm that the pressure is venous before using the dilator.

To position the tip of the catheter at the junction of the superior vena cava and right atrium, the length should be equal to the distance from skin penetration to a point 2 cm below the upper border of the manubrium.

The tip of the guidewire, accurately placed to just protrude from the catheter, may be used as an internal ECG electrode to position the catheter. A biphasic P wave is seen if the catheter is correctly placed.

Always check the position of the tip of the catheter on the radiograph if the catheter is to be left in place postoperatively. Catheters that extend too far into the right atrium may perforate the heart.

If IJV puncture cannot be performed and the external jugular vein is visible, it may be a useful alternative route for CVP monitoring.

External Jugular Vein Cannulation

1. Position the patient with a 15° head-down tilt and a small pillow under the shoulders.
2. Locate the external jugular vein, and prepare and drape the area.
3. Puncture the vein and insert a 22-gauge intravenous catheter.
4. Feed a J-wire through the catheter and advance it centrally, rotating as necessary. A 6-mm-diameter J-wire is most likely to pass easily. The catheter must be manipulated gently to avoid the possibility of damage. It may be advantageous to move the patient's arm and shoulder if the wire does not advance.
5. When the wire has advanced, a dilator may be gently used, but do not pass it further than just into the external jugular vein or a tear at the junction with the subclavian vein may result.
6. Advance the soft central venous catheter over the guidewire until it is sited at the junction of the superior vena cava and right atrium. This distance can be judged by measuring the distance from skin puncture to manubriosternal junction.
7. The position of long-indwelling CVP lines should be checked by radiography. Complications (including perforation) may occur if the line is too long.

Other Important Forms of Monitoring

Blood Glucose. Infants, especially preterm or small-for-gestational-age infants, are prone to hypoglycemia; their blood glucose levels should be checked frequently. This is simply accomplished in the OR by using an inexpensive handheld glucometer. The results obtained are accurate enough to detect important abnormalities. Hypoglycemia (less than 40 mg/dl) should be corrected by infusions of glucose (6 mg/kg/min).

Avoid excessive glucose administration, however, because it may result in hyperglycemia, glycosuria, and dehydration and may increase the risk of cerebral damage should a hypoxic episode occur.

Fluid Administration. The intravenous administration of fluids must be very carefully monitored to avoid overload. Syringe pumps or controlled intravenous infusion pumps should always be used. Total all fluids given, including those given with drugs. The use of a low-volume remote injection site* or an injection cap at the infusion line site minimizes the need for large volumes of flushing fluid. Small-size (tuberculin) syringes should be used to measure small doses accurately, avoiding the need to dilute drugs to give accurate doses.

Anesthesia Chart. The anesthesia chart is an important monitor and, if well kept, permits the anesthesiologist to detect important trends in the patient's progress.

Suggested Additional Reading

Pulse Oximetry

Broome IJ, Harris RW, and Reilly CS: The response times of pulse oximeters measuring oxygen saturations during hypoxemic events. Anaesthesia 47:17–19, 1992.

Cote CJ, Goldstein EA, Cote MA, et al.: A single blind study of pulse oximetry in children. Anesthesiology 68:184–188, 1988.

Deckhart R and Steward DJ: Continuous transcutaneous arterial oxygen saturation measurement: II. Arterial hemoglobin saturation versus oxygen tension monitoring in the preterm infant. Crit Care Med 12:935–939, 1984.

Murphy KG, Secunda JA, and Rockoff MA: Severe burns from a pulse oximeter. Anesthesiology 73:350–352, 1990.

O'Leary RJ, Landon M, and Benumoff JL: Buccal pulse oximeter is more accurate than finger pulse oximeter in measuring oxygen saturation. Anesth Analg 75:495–498, 1992.

Tremper KK and Barker SJ: Pulse oximetry. Anesthesiology 70:98–108, 1989.

Versmold HT, Lindekamp O, Holzmann M, et al.: Hyperbilirubinemia does not interfere with hemoglobin saturation measured by pulse oximetry. Anesthesiology 70:118–122, 1989.

End-Tidal Carbon Dioxide Monitoring

Badgwell JM, Heavner JE, May WS, et al.: End tidal PCO_2 monitoring in infants and children ventilated with either a partial rebreathing or a non-rebreathing circuit. Anesthesiology 66:405–410, 1987.

Badgwell JM, Mcleod ME, Lerman J, and Creighton RE: End-tidal PCO_2 measurements in infants and children ventilated with the Sechrist ventilator. Anesthesiology 67:A511,1987.

Badgwell JM, Mcleod ME, Lerman J, and Creighton RE: End-tidal PCO_2 monitoring in infants and children during ventilation with the Air Shields Ventimeter ventilator. Anesthesiology 65:A418, 1986.

Badgwell JM, Mcleod ME, Lerman J, et al.: End-tidal PCO_2 measurements

---

*Sims North America, Keene, NH.

sampled at the distal and proximal ends of the endotracheal tube in infants and children. Anesth Analg 66:959–964, 1987.

Burrows FA: Physiologic dead space, venous admixture, and the arterial to end-tidal carbon dioxide difference in infants and children undergoing cardiac surgery. Anesthesiology 70;219–225,1989.

Cote CJ, Rolf N, Lui LMP, et al.: A single blind study of combined pulse oximetry and capnography in children. Anesthesiology 74:980–987, 1991.

Markovitz BP and Silverberg M: Unusual cause of an absent capnogram. Anesthesiology 71:992–993, 1989.

Hemodynamic Monitoring

Alderson PJ, Burrows FA, Stemp LI, and Holtby HM: Use of ultrasound to evaluate internal jugular vein anatomy and to facilitate central venous cannulation in paediatric patients. Br J Anaesth 70:145–148, 1993.

Damen J: Positive bacterial cultures and related risk factors associated with percutaneous internal jugular vein catheterisation in pediatric cardiac patients. Anesthesiology 66:558–562, 1987.

Glenski JA, Beynen FM, and Brady J: A prospective evaluation of femoral artery monitoring in pediatric patients. Anesthesiology 66:227–229, 1987.

Hill GE and Machin RH: Doppler determined blood pressure recordings: the effect of varying cuff sizes in children. Can Anaesth Soc J 23:323, 1976.

Lowenstein E, Little JW, and Lo HH: Prevention of cerebral embolization from flushing radial artery cannulas. N Engl J Med 285:1414, 1971.

Lum LG and Jones MD: The effect of cuff width on systolic blood pressure measurements in neonates. J Pediatr 91:963, 1977.

Miyasaka K, Edmonds JF, and Conn AQ: Complications of radial artery lines in the paediatric patient. Can Anaesth Soc J 23:9, 1976.

Nordstrom L and Fletcher R: A comparison of two different J-wires for central venous cannulation via the external jugular vein. Anesth Analg 62:365, 1983.

Simon L, Teboul A, Gwinner G, et al.: Central venous catheter placement in children: evaluation of electrocardiography using J wire. Paediatr Anaesth 9:501–504, 1999.

Verghese ST, Patel RI, and Hannallah RS: Central venous cannulation in infants and children: a comparison of internal and external jugular vein approaches. Paediatr Anaesth 3:95–99, 1993.

Verghese ST, McGill WA, Patel RI, et al.: Ultrasound guided internal jugular venous cannulation in infants: a prospective comparison with the traditional palpation method. Anesthesiology 91:71–77, 1999.

MANAGEMENT OF BODY TEMPERATURE

Monitoring

Continuous monitoring of body temperature with a thermistor probe is essential for all patients undergoing general anesthesia. In larger children having minor surgery, the temperature is usually recorded from the axilla. This reflects body core temperature accurately provided that the tip of the probe is close to the axillary artery and the patient's arm is adducted. Adhesive skin temperature sensors (e.g., on the forehead) do not provide an accurate estimate of core temperature. In smaller children and infants and in children undergoing major surgery, the temperature should be monitored in the esophagus or rectum. Esophageal temperatures should be recorded in the lower third of the esophagus to avoid falsely low readings caused by gas flowing into the trachea. When using an esophageal stethoscope with thermistor, adjust the position until the heart sounds are best heard; the thermistor is then optimally placed behind the left atrium.

Tympanic membrane probes have been used to monitor core temperature. The tympanic membrane temperature closely follows lower esophageal temperature, but care must be taken not to damage the ear. We prefer to take the safe and easy course and monitor the esophageal temperature.

Conservation of Body Heat in Neonates

The objective of body heat conservation is to prevent cold stress and to avoid hypothermia, which affects recovery from anesthetic and relaxant drugs, impairs coagulation, may depress ventilation, may result in arrhythmias, and increases postoperative oxygen consumption.

Preoperatively. Adjust the OR ambient temperature to 24°C (75°F) or higher. Ensure that a heating blanket set at 40°C and covered by two layers of flannelette is in place on the OR table. Prepare a Bair Hugger* or similar forced air heater and mattress. Keep the patient in the heated transport incubator until you are ready to induce anesthesia.

Perioperatively. Position an infrared heating lamp at the correct distance over the patient during induction and preparation for surgery. Keep a woolen cap on the infant's head whenever possible. Use warmed intravenous solutions and heated humidified anesthetic gases (at 36°C). Warmed (40°C) skin preparation solution should be used, and any excess should be dried from the skin to prevent cooling by evaporation. The use of a hot air blanket (e.g., Bair Hugger) may be advantageous in some cases.

Postoperatively. Use the infrared heater during extubation and other procedures at the end of anesthesia. Place the infant in a warmed incubator and return the infant promptly to the postanesthesia room, intensive care unit, or neonatal unit.

Hyperthermia During Surgery

Hyperthermia sometimes develops during surgery if all of the described heat-conserving procedures are followed. If this occurs, the temperature of the inspired gases should be reduced or the heating blanket switched off. Other causes for hyperthermia during surgery include pyrexial reactions (e.g., from manipulation of an infected organ or a blood transfusion reaction); very rarely, it is caused by the malignant hyperpyrexia syndrome.

---

*Augustine Medical Inc., Eden Prairie, MN.

Suggested Additional Reading

Bennett EJ, Patel KP, and Grundy EM: Neonatal temperature and surgery. Anesthesiology 46:303, 1977.

Bissonette B, Sessler DI, and LaFlamme P: Intraoperative temperature monitoring sites in infants and children and the effect of inspired gas warming on esophageal temperature. Anesth Analg 69:192–196, 1989.

Engelman DR and Lockhart CH: Comparisons between temperature effects of ketamine and halothane anesthesia in children. Anesth Analg 51:98, 1972.

Kurz A, Kurz M, Poeschl G, et al.: Forced air warming maintains intraoperative normothermia better than circulating water mattresses. Anesth Analg 77:89–95, 1993.

Sessler DI: Consequences and treatment of perioperative hypothermia. Anesthesiol Clin North Am 12:425–456, 1994.

INTRAVENOUS THERAPY

1. For all children weighing less than 20 kg, insert a Buretrol or similar graduated reservoir between the intravenous bag and the administration set; this prevents accidental fluid overload and permits an accurate check of infused volumes.
2. Always use an infusion pump (e.g., intravenous accurate control device [IVAC]). This allows accurate control of the rate of infusion and easy monitoring of volumes administered, and it provides a warning if the infusion becomes obstructed.
3. Percutaneous insertion of a plastic cannula into a vein is considered optimal. If this is to be done with the child awake, apply EMLA* cream to the site (60 to 90 minutes in advance if possible!). Amethocaine gel (Ametop), if available, provides more rapid skin anesthesia. Use a 22-gauge cannula or larger if blood transfusion may be required. Observe strict asepsis when performing cannulation; use Betadine skin preparation solution, and cover the puncture site with a sterile dressing. Label the intravenous line with the size of the cannula and the date of insertion.
4. For major abdominal surgery, the intravenous lines must be placed in the upper limbs.
5. Before surgery commences, ensure that the intravenous line is working well. Do not embark on any procedure with a doubtful intravenous line.

Venipuncture and Insertion of Intravenous Cannulas

The ability to perform a venipuncture painlessly and to cannulate small veins successfully is essential for the pediatric anesthesiologist. Some tips that may help follow.

1. For venipuncture (e.g., with a small butterfly needle):
   a. Apply EMLA cream 90 minutes in advance (or Ametop 45 minutes in advance) whenever possible. Alternatively, nitrous

---

*Astrazeneca, Wayne, PA.

oxide may be administered (50%–75% inspired concentration) to sedate the child during venous cannulation. Make sure that you have a skilled assistant who can distract the child while gently restraining him.

b. Never use a rubber tourniquet on a young child; have your assistant grasp the arm to gently impede venous return and thereby fill the veins. Do not attempt venipuncture unless the vein is obviously well filled: filling can be facilitated by having the assistant hold the hand below the patient's body level and apply gentle manual constriction to the limb.

c. Never inject drugs into veins of the antecubital fossa. Accidental intra-arterial injection is more common here than at any other site. The risk is higher in children because of the close proximity of vessels and the possibility that the child might move during the injection.

d. Usually a vein on the dorsum of the hand is most suitable. Look and palpate across the back of the hand opposite the fourth digit.

e. Use the smallest size needle and syringe possible, and keep the equipment from the child's view at all times.

f. Hold the needle and syringe firmly, and avoid accidentally touching the skin with the needle until ready to puncture the vein.

g. When ready, puncture the skin and vein firmly with one rapid movement, and then hold the needle firmly in place until the injection is completed.

2. Cannulation of a vein may be performed after induction of anesthesia; otherwise, apply a surface analgesic (e.g., EMLA cream or Ametop) well in advance of the procedure.

a. Select a suitable vein. The best sites usually are the dorsum of the hand, the medial aspect of the ankle, the lateral aspect of the foot, a scalp vein (in infants), or the lateral aspect of the wrist (in older children). Consider which sites are appropriate; for example, patients with abdominal trauma or tumor must have an intravenous line in the upper limb. Those patients who will be using crutches should not have an intravenous line inserted in the back of the hand.

b. Use careful aseptic technique and prepare the skin with Betadine solution.

c. Make sure the vein selected is well filled, and make a small incision over it with an 18-gauge needle.

d. Note the direction of the bevel on the cannula needle. After the initial venous puncture is made, turn the bevel face down before attempting to advance the cannula into the vein. This ensures that the point of the needle is unlikely to be in the distal wall of a small vein and that the cannula will advance unimpeded into the vein (*see* Fig. 4–2).

e. When the cannula is in place, apply antibiotic spray or ointment to the puncture site and cover it with a sterile dressing. Tape the cannula firmly in place, and immobilize the limb on a splint.

f. When inserting a cannula into a very small, fine vein it may help to pass a fine guidewire into the cannula before attempting to advance it:

i. A 22-gauge Angiocath is inserted toward the vein at a shallow angle.

ii. As soon as there is a "flashback" of blood into the hub of the needle, the cannula is held absolutely still and the needle is very gently removed. Blood is usually seen flowing back into the cannula.

iii. A 0.018-inch (0.46-mm) diameter spring wire guide* is then gently advanced through the cannula into the vein. In most instances this guidewire is easily inserted, even into very small veins, and can be seen tracking inside the vein for some distance up the limb. The cannula is now advanced over the guidewire with full confidence that it will end up lying freely within the lumen of the vein and will provide a very reliable intravenous route.

This technique should be considered for all very small infants and especially for those in whom all the "good veins" have already been used and/or traumatized.

Intraosseous Infusions

When venipuncture is impossible and urgent fluid or drug therapy is indicated, the intraosseous route should be employed. Any drug or solution that can be given intravenously can also be given by this route. Continuous infusions can be given. In "shock" or "arrest" states, absorption from the intraosseous site may be more rapid than from a peripheral intravenous line.

The usual insertion sites are the distal femur (midline 1 cm above the patella) and the proximal tibia (medial on the tibial plateau 1 cm below the tuberosity); accidental injections into the epiphysis do not usually cause any harm. A bone marrow needle† or a strong large-bore spinal needle is firmly advanced through the bone until a "give" is noted and the needle stands rigidly. At this point bone marrow can be aspirated and fluid can be injected with very little resistance and with no swelling or extravasation. After initial fluid resuscitation by this route, it is often possible to start an intravenous infusion into a peripheral vein.

Preoperative Fluid Replacement

Preoperative dehydration can be classified by the size of the deficit as mild, moderate, or severe:

Mild: 50 ml/kg (5% body weight loss)
Moderate: 100 ml/kg (10% body weight loss)
Severe: 150 ml/kg (15% body weight loss)

---

*0.45 mm × 25 cm spring wire guide (Ref # AW-04018), Arrow International Inc., Reading, PA.

†Cook Critical Care, Bloomington, IN.

Replacement of water and electrolytes should proceed in three phases:

1. **Treatment of overt or impending shock** (severe dehydration and hypovolemia): Order an initial infusion of whole blood (10 ml/kg); if this is not available, give plasma or 5% albumin (20 ml/kg).
2. **Replacement of extracellular water and sodium:** Half the estimated fluid deficit can be replaced over the initial 6–8 hours as 0.3 N saline. If the deficit is severe, give an initial infusion of 1 N saline (20 ml/kg). The degree of success of this therapy can be gauged from the clinical signs (heart rate, arterial and venous pressures, and urine output). The following formula is useful in correcting sodium deficiency:

$$Na^+ \text{ deficit (mEq)} = normal\ Na^+ \text{ (mEq)} - measured\ Na^+ \text{ (mEq)} \times 0.6 \times weight\ (kg)$$

   where 0.6 = diffusion constant.

   Metabolic acidosis should be treated simultaneously, using the formula:

$$Dose\ required\ (mEq\ of\ HCO_3^-) = base\ deficit \times weight\ (kg) \times 0.3\ (0.4\ for\ infants)$$

   Give half the calculated requirement, then reassess the acid-base status.
3. **Replacement of potassium:** Potassium (K^+) replacement should be initiated when a good urinary output has been established, according to the following general guidelines:
   a. Replace a maximum of 3 mEq/kg of potassium per 24 hours.
   b. The rate of administration should not exceed 0.5 mEq/kg/hr.
   c. Complete correction of severe K^+ deficiency should take 4–5 days.

   These figures are only a guide and must be adjusted for changes in metabolic activity, clinical conditions, and extrarenal losses (e.g., gastric suction).

   N.B. A neonate's insensible water loss decreases by 30%–35% when nursed in a high-humidity atmosphere or ventilated with humidified gases. Insensible water loss is increased by crying, sweating, hyperventilation, and the use of a radiant heater or "bili" lights. Pyrexia increases water loss by 12% per 1°C.

Perioperative Fluid Management

Calculation of the volume and type of fluid required must take the following aspects into consideration:

1. Dehydration present *before* preoperative fasting.
2. Fluid deficit incurred *during* preoperative fasting.
3. Maintenance fluid requirement during surgery.
4. Estimated extracellular fluid loss resulting from surgical trauma.
5. Alterations in body temperature.

For brief surgical procedures (less than 30 minutes) in otherwise healthy children, intravenous fluids usually are not needed perioperatively if the preoperative deficit was small, the fasting period was short, and blood loss or tissue trauma was minimal. Oral intake is likely to be reestablished early in the postoperative period (e.g., myringotomy and tubes).

For surgical procedures of greater duration, when reestablishment of oral intake may be delayed:

1. An intravenous infusion is established.
2. Fluid is administered perioperatively and postoperatively until oral intake is reestablished.
3. Lactated Ringer's solution is usually given for simple procedures; 5% dextrose in lactated Ringer's solution may cause hyperglycemia during longer procedures, and plain lactated Ringer's solution is more appropriate.
4. For extensive surgery, especially in infants, it is advantageous to separate the administration of dextrose from other fluid therapy. An infusion of 5% or 10% dextrose can be established at a rate that will deliver 4–6 mg/kg/min. Blood glucose levels should be checked periodically. Other isotonic fluids given to replace losses should be free of dextrose.

The hourly rate of infusion is based on daily maintenance requirements (Table 4–6). Adjust the hourly rate if (1) factors affecting insensible fluid loss are present (e.g., increased body temperature) or (2) there are extrarenal losses (e.g., gastrointestinal).

Sufficient fluid should be given to compensate for preoperative fasting. The total volume to be administered during surgery is calculated by multiplying the number of hours (fasting + surgery) by the hourly maintenance requirement. For example, for a 10-kg child fasting for 4 hours and then undergoing an estimated 4-hour operative procedure, replacement and maintenance requirements would total 160 + 160 = 320 ml (i.e., 8 ml/kg/hr).

Additional Fluids

For surgical procedures causing significant tissue trauma and/or blood loss, give additional fluids to replace extracellular fluid lost in blood or

Table 4–6. Daily Maintenance Requirements

Weight (kg)	Maintenance Fluid Requirement (ml/kg/hr)
Newborn	3
4–10	4
11–20	3
21–40	2.5–3.0
41+	2.0–2.5

Table 4–7. Composition of Electrolyte Solutions

Solution	Concentration (mEq/L)					Concentration HCO₃⁻ (mEq/L)		
	Na⁺	K⁺	Mg⁺⁺	Ca⁺⁺	Cl⁻	Acetate	Gluconate	Lactate
Normal saline (0.9%)	154	—	—	—	154	—	—	—
0.3 N saline in D₅W	51	—	—	—	51	—	—	—
0.2 N saline in D₅W	34	—	—	—	34	—	—	—
Normosol-M	40	13	3	—	40	16	—	—
Normosol-R	140	5	3	—	98	27	23	—
Lactated Ringer's solution	130	4	—	3	109	—	—	28

Magnesium sulfate (2 ml amp., 50% w/v): 4.0 mEq Mg⁺⁺/ml
Sodium bicarbonate (50 ml amp., 7.5% w/v): 0.9 mEq HCO₃⁻/ml
Calcium gluconate (10 ml amp., 10% w/v): 0.447 mEq Ca⁺⁺/ml
Calcium chloride (10 ml amp., 10% w/v): 1.36 mEq Ca⁺⁺/ml

D₅W, 5% dextrose in water.

sequestered into damaged tissue. This deficiency should be replaced with a multiple-electrolyte solution (e.g., lactated Ringer's solution) in which the electrolyte concentrations are similar to those in extracellular fluid (Table 4–7). Abdominal surgery and surgery of the spine are associated with large fluid losses into the tissues and may require similarly large volumes of additional fluid (6–10 ml/kg or more). Thoracotomy is associated with much less translocation of fluid, so lesser volumes are required.

Adequacy of fluid replacement is best judged by continuous monitoring of the cardiovascular indices and urine output. If there is less than 0.5–1 ml/kg/hr of urine, the fluid infusion rate should be increased.

Postoperative hyponatremia is a danger in children. It is usually associated with the intraoperative and postoperative use of hypotonic fluids and occasionally with inappropriate secretion of antidiuretic hormone. Children are much more susceptible than adults to brain damage from hyponatremia. Do not use hypotonic solutions during surgery or order them postoperatively. Monitor serum electrolytes during and after major surgery.

Suggested Additional Reading

Arieff AI: Postoperative hyponatraemic encephalopathy following elective surgery in children. Paediatr Anaesth 8:1–4, 1998.

Berry FA: Practical aspects of fluid and electrolyte therapy. In Berry FA (ed.): Anesthetic Management of Difficult and Routine Pediatric Patients, 2nd ed. Churchill Livingstone, New York, 1990, pp 89–120.

Filston HC and Johnson DG: Percutaneous venous cannulation in neonates and infants: a method for catheter insertion without cutdown. Pediatrics 48:896, 1971.

Freeman JA, Doyle E, Tee NG, and Morton NS: Topical anaesthesia of the skin: a review. Paediatr Anaesth 3:129–138, 1993.

Orlowski JP: Emergency alternatives to intravenous access. Pediatr Clin North Am 41:1183–1199, 1994.

Rice HE, Caty MG, and Glick PL: Fluid therapy for the pediatric surgical patient. Pediatr Clin North Am 45:719–727, 1998.

Shepard FM, Arango LM, and Berry FA: Acid-base response of the newborn to major surgery. Anesth Analg 50:31, 1971.

Steward DJ: Venous cannulation in small infants: a simple method to improve success. Anesthesiology 90:930–931, 1999.

Tobias JD: Shock in children: the first 60 minutes. Pediatr Ann 25:330–338, 1996.

Wellborn LG, Hannalah RS, McGill WA, et al.: Glucose concentrations for routine intravenous infusion in pediatric outpatient surgery. Anesthesiology 67:427–430, 1987.

BLOOD REPLACEMENT

Preoperative Assessment

A normal Hb level (Table 4–8) is desirable in every case of major elective surgery. If the patient is anemic, elective surgery is sometimes delayed until the anemia has been investigated and treated. In other cases, surgery is more urgent; anesthesia for these patients must be administered with a technique that is compatible with their anemia (*see* page 156). When surgery cannot be delayed despite a very low Hb value, packed cells should be infused preoperatively. Approximately 4 ml/kg of packed cells (6 ml/kg whole blood) is required to raise the Hb level 1 g/dl.

The hemoglobin content of stored whole blood is 12 g/dl; that of packed cells is 24 g/dl; and that of buffy-coat-poor washed cells is 28 g/dl.

When significant blood losses (10% of the estimated blood volume [EBV] or greater) are expected, the patient's blood group should be determined and an appropriate number of units cross-matched. Insert a

Table 4–8. Normal Hemoglobin Levels

Age	Normal Hb Values[a] (g/dl)
1st day of life	20 (18–22)
2nd wk	17
3 mo	10–11
2 yr	11
3–5 yr	12.5–13.0
5–10 yr	13.0–13.5
10+ yr	14.5

[a]The Hb concentration declines gradually to about 10–11 g/dl during the first few months of life as fetal Hb is replaced. It then gradually increases and is maximal at about 14 years.

CVP line preoperatively in patients who are hypovolemic and/or may require extensive blood replacement during surgery.

Perioperative Management

At commencement of the operation, record on the anesthesia chart the EBV and the preoperative Hb level.

Assessment of Blood Loss

Accurate estimates of blood loss must be maintained throughout the operation.

1. Monitor cardiovascular system indices; in infants, the systolic BP is the most reliable indicator of blood volume.
2. Measure blood loss from the surgical site:
   a. All sponges must be weighed before they dry out. This method is simple and accurate (assume 1 g = 1 ml blood and subtract the known dry weight).
   b. Measure blood from suction (in graduated flasks).
   c. Estimate blood on drapes.
3. Chart the running total continually.
4. Be aware of the possibility that blood losses may accumulate in body cavities (e.g., peritoneum, pleura).

Blood Transfusion

The decision whether to transfuse blood must be based on the preoperative Hb level, the measured surgical blood loss, and the patient's cardiovascular response. As a rough guide, in otherwise healthy children blood replacement may be necessary after loss of 15% of the EBV. The need for blood transfusion can be determined more accurately from serial hematocrit (Hct) measurements. Normally the Hct should be maintained at or higher than 30%–40% in infants and in those patients with significant cardiac or respiratory disease, and higher than 25% in other patients.

Check each unit of blood against the patient's identity bracelet and mix it well by repeated inversion of the bag. Blood should be warmed to 37°C before administration; it should not be heated to more than 38°C or it may be damaged. Packed red blood cells are commonly diluted in saline before administration. If larger volumes of blood are going to be required for smaller children, it is preferable to dilute cells in fresh-frozen plasma or a dilutional coagulopathy may result.

Calcium is rarely necessary during massive transfusion in children but should be given if persistent hypotension follows apparently adequate volume replacement in infants. (Give 0.2–0.3 ml of a 10% solution of calcium gluconate per kilogram or 0.1–0.2 ml of a 10% solution of calcium chloride per kilogram.) In severely shocked patients who require rapid massive transfusion, be prepared to give sodium bicarbonate if indicated by serial acid-base determinations.

Massive Blood Transfusion

If it becomes apparent that massive blood transfusion will be required (i.e., more than 75% of the EBV), institute monitoring of coagulation indices. Platelet counts, prothrombin time, and partial thromboplastin time together with tests for fibrinolysis (determination of fibrin split products) should be repeated at least after every 50% blood volume replacement. It is helpful to have a preoperative platelet count if massive transfusion is a possibility. A low initial count indicates the need for early platelet transfusion. Platelet counts of less than 65,000/mm³ increase clinical bleeding and should be corrected. In practice, if platelets are being monitored during a continuing massive replacement, platelets should be ordered as the count falls below 100,000/mm³. Infusion of 1 unit of platelet concentrate per 5 kg body weight increases the platelet count by 30,000–40,000/mm³. Platelets must be stored at room temperature, not refrigerated, and they should be rocked periodically. Other deficiencies that become apparent should be dealt with by appropriate therapy (e.g., fresh-frozen plasma, appropriate blood component therapy).

Cryoprecipitate may be required if bleeding persists despite all other measures in small infants. Remember that fresh-frozen plasma, cryoprecipitate, and platelet solutions contain more citrate per unit volume than does whole blood. Therefore, calcium infusions may be required if hypotension occurs as these products are given rapidly.

Alternatives to Blood Transfusion

The risk of infection through transfusion has prompted the search for alternatives, many of which may be applicable in children:

1. **Blood conservation:** Blood losses are minimized through the use of proper positioning, infiltration of vasoconstrictors, induced hypotension, and meticulous surgical technique.
2. **Autologous transfusion of blood donated preoperatively:** Suitable size donations may be collected at 4- to 5-day intervals preoperatively. If blood donation is combined with measures to increase erythropoiesis (oral iron, erythropoietin), significant volumes may be collected for intraoperative transfusion even in quite small children.
3. **Acute intraoperative normovolemic hemodilution:** Blood is withdrawn after anesthesia but before surgery commences, and it is replaced with three times the volume of warmed lactated Ringer's solution. It has been suggested that hemodilution to a Hct of 20% is acceptable in otherwise healthy children. Blood is then reinfused as the surgery proceeds, saving the first collected unit of blood to be

transfused last. The volume to be collected can be calculated from the following formula*:

Volume = EBV × [(initial Hct − final Hct) ÷ average Hct]

4. **Intraoperative autotransfusion of shed blood using a "cell saver":** This technique has limited application, but it may be useful in orthopedic surgery. Shed red cells may be collected by suction, washed, and reinfused. However, coagulation factors are discarded in the washing process, and extensive reinfusion of washed cells may lead to dilution of these factors and coagulopathy.

Suggested Additional Reading

Bourke DL and Smith TC: Estimating allowable hemodilution. Anesthesiology 41:609, 1974.

Consensus Conference: Perioperative red blood cell transfusion. JAMA 260:2700–2703, 1988.

Cote CJ, Liu LMP, Szyfelbein SK, et al.: Changes in serial platelet counts following massive blood transfusions in pediatric patients. Anesthesiology 62:197–201, 1985.

Davenport HT and Barr MN: Blood loss during pediatric operations. Can Med Assoc J 89:1309, 1963.

Furman EB, Roman DG, Lemmer LAS, et al.: Specific therapy in water, electrolyte and blood-volume replacement during pediatric surgery. Anesthesiology 42:187, 1975.

Jacobs RG, Howland WS, and Goulet AH: Serial microhematocrit determinations in evaluating blood replacement. Anesthesiology 22:342, 1961.

Murray DJ, Pennell BJ, Weinstein SLM, and Olson JD: Packed red cells in acute blood loss: dilutional coagulopathy as a cause of surgical bleeding. Anesth Analg 80:336–342, 1995.

SPECIAL CONSIDERATIONS FOR THE PRETERM INFANT

1. **Infection:** The immune system is immature, and the preterm infant is particularly prone to infection. Use careful aseptic technique for all invasive procedures.
2. **Intraventricular hemorrhage:** The preterm infant is prone to intraventricular hemorrhage. Avoid causing fluctuations in blood pressure, ensure adequate anesthesia, avoid overtransfusion, infuse hypertonic solutions slowly (e.g., dextrose, sodium bicarbonate), treat anemia and coagulopathy.
3. **Apneic spells:** These are common in preterm infants, who must be monitored closely at all times and especially during and after anesthesia. Risk factors for perioperative apnea include
   a. Low postconceptual age—infants of less than 45 weeks'

---

*Gross JB: Estimating allowable blood loss: correction for dilution. Anesthesiology 58:277–280, 1983.

postconceptual age are the most likely to experience significant episodes of apnea.

b. Low gestational age at birth—infants born before 34 weeks' gestation are at greater risk.

c. Anemia increases the risk of apnea.

d. A history of apnea episodes and use of an apnea monitor indicate higher risk.

e. The presence of chronic lung disease increases the risk of apnea.

In very small infants, the risk of apnea may extend for as long as 72 hours into the postoperative period. The following are general recommendations:

f. It is usual practice to admit all preterm infants of less than 50 weeks' postconceptual age after any general or regional anesthesia.

g. Infants born at less than 34 weeks' gestation and those with anemia (Hb less than 10 g/dl) should be admitted if still less than 60 weeks' postconceptual age.

h. Older infants should also be admitted and observed if there is any evidence of ventilatory disturbance in the perioperative period.

N.B. Apnea may be less common after surgery performed under spinal analgesia, but it may still occur, so the patient must be admitted and monitored. Caffeine therapy (10 mg/kg IV administered slowly after induction) may prevent apnea, but monitoring is still advised.

4. **Temperature control:** The preterm infant is extremely vulnerable to heat loss—even more so than the full-term newborn. The surface area is even larger relative to body mass, and there are no insulating subcutaneous tissues. Be especially alert to prevent heat loss at all times.

5. **Oxygenation:** This must be very carefully controlled if hyperoxia is to be avoided and the risk of retrolental fibroplasia minimized. Inspired concentrations must be kept to the minimum that will allow safe conduct of general anesthesia. Monitor with a pulse oximeter and attempt to keep the saturation between 90% and 95%.

a. Ascertain the FiO_2 required preoperatively that ensures satisfactory oxygenation. During nonthoracic surgery with controlled ventilation, continue with this FiO_2 and check saturation.

b. Whenever N_2O is contraindicated, use an air-O_2 mixture to achieve the desired FiO_2 and saturation.

c. During intrathoracic surgery it is often essential to increase the FiO_2; monitor saturation and limit the O_2 concentration as far as possible while avoiding the possibility of inducing hypoxemia.

6. **Hypoglycemia and hyperglycemia:** Preterm infants are prone to hypoglycemia. Blood sugar levels should be checked frequently, and hypoglycemia (less than 40 mg/dl) should be corrected by infusions of glucose. The preterm infant is also subject to hyperglycemia, which is usually iatrogenic but may also be caused by poor insulin

response and continued glycolysis. Hyperglycemia leads to glycosuria, osmotic diuresis, and dehydration and should be avoided by frequent blood sugar determinations and limited intravenous glucose administration.

7. **Fluid administration:** Avoid overload by very careful control of intravenous fluids. Determine the total intravenous fluids given, including those given with drugs. Use small (1-ml) syringes to accurately measure small volumes of drugs. Syringe pumps and controlled infusion lines are essential.

8. **Benzyl alcohol:** This is used as a preservative in multidose vials of some medications and has been linked with kernicterus, intraventricular hemorrhage, and mortality in preterm infants. Preparations containing this substance should be avoided.

9. **Coagulation:** The preterm infant is subject to coagulopathy associated with shock and sepsis. Thrombocytopenia is common. Perform coagulation studies on all seriously ill preterm infants. Platelet concentrates, fresh-frozen plasma, or exchange transfusion may be required.

Suggested Additional Reading

Betts EK, Downes JJ, Schaffer DB, and Johns R: Retrolental fibroplasia and oxygen administration during general anesthesia. Anesthesiology 47:518, 1977.

Cote CJ, Zavlavski A, Downes JJ, et al.: Postoperative apnea in former preterm infants after inguinal herniotomy: a combined analysis. Anesthesiology 82:809–822, 1995.

Friesen RH, Honda AT, and Thieme RE: Perianesthetic intracranial hemorrhage in preterm neonates. Anesthesiology 67:814–816, 1987.

Gerber A CH, Baitella LC, and Dangel PH: Spinal anaesthesia in former preterm infants. Paediatr Anaesth 3:153–156, 1993.

Gross SJ and Stuart MJ: Hemostasis in the premature infant. Clin Perinatol 4:259, 1977.

Maze A and Samuels SI: Hypoglycemia-induced seizures in an infant during anesthesia. Anesthesiology 52:77, 1980.

Phibbs RH: Oxygen therapy: a continuing hazard to the premature infant. Anesthesiology 47:486, 1977.

Reynolds P and Wilton N: Inadvertent benzyl alcohol administration to neonates: do we contribute? Anesth Analg 69:855–856, 1989.

Spaeth JP, O'Hara IB, and Kurth CD: Anesthesia for the micropremie. Semin Perinatol 22:390–401, 1988.

Stow PJ, Mcleod ME, and Burrows FA: Anterior fontanel pressure response to endotracheal intubation in neonates and young infants. Anesth Analg 66:S169, 1987.

Welborn LG, Hannalah RS, Fink R, and Hicks JM: The role of caffeine in the prevention of postoperative apnea in former premature infants: if some is good, is more better? Anesthesiology 69:A753, 1988.

ANESTHESIA FOR OUTPATIENT SURGERY

Advantages of Outpatient Surgery

1. The child's psychological upset is minimized.
2. There is less risk of hospital-acquired infection.

3. Cost of care is reduced; hospital beds are available for others.

Selection of Cases

1. The child must be healthy or have any chronic disease under good control.
2. The child's parents must be reliable and willing to follow instructions concerning preoperative and postoperative care.
3. The operation should be associated with minor physiologic upset, with no complex postoperative care or pain management required.
4. Infants who were born preterm and are still less than the minimal postconceptual age should be admitted.

Preoperative Preparation

Preoperative preparation is the same as for inpatient surgery. The parents should be given written instructions concerning preoperative fasting and methods to prepare their child for a visit to the hospital. They should also be given a health questionnaire to complete and bring with them to facilitate obtaining a medical history for the child (Fig. 4–3).

On the day of the operation, the child is brought to the outpatient department surgical unit. Routine Hb determination is not usually required for healthy children but should be obtained when indicated; if indicated, a sickle cell preparation is obtained. The parent's or legal guardian's consent for operation must be properly obtained.

The anesthesiologist makes a preoperative assessment by taking the history, examining the patient, and noting any laboratory and other data.

Selection of Anesthetic Techniques

Premedication is not routinely given to outpatients, so that the recovery phase is not prolonged. Many properly prepared children attending for outpatient surgery with their parents are not very upset, and premedication may not be necessary. In the event that the child is apprehensive, premedication may be administered, as described earlier (*see* page 77).

Use simple general anesthesia techniques that are likely to result in rapid recovery. Do not give unnecessary drugs that might increase postoperative morbidity (a single dose of any narcotic analgesic increases the incidence of postoperative nausea and vomiting). Volatile agents have been widely used for pediatric outpatients, sevoflurane or halothane being the agents of choice for short procedures. Simple inhalation anesthesia for short procedures in children is followed by relatively rapid and complete recovery.

It is preferable, whenever possible, to supplement a light general anesthetic with the appropriate regional analgesia technique. This, if established before surgery, provides analgesia during and after surgery. Regional block before surgery may also reduce the total pain experienced after surgery (preemptive analgesia).

The introduction of propofol has provided the alternative of using an

AMBULATORY SERVICES
OUT-PATIENT SURGERY

INSTRUCTIONS:
— CHECK ONE ANSWER TO EACH QUESTION
— PLEASE COMPLETE THIS SIDE ONLY
— PLEASE BRING THIS FORM WITH YOU ON THE DAY OF SURGERY

	YES	NO	DON'T KNOW			YES	NO	DON'T KNOW
1. HAS YOUR CHILD EVER BEEN IN HOSPITAL?	☐	☐	☐		12. IS THERE ANYONE IN THE FAMILY WITH A BLEEDING PROBLEM?	☐	☐	☐
2. HAS HE BEEN IN THIS HOSPITAL BEFORE?	☐	☐	☐		13. HAS THE PATIENT HAD ANY MINOR INJURIES, OPERATIONS, OR TOOTH EXTRACTION FOLLOWED BY AN UNUSUAL AMOUNT OF BLEEDING?	☐	☐	☐
3. HAS YOUR CHILD EVER HAD AN ANAESTHETIC?	☐	☐	☐					
4. DID YOUR CHILD HAVE ANY PROBLEMS WITH THE ANAESTHETIC?	☐	☐	☐		14. DOES THE CHILD BRUISE EASILY ON BODY AREAS OTHER THAN THE LEGS?	☐	☐	☐
5. DOES YOUR CHILD HAVE ANY ALLERGIES?	☐	☐	☐		15. HAS YOUR CHILD BEEN EXPOSED TO ANY INFECTIOUS DISEASE WITHIN THE PAST MONTH?	☐	☐	☐

6. WAS THE ALLERGY DUE TO:
 a) A DRUG OR MEDICINE? ☐ ☐ ☐
 b) ANY TYPE OF FOOD? ☐ ☐ ☐
 c) OTHER THINGS? ☐ ☐ ☐

7. IF HE HAD AN ALLERGY, DID HE HAVE:
 a) A SKIN RASH OR HIVES? ☐ ☐ ☐
 b) WHEEZING OR TROUBLE BREATHING? ☐ ☐ ☐
 c) HAY FEVER OR A RUNNY NOSE? ☐ ☐ ☐
 d) A HIGH FEVER? ☐ ☐ ☐

8. HAS THIS CHILD HAD A HEAD COLD OR COUGH WITHIN THE PAST WEEK? ☐ ☐ ☐

9. DOES YOUR CHILD WEAR A DENTAL PLATE OR BRIDGE? ☐ ☐ ☐

10. HAS YOUR CHILD HAD A CORTISONE TYPE DRUG WITHIN THE PAST TWO YEARS? ☐ ☐ ☐

11. IS YOUR CHILD RECEIVING ANY MEDICINE JUST NOW? ☐ ☐ ☐

16. HAS YOUR CHILD EVER HAD:
 DIABETES ☐ ☐ ☐
 ASTHMA ☐ ☐ ☐
 CYSTIC FIBROSIS ☐ ☐ ☐
 TUBERCULOSIS ☐ ☐ ☐
 RHEUMATIC FEVER ☐ ☐ ☐
 RHEUMATISM ☐ ☐ ☐
 HEART DISEASE ☐ ☐ ☐
 LIVER DISEASE ☐ ☐ ☐
 ANEMIA ☐ ☐ ☐
 CONVULSIONS OR FITS ☐ ☐ ☐
 GLAUCOMA ☐ ☐ ☐
 JAUNDICE ☐ ☐ ☐

17. IS THERE ANY PROBLEM ABOUT YOUR CHILD NOT MENTIONED SO FAR? ☐ ☐ ☐

18. HAS ANYONE IN YOUR FAMILY EVER HAD A PROBLEM WITH AN ANAESTHETIC? ☐ ☐ ☐

IF ANY QUESTIONS ABOVE RECEIVED A "YES" ANSWER GIVE DETAILS BELOW:

_____
_____
_____
_____
_____
_____
_____
_____
_____

DATE COMPLETED:_____ SIGNATURE OF PARENT:_____

Figure 4–3. Questionnaire for outpatients.

infusion technique that is also followed by a rapid recovery and minimal morbidity. Propofol infusion may be used to supplement regional analgesia, or it may be combined with a short-acting narcotic drug (e.g., alfentanil) and a short-acting relaxant drug (e.g., rapacuronium or cisatracurium), depending on the surgical procedure. A suitable regimen for total intravenous anesthesia for children undergoing relatively short procedures would be the following:

Propofol: 2.5–3.5 mg/kg for induction, then infusion of
    250 μg/kg/min for 10 minutes
    200 μg/kg/min for next 10 minutes
    150 μg/kg/min for remainder of operation
Alfentanil: 20 μg/kg at induction, then infusion of 1 μg/kg/min

Intubation should be used whenever indicated; postintubation complications can be avoided by gentle laryngoscopy and by using a tube that passes easily through the glottis and subglottic space. A small leak should be present when the circuit is pressurized to 20 cmH$_2$O. In many cases the LMA is a suitable alternative for the healthy outpatient.

For dental surgery a nasotracheal tube is used. If the distal end is warmed before insertion, it is less likely to traumatize the nose. At the end of the procedure, always perform a laryngoscopy, suction the pharynx well, and ensure that all throat packs and other items have been removed.

For strabismus surgery, it has been demonstrated that a technique employing an infusion of propofol is followed by less nausea and vomiting than when volatile inhalation agents are used.

Some procedures in older children may be performed under regional analgesia; when possible, this is ideal for the outpatient. For example, for superficial surgery on the limbs, an intravenous block may provide excellent results.

Tonsillectomy in the Day Surgery Unit

Tonsillectomy is now frequently performed in the day care unit. It is important that patients are well hydrated during and after the operation, because a return to adequate oral fluid intake may be delayed. We suggest that intravenous fluids be given to fully replace the preoperative deficit and to "load" the patient slightly before discharge home. Careful surgical technique and follow-up for bleeding are obvious requirements.

Special consideration must be given to the child with a history of obstructive sleep apnea; such patients should be admitted for postoperative monitoring. Other patients who should be admitted, as suggested by the American Association of Otolaryngology–Head and Neck Surgery,* include the following:

---

*Brown OE and Cunningham MJ: Tonsillectomy and Adenoidectomy Inpatient Guidelines: Recommendations of the AAO-HNS Pediatric Otolaryngology Committee. AAO-HNS Bulletin, September 1996, pp 13–15.

1. All patients younger than 3 years of age *(This is controversial!)*
2. Patients with any evidence of coagulopathy
3. Patients with obstructive sleep apnea
4. Patients with systemic diseases that may increase risk
5. Patients with craniofacial or airway disorders (including Down syndrome)
6. Patients with peritonsillar abscess
7. Patients with geographic or social factors that might compromise their management or emergency return to the hospital

Postoperative Care for the Outpatient

Many patients require no analgesics immediately after surgery, especially if a regional block has been performed (e.g., for hernia; *see* page 140), but beware of the "analgesic window," which may occur later at home as the block wears off. Analgesics should be ordered in anticipation of pain and should be administered by the clock rather than waiting for pain to occur. Plan for adequate continuing analgesia, and thoroughly instruct the parents on how to dose their child. Acetaminophen and/or acetaminophen with codeine can be given in the usual dosage depending on the surgery. More potent analgesics are only very rarely indicated for outpatients.

Many patients take and retain oral fluids well before discharge, but it is unwise to "push" fluids before the child is ready to drink; doing so increases the incidence of postoperative vomiting. A useful method of fluid administration is to offer Popsicles* ad lib, especially to children who have undergone tonsillectomy or adenoidectomy (*see* page 187).

Every patient must be examined and discharged by an anesthesiologist. Infants may be taken home when they are obviously fully recovered. Children should be tested for street fitness and should be able to walk out; if dizzy or nauseated, they must stay longer. If the anesthesiologist considers a patient unfit for discharge within 4 hours, overnight admission is recommended.

Children must be accompanied home by an adult, who preferably should not also be the driver of the vehicle. Warn the parents that their child must not ride a bicycle or engage in dangerous activities for 24 hours. A brochure containing basic information and a follow-up service should be provided. Parents must be encouraged to seek advice from the hospital if problems develop during the postoperative period.

Complications After Pediatric Outpatient Surgery

Complications are rare after pediatric outpatient surgery, and fewer than 1% of children need to be admitted overnight after a planned day care procedure. The most common reasons for admission are protracted vomiting or a complication of surgery. Nausea and vomiting are a predictable consequence of some types of surgery (e.g., correction of strabis-

---

*Popsicle Industries Canada, Burlington, Ontario.

mus, tonsillectomy). In such cases the choice of anesthesia techniques (e.g., propofol) or the preemptive administration of effective antiemetic drugs should be considered.

Complications that may occur at home include vomiting, cough, sleepiness, sore throat, and hoarseness. If the parents are well prepared, these can usually be treated effectively in the home.

Suggested Additional Reading

Gabalski EC, Mattucci KF, Setzen M, and Moleski P: Ambulatory tonsillectomy and adenoidectomy. Laryngoscope 106:77–80, 1996.

Gurkan Y, Kilickan L, and Toker K: Propofol nitrous oxide versus sevoflurane-nitrous oxide for strabismus surgery in children. Paediatr Anaesth 9:495–500, 1999.

Hannallah RS and Patel RI: Pediatric considerations. In Twersky RS (ed.): The Ambulatory Anesthesia Handbook. Mosby, St Louis, 1995, pp 145–170.

Mitchell RB, Pereira KD, Friedman NR, and Lazar RH: Outpatient adenotonsillectomy: is it safe in children younger than 3 years? Arch Otolaryngol Head Neck Surg 123:681–683, 1997.

Patel RI and Hannallah RS: Anesthetic complications following pediatric ambulatory surgery. Anesthesiology 69:1009–1012, 1988.

Schreiner MS, Nicholson SC, Martin T, and Whitney L: Should children drink before discharge from day surgery? Anesthesiology 76:528, 1992.

Chapter **5**

Regional Analgesia Techniques

REGIONAL ANALGESIA FOR PAIN CONTROL

Regional analgesia techniques alone are of limited value during pediatric surgical procedures; the overall nonacceptance and lack of cooperation in the awake young patient result in the need for such large doses of sedatives that general anesthesia usually becomes preferable. However, in the management of postoperative pain, regional analgesic techniques have become an indispensable part of our pediatric anesthesia practice (*see* page 188).

Regional analgesia may provide satisfactory pain control intraoperatively for some selected pediatric patients. Spinal anesthesia is useful for small infants, especially for the ex-preterm infant with residual lung disease who has a hernia or other abdominal lesion. Epidural analgesia may be a suitable alternative to general anesthesia in some older children (e.g., those with cystic fibrosis), and it may then usefully be continued into the postoperative period. Some older children (5 years of age and older) can be charmed into cooperation and have their upper limb fractures reduced under a regional block. Intravenous regional analgesia (Bier block) can be used for some older children having superficial surgery to lesions on the distal limbs. The possibility of using regional or local infiltration analgesia (Table 5–1) should also be considered for any minor procedure in a high-risk patient (e.g., skeletal muscle biopsy in a child with cardiomyopathy, lymph node biopsy in a patient with a mediastinal mass).

Rarely, regional blocks are also indicated for chronic pain therapy and/or diagnostic purposes.

Basic rules for regional analgesia are as follows:

1. Calculate the allowable dose of the local analgesic agent for each child and do not exceed that dose.
2. Use as much of the allowable dose of agent as is necessary to ensure a good block.
3. Use careful aseptic technique; beware of intravascular injection. Test by aspirating frequently.

Table 5–1. Suggested Maximum Doses of Local Anesthetic Drugs

Drug	Maximum Dose (mg/kg)
For epidural or peripheral nerve block	
Bupivacaine (plain or with epinephrine)	3
Ropivacaine	3
Lidocaine	5
With 1:200,000 epinephrine	8
Mepivacaine or prilocaine	5
With 1:200,000 epinephrine	7
For spinal block	
Tetracaine	0.4–0.6

4. Plan ahead; allow a generous period for the block to become well established before allowing the surgeon to approach the patient.
5. Remember the special considerations for the use of local analgesic drugs in infants and young children (*see* page 66).
6. Always be prepared to deal with the complications of regional analgesia. Drugs and equipment to induce general anesthesia, secure the airway, and ventilate the patient must be immediately available. Establish IV access before the block.
7. Be prepared; unsatisfactory regional analgesia may require administration of general anesthesia to permit completion of the surgical procedure.
8. If possible, 90 minutes preoperatively, apply topical anesthetic cream over the site of the proposed initial needle insertion point (*see* page 111).
9. Children are generally upset by paresthesias; techniques that do not rely on eliciting these effects are preferred.
10. Supplement your regional technique with age-appropriate sedation (e.g., midazolam orally), systemic analgesics (e.g., fentanyl intravenously), and distraction (e.g., video or transistor radio and earphones).
11. The consensus of pediatric anesthesiologists is that it is acceptable standard practice to perform an epidural puncture with passage of a catheter in an anesthetized patient. Pediatric patients will not lie still to have the catheter inserted while they are awake. In pediatric patients the risks of insertion under general anesthesia are considered to be less than those in a distressed and mobile awake patient.

For more detailed descriptions of the anatomic considerations and techniques of regional nerve blocks, the reader is referred to standard textbooks.

Suggested Additional Reading

Broadman LM: Regional analgesia for the pediatric outpatient. Anesth Clin North Am 5:53, 1987.

Dalens B (ed.): Regional Analgesia in Infants, Children, and Adolescents. Williams & Wilkins, Waverley Europe, London, 1995.

Krane EJ, Dalens BJ, Murat I, and Murrell D: The safety of epidurals placed during general anesthesia [Editorial]. Reg Anesth Pain Med 23:433–438, 1998.

Raj PP: Clinical Practice of Regional Anesthesia. Churchill Livingstone, New York, 1991.

Saint-Maurice C and Schulte-Steinberg O: Regional Anaesthesia in Children. Appleton & Lange, Norwalk, CT, 1990.

Yaster M and Maxwell LG: Pediatric regional anesthesia. Anesthesiology 70:324–338, 1989.

SPINAL ANALGESIA FOR INFANTS

In infants spinal analgesia is most commonly indicated for surgery at or below the umbilicus, but it has also been used for upper abdominal surgery in small infants with a history of respiratory disease. It avoids the necessity to intubate and ventilate the patient and therefore also the risk of further airway damage or ventilator dependence. Very little change in blood pressure occurs in infants or children after spinal block. Postoperative apnea of the ex-preterm infant may be less common after spinal analgesia but has been reported.

Special Considerations

1. The spinal cord may extend to as low as L3 in the infant (compared with L1–2 in the older child or adult), so perform the lumbar puncture at L4–5.
2. The dural space extends to S3–4 in the neonate.
3. The volume of cerebrospinal fluid (CSF) is relatively higher in infants (4 ml/kg) than in adults (2 ml/kg).

Contraindications

1. Sepsis or infected lumbar puncture site.
2. Coagulopathy.
3. Lack of enthusiastic parental consent.

Anesthesia Management

Preoperative

1. The patient should be fasted as for general anesthesia.
2. No premedication is necessary for small infants.

Perioperative

1. Observe all special precautions for infants, both term and preterm. Prepare the anesthesia machine, endotracheal tubes, and so on.
2. A brandy-and-sugar soother is often useful to settle the infant. The use of more sedation (e.g., ketamine) may negate the advantages of spinal analgesia.
3. Establish a reliable intravenous infusion using local analgesia.
4. Scrub, gown, and glove.
5. Instruct your assistant to gently but firmly restrain the patient in the chosen lateral or sitting position, but avoid neck flexion, which may compromise the airway.
6. Prepare and drape the patient. Infiltrate the skin over the L4–5 interspace with 1% lidocaine.
7. Prepare a neonatal spinal needle (e.g., 22-gauge, 1 inch [26 mm] long) and measure the dead space of this needle with the use of a tuberculin syringe.
8. Prepare a syringe containing 0.4–0.6 mg/kg of 1% tetracaine mixed with an equal volume of 10% dextrose, plus a volume of this mixture equal to the dead space of the needle (approximately 0.2

ml). For upper abdominal surgery, 1 mg/kg of tetracaine has been used.

9. Insert the needle at L4–5 with the bevel facing laterally until CSF is obtained.
10. Slowly inject the local analgesic solution.
11. Turn the patient to a supine horizontal position. Motor function in lower limbs usually ceases immediately. Do not allow the patient's legs to be raised (e.g., to apply the cautery pad) or an excessively high block may result.
12. Duration of anesthesia is usually about 1.5 hours.
13. **N.B.** Total spinal anesthesia in infants is heralded by apnea with little change in blood pressure. Treat by controlled ventilation until recovery occurs.

Postoperative

1. Continue to nurse the patient in the horizontal position until motor function in the legs returns.
2. Monitor the ex-term infant carefully for apnea; it is less common than after general anesthesia but may occur.

Suggested Additional Reading

Abajian JC, Mellish RW, Browne AF, et al.: Spinal anaesthesia for surgery in the high risk infant. Anesth Analg 63:359–362, 1984.

Gerber ACH, Baitella LC, and Dangel PH: Spinal anaesthesia in former preterm infants. Paediatr Anaesth 3:153–156, 1993.

Gingrich BK: Spinal anesthesia for a former premature infant undergoing upper abdominal surgery. Anesthesiology 79:189–190, 1993.

Harnick E, Hoy GR, Potoliccchio S, et al.: Spinal anesthesia in premature infants recovering from respiratory distress syndrome. Anesthesiology 64:95–99, 1986.

CAUDAL BLOCK

The caudal block is very useful in infants and children; it provides good postoperative analgesia after abdominal, lower limb, or perineal surgery. Caudal analgesia has also been used as an alternative to spinal analgesia for lower abdominal surgery in infants. In young patients, the contents of the epidural space offer little resistance to the spread of local analgesic solutions. In this age group, epidural analgesia is accompanied by very little change in blood pressure or cardiac output. Continuous caudal catheters have been used intraoperatively for more prolonged surgery, and they may safely be threaded to a surprising distance cephalad (T6). Local infection has not been a problem when catheters were left in situ for up to 2 days.

Narcotic analgesics administered via the caudal route provide analgesia for thoracic and abdominal procedures and reduce the need for systemic analgesic drugs.

Preferred Technique

For postoperative analgesia, the block should be performed after general anesthesia has been induced but before the surgery commences. This allows for the block to become well established during surgery and offers the potential for preemptive analgesia. The child is placed in a lateral position with the upper knee well flexed. The landmarks are then identified (Fig. 5–1): the tip of the coccyx to fix the midline and the sacral cornua bounding the sacral hiatus. These lie at the apex of an inverted equilateral triangle, the base of which is a line drawn between the posterior superior iliac spine. The patient is carefully prepared and draped, and the operator wears gloves. The skin over the sacral hiatus is nicked with an 18-gauge needle, after which a 22- or 20-gauge angiocatheter (for patients younger or older than 2 years of age, respectively) is advanced cephalad at an angle of 45° to the skin with the bevel facing anteriorly. A distinctive sudden "give" is felt as the needle passes through the sacrococcygeal membrane. At this point the angle of the needle is reduced slightly as it is advanced (Fig. 5–2). The needle can then be withdrawn, leaving the intravenous catheter in the epidural space. The catheter should be observed for passive reflux of blood or CSF. If there is no evidence of blood or CSF, the local anesthetic is injected slowly while the electrocardiogram is observed. Changes in QRS pattern and/or T-wave elevation may be an early sign of intravascular injection. A finger should be placed over the sacrum to detect inadvertent subcutane-

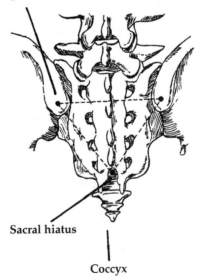

Posterior superior iliac spine

Sacral hiatus

Coccyx

Figure 5–1. Caudal block: landmarks.

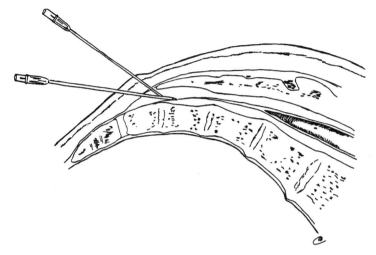

Figure 5–2. Caudal block: direction of needle insertion.

ous injection. The use of an intravenous catheter rather than a needle diminishes the risk that any movement made during injection will result in an intravascular or intraosseous administration.

Drugs, Concentrations, and Volumes

For single-shot caudal analgesia in outpatients, 0.175% bupivacaine with epinephrine provides analgesia as effective as that of 0.25% bupivacaine with less motor block. (The 0.175% bupivacaine can be prepared by adding 3 ml of preservative-free saline to 7 ml of 0.25% bupivacaine with epinephrine.) Ropivacaine 0.2% appears to provide similar analgesia and duration of action to bupivacaine and may be less cardiotoxic.

The addition of clonidine (1–2 µg/kg) to bupivacaine extends its duration of action significantly. Other drugs that have been used to enhance caudal analgesia include midazolam and ketamine; however, suitable approved preparations are not currently available.

The following are volumes to be injected via the caudal route:

Perineal surgery (e.g., hypospadias repair): 0.5 ml/kg
Lower abdominal surgery (e.g., orchidopexy): 1.0 ml/kg
Upper abdominal surgery (e.g., pyloromyotomy): 1.25 ml/kg

Caudal Morphine. Caudal morphine in a dose of 75–100 µg/kg, diluted in preservative-free saline to a volume of 0.5 ml/kg and administered as a single shot preoperatively, provides analgesia for up to 24 hours and reduces the need for other analgesic drugs.

Suggested Additional Reading

Gunter JB, Dunn CM, Bennie JB, et al.: Optimum concentration of bupivacaine for combined caudal-general anesthesia in children Anesthesiology 75:57–61, 1991.

Ivani G, De Negro P, and Conio A: Paediatric regional analgesia for surgical procedures: a guide to drug choice. CNS Drugs 12:357–368, 1999.

Ivani G, Lampugnani E, and Torr MA: Comparison of ropivacaine with bupivacaine for paediatric caudal block. Br J Anaesth 81:247–248, 1998.

Jamali S, Monin S, Begon C, et al.: Clonidine in pediatric caudal anesthesia. Anesth Analg 78:663–666, 1994.

Krane EJ, Tyler DC, Jacobson LE: The dose response of caudal morphine in children. Anesthesiology 71:48–52, 1989.

Payen D, Ecoffey C, Carli P, and Dubosset A: Pulsed Doppler ascending aortic, carotid, brachial, and femoral artery blood flows during caudal analgesia in infants. Anesthesiology 67:681, 1987.

Single-Shot Caudal Analgesia for Lower Abdominal Surgery in Small Infants

As an alternative to spinal analgesia, 1 ml/kg of a 0.375% or 1–1.25 ml of a 0.25% solution of bupivacaine produces very effective analgesia plus a motor block lasting up to 90 minutes. In small patients, a caudal block can be readily performed while an assistant supports the infant over a shoulder ("burping" position). The dose of bupivacaine given when these techniques are used may reach 3.75 mg/kg, but has been considered acceptable because of the larger volume of distribution of the drug in the very small infant and has proven safe in practice.

Suggested Additional Reading

Gunter JB, Watcha MF, Watcha JE, et al.: Caudal epidural anesthesia in conscious premature and high risk infants. J Pediatr Surg 26:9–14, 1991.

Spear RM, Despande JK, and Maxwell LG: Caudal anesthesia in the awake, high risk infant. Anesthesiology 69:407–409, 1988.

Continuous Caudal Analgesia

In neonates and small infants, prolonged intraoperative and postoperative analgesia can be provided by means of continuous caudal block. With the use of careful aseptic precautions, a 20-gauge catheter may be threaded through an 18-gauge cannula and advanced to the desired level. In most infants it is possible to pass the catheter to the thoracic level. If resistance is felt and is not relieved by slight flexion or extension of the patient's spine, no attempt should be made to advance the catheter further. A transparent occlusive dressing should be applied to the puncture site, which should be regularly inspected.

A continuous infusion of bupivacaine may be given at a rate of 0.1–0.3 ml/kg/hr in a concentration that is calculated to deliver a safe dose.

The maximum safe dose range for epidural bupivacaine is 0.15–0.2 mg/kg/hr in neonates and 0.2–0.3 mg/kg/hr in infants.

Neonates and small infants metabolize bupivacaine less rapidly; hence the blood level of the drug may increase dangerously during a continuous infusion unless it is infused at an appropriately slow rate. Be very cautious if the infusion is continued for longer than 36 hours.

Some centers are using continuous infusions of lidocaine for continuous epidural analgesia. This technique has the advantage that blood levels of lidocaine can easily be monitored in a routine laboratory and toxic levels avoided.

Suggested Additional Reading

Bosenberg AT, Bland BAR, Schulte-Steinberg O, and Downing JW: Thoracic epidural analgesia via the caudal route in infants and children. Anesthesiology 69:265, 1988.

Luz G, Innerhofer P, Bachmann B, et al.: Bupivacaine concentrations during continuous epidural anesthesia in infants and children. Anesth Analg 82:231–234, 1996.

Peutrell JM, Holder K, and Gregory M: Plasma bupivacaine concentrations associated with continuous extradural infusions in babies. Br J Anaesth 78:160–162, 1997.

EPIDURAL BLOCKS

Lumbar epidural block has been widely used for postoperative pain relief in children and occasionally for surgery in older patients with special indications. The technique used is similar to that for adults; the "loss of resistance method" using saline is recommended to identify the epidural space. Air should not be used to test for loss of resistance, because this procedure has been associated with increased complications in children.

Thoracic epidural block may be performed in children using a technique similar to that used in adults. A midline approach is preferred, and the needle must be advanced at an angle determined by the configuration of the vertebral spine at the level selected. (Examination of the lateral chest radiograph is helpful before performing this block.)

Special Considerations

In children weighing more than 10 kg, the distance from skin to lumbar epidural space in millimeters is approximately numerically similar to the child's weight in kilograms (i.e., the distance in a 20-kg child is about 20 mm).

A 19-gauge Tuohy needle and a 21-gauge catheter are usually used in children younger than 5 years of age. In older children, an 18-gauge Tuohy needle and a 20-gauge epidural catheter are used.

Dose requirements for local analgesic solutions are less predictable when the lumbar (or thoracic) route is used, as opposed to the caudal route.

Epidural block is associated with little change in hemodynamic parameters.

Initial Volume to be Injected

Bupivacaine 0.25% with 1:200,000 epinephrine is used in a dose of 0.5 ml/kg (0.75 ml/kg for infants), supplemented with a dose of 0.2 ml/kg to achieve the level of block required.

For surgery, bupivacaine 0.5% may be required to achieve motor block.

Continuous Infusion Epidural Analgesia

A solution of 0.1%–0.125% bupivacaine is usually used, to which fentanyl (0.5–2 μg/ml) may be added. The infusion may be administered at a rate of 0.1 to 0.3 ml/kg/hr and adjusted to provide optimal analgesia. The maximum rate of bupivacaine administration should not exceed 0.4–0.5 mg/kg/hr in children.

Beware of toxic effects of local analgesics when children are receiving continuous infusions, especially when the infusion is continued for longer than 48 hours. Recognize that children may not report the early symptoms of tinnitus, lightheadedness, and visual effects. Some authorities consider that intermittent "top-up" doses are safer than continuous infusions in young children.

The narcotic analgesics morphine and fentanyl have been used to provide epidural analgesia without motor block. For children, morphine may be given in a loading dose of 75 μg/kg (to a maximum of 3 mg), followed by a daily bolus of a similar dose. Fentanyl may be administered in an initial dose of 2 μg/kg (maximum, 100 μg), followed by an infusion of 5 μg/kg/day (maximum, 300 μg/day). Both regimens result in similar analgesia, but the side effects of nausea, vomiting, and pruritus are less frequent with fentanyl. Patients receiving extradural narcotics should be monitored for ventilatory depression during and for 24 hours after therapy. Urinary retention may be more common in children than in adults.

Suggested Additional Reading

Berde CB: Convulsions associated with pediatric regional anesthesia. Anesth Analg 75:164–166, 1992.

Dalens B, Tanguy A, and Haberer JP: Lumbar epidural analgesia for operative and postoperative pain relief in infants and young children. Anesth Analg 65:1069, 1986.

Ecoffey C, Dubosset AM, and Samii K: Lumbar and thoracic epidural anesthesia for urologic and upper abdominal surgery in infants and children. Anesthesiology 65:87, 1986.

Lejus C, Roussiere G, Testa S, et al.: Postoperative extradural analgesia in children: comparison of morphine with fentanyl. Br J Anaesth 72:156–159, 1994.

Uemura A and Yamashita M: A formula for determining the distance from the skin to the lumbar epidural space in infants and children. Paediatr Anaesth 2:305–307, 1992.

INTERCOSTAL NERVE BLOCK

Intercostal nerve blocks may be performed to relieve pain after thoracotomy or some upper abdominal procedures. For example, a bilateral T10 block provides good pain relief after umbilical hernia repair.

Special Considerations

1. Systemic absorption of local analgesics from the very vascular intercostal space can be extremely rapid, with a commensurate risk of toxic effects; take care not to exceed a total dose of 2 mg/kg of bupivacaine.
2. The risk of pneumothorax is high, especially in small children, in whom the distance from nerve to pleura is very small.
3. The intercostal nerves are sheathed in a dural layer posteriorly; injection near their origin can result in a total spinal block.

Preferred Technique

In infants and small children, the nerve in the intercostal space can be more precisely approached by angling the needle posteromedially, so that it lies almost parallel to the rib, rather than at right angles to it (Fig. 5–3).

Suggested Additional Reading

Rothstein P, Arthur GR, Feldman HS, et al.: Bupivacaine for intercostal nerve blocks in children: blood concentrations and pharmacokinetics. Anesth Analg 65:625–632, 1986.

Shelley MP: Intercostal nerve blockade for children. Anaesthesia 42:591–592, 1987.

ILIOINGUINAL AND ILIOHYPOGASTRIC NERVE BLOCK

The ilioinguinal and iliohypogastric nerve block provides skin analgesia over the inguinal region and is useful for providing postoperative analgesia after herniotomy. The block should preferably be performed immediately after induction of general anesthesia, before the operation commences. The nerves run beneath the internal oblique muscle just medial to the anterior superior iliac spine and may be blocked by a fan-shaped infiltration of the abdominal wall in this region (Fig. 5–4). Bupivacaine 0.25% or 0.5% (up to 2 mg/kg) may be used; more complete analgesia may be obtained with the use of the 0.5% solution, but very occasionally this concentration produces a transient motor block of the femoral nerve, with leg weakness.

Posterior

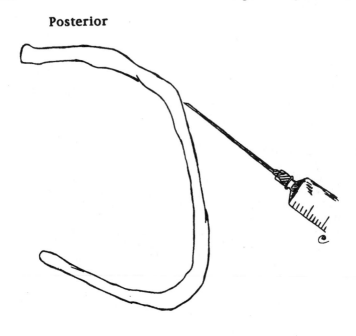

Anterior

Figure 5–3. Intercostal nerve block: direction of needle insertion in relation to rib.

Suggested Additional Reading

Hannallah RS, Broadman LM, Bellman AB, et al.: Comparison of caudal and ilioinguinal/iliohypogastric blocks for control of post orchidopexy pain in pediatric ambulatory surgery. Anesthesiology 66:832–834, 1987.

Shandling B and Steward DJ: Regional analgesia for postoperative pain in pediatric outpatient surgery. J Pediatr Surg 15:477–480, 1980.

PENILE BLOCK

The paired dorsal nerves pass inferior to the pubic bones on either side of the midline and supply the dorsal aspect of the penis and foreskin. A block of these nerves provides good pain relief after circumcision but does not provide adequate analgesia after hypospadias repair. Epinephrine-containing solutions should not be used, because vasoconstriction might result in damaging ischemia. Complications have been very rare after properly performed penile block; however, it has been suggested that a subcutaneous ring block at the base of the penis is safer.

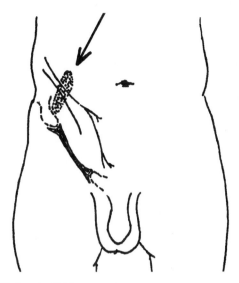

Figure 5–4. Iliolinguinal-iliohypogastric nerve block: area to be infiltrated with local anesthetic solution.

Volume to be Injected

Up to 2 mg/kg of 0.5% bupivacaine without epinephrine is injected, to a maximum volume of 1 ml in the small infant or 6 ml in the large child.

Preferred Technique

With careful aseptic technique, bilateral injections are made beneath the pubis at the base of the penis at the 11 o'clock and 1 o'clock positions (Fig. 5–5). The needle should be felt to pass through Buck's fascia to deposit an equal volume adjacent to each nerve. Alternatively, a ring block at the base of the penis may be performed (Fig. 5–6).

Suggested Additional Reading

Broadman LM, Hannallah RS, Belman AB, et al.: Post circumcision analgesia: a prospective evaluation of subcutaneous ring block of the penis. Anesthesiology 67:399–402, 1987.

Soliman MG and Tremblay NA: Nerve block of the penis for postoperative pain relief in children. Anesth Analg 57:495–498, 1978.

HEAD AND NECK AND UPPER LIMB BLOCKS

Infraorbital Nerve Block

The infraorbital nerve block is simple to perform and provides good analgesia for infants and children after cleft lip repairs.

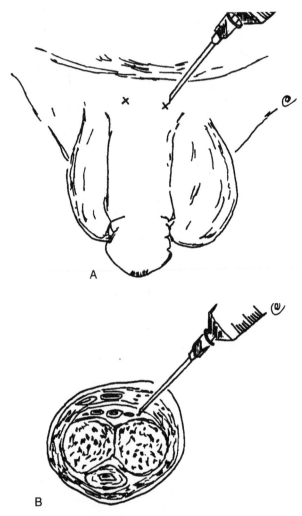

Figure 5–5. Block of the dorsal nerves of the penis. **(A)** Injection sites. **(B)** Position of nerves at base of penis.

In adults and older children, the site of the infraorbital foramen can be palpated 1–1.5 cm below the infraorbital rim in line with the supraorbital notch and the pupil. A needle can be inserted at this point and 1–1.5 ml of local analgesic injected.

In infants the foramen cannot be palpated, and its position must be estimated by using the following landmarks: The infraorbital nerve has been demonstrated to lie approximately under the midpoint of a line

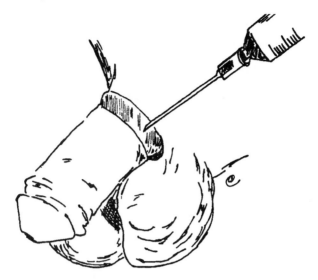

Figure 5–6. Ring block of the penis.

drawn between the middle of the palpebral fissure and the angle of the mouth.

Preferred Technique

Once the estimated position of the infraorbital foramen has been identified, a needle is passed vertically through the skin and gently advanced until bony resistance is felt. The needle is then withdrawn very slightly, an aspiration test is performed, and 1 ml of 0.25% bupivacaine with epinephrine is injected.

Suggested Additional Reading

Bosenberg AT and Kimble FW: Infraorbital nerve block in neonates for cleft lip repair: anatomical study and clinical application. Br J Anaesth 74:506–508, 1995.

Brachial Plexus Block

Axillary Approach

The axillary approach is recommended because of its simplicity and lack of serious complications (e.g., pneumothorax); it is easy to perform if the patient can abduct the arm and is further simplified by placing the hand behind the head. It is useful for forearm fractures, plastic surgery procedures, and insertion of shunts for dialysis, but the block does not include the area of the upper arm and sometimes not the area supplied by musculocutaneous nerves.

Preferred Technique

With careful asepsis, after skin analgesia, a 1 inch long, 25-gauge small-vein needle is advanced cephalad, at a 45° angle to skin, alongside and parallel to the axillary artery (Fig. 5–7). A slight "give" or "pop" should be felt as the neurovascular sheath is entered, and the arterial pulsations will be seen rocking the needle. The needle is supported gently, the plastic extension is connected to the syringe, and after aspiration the drug is carefully injected, with periodic aspiration. Pressure distally over the axillary artery may encourage proximal spread of the local analgesic solution and a more complete block.

Volume to be Injected

Use 0.3–0.5 ml/kg of 1% lidocaine with 1:200,000 epinephrine or 0.5 ml/kg of 0.25% bupivacaine. For the older child, a maximum volume of 20 ml is usually satisfactory.

Interscalene Approach

The interscalene approach may also be used in children and provides additional analgesia of the shoulder and upper arm. Paresthesias are usually felt; they are most useful to aid the correct placement of the needle but may upset the child. Possible complications with this route include block of the phrenic or recurrent laryngeal nerve, stellate ganglion block (Horner syndrome), total spinal block, and pneumothorax.

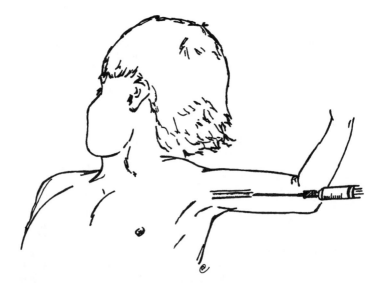

Figure 5–7. Brachial plexus block, axillary route: direction of needle in relation to artery.

Preferred Technique

The interscalene groove is palpated at the level of the cricoid (C6). In thin patients, the trunks of the plexus at this level can often be palpated through the skin as tight cords if the head is turned to the opposite side and slight downward traction is exerted on the arm to be blocked. After suitable skin preparation and analgesia, a 22-gauge needle is advanced perpendicularly into the groove until paresthesias are obtained in the elbow or hand. Injection of bupivacaine must be preceded by careful aspiration for blood or CSF.

Volume to be Injected

Use 0.25 ml/kg of bupivacaine 0.25% with 1:200,000 epinephrine.

LOWER LIMB BLOCKS

Femoral Nerve Block

The femoral nerve block is useful for fractures of the shaft of the femur and for muscle biopsy in patients with suspected myopathy (in which case it should be combined with a lateral femoral cutaneous nerve block).

For patients with fracture of the femur, a continuous femoral nerve block may give very good continuing analgesia and also relieves the muscle spasm in the thigh.

Preferred Technique

The femoral artery is identified by palpation just below the inguinal ligament. After skin analgesia has been established, a 1-inch-long, 21-gauge small-vein needle is advanced slowly just lateral to the artery at an angle of 45° to skin (Fig. 5–8). Slight resistance should be felt at two separate levels, the fascia lata and the fascia iliaca, after which the needle lies within the femoral canal. The needle should then be gently supported, aspirated, and injected, with periodic aspiration.

Volume to Be Injected

Use 0.3 ml/kg of 1% lidocaine with 1:200,000 epinephrine or 0.5% bupivacaine.

Continuous Femoral Nerve Block

With careful asepsis, after skin analgesia, a Tuohy needle with obturator is advanced, as outlined previously, through the two identified layers of resistance. The needle is positioned with the opening facing cephalad, and a standard epidural catheter is advanced proximally for 5–10 cm within the femoral sheath. When the Tuohy needle is correctly placed, the catheter should advance very easily with very little resistance. The Tuohy needle can then be withdrawn and the catheter left in situ, as

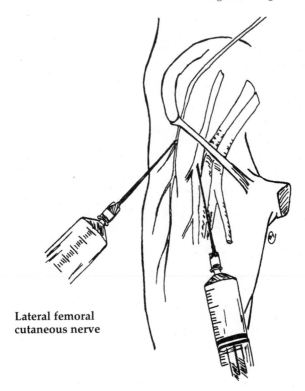

Lateral femoral cutaneous nerve

Femoral nerve

Figure 5–8. Femoral nerve block and block of the lateral femoral cutaneous nerve of the thigh.

when inserting an epidural catheter. *Never attempt to withdraw the catheter through the needle, because the tip may be sheared off and remain in the patient.*

Volume to be Injected

Intermittent top-up doses of bupivacaine 0.25% (0.4 ml/kg) may be given every 8–12 hours as required, or a continuous infusion may be used at a rate of 0.1 ml/kg/hr.

Lateral Femoral Cutaneous Nerve Block

Block of the lateral femoral cutaneous nerve provides analgesia over the lateral aspect of the thigh.

Preferred Technique

The needle is inserted medial and inferior to the anterior superior iliac spine, just superior to the inguinal ligament, and advanced superiorly and laterally until it impinges on the iliac bone (*see* Fig. 5–8). The local analgesic solution is injected as the needle is slowly withdrawn.

Volume to be Injected

Use 2–5 ml of 1% lidocaine with 1:200,000 epinephrine or 0.5% bupivacaine.

Intravenous Regional Analgesia

The Bier block may be useful in older children having excision of lesions on either of the limbs (e.g., ganglion). Intravenous blocks are not generally suitable for reduction of fractures, because it is difficult to apply an optimally tight cast to an ischemic limb.

Preferred Technique

Insert a small intravenous cannula in the hand or foot. Use a reliable double pneumatic tourniquet. The success of the block varies with the degree of limb exsanguination, which can be achieved before injection of the local analgesic; use an elastic bandage or air splint if possible. Inflate the proximal cuff and inject the local analgesic solution. Do not exceed 5 mg/kg of 0.25% lidocaine or 3 mg/kg of prilocaine. *Bupivacaine should never be used for an intravenous block.* When the block is established (5 minutes), inflate the distal cuff and then deflate the proximal cuff. Do not release the remaining cuff until at least 30 minutes has elapsed, even if the operation is finished sooner.

Suggested Additional Reading

Fleming SA, Veiga-Pires JA, McCutcheon RM, and Emanuel CI: A demonstration of the site of action of intravenous lignocaine. Can Anaesth Soc J 13:21, 1966.

Rose RJ: Use of an air splint to provide limb exsanguination during intravenous regional anaesthesia in children. Reg Analg 12:8, 1987.

Chapter **6**

Medical Conditions Influencing Anesthesia Management

UPPER RESPIRATORY TRACT INFECTION

Pediatric patients often have or are recovering from a runny nose or other manifestations of upper respiratory tract infection (URTI) when they are seen for evaluation before general anesthesia. Indiscriminate cancellation of children with any symptom of URTI causes emotional and financial problems for patients and their families; each case needs to be carefully considered. Some children seem to have a runny nose most of the time, possibly because of allergies or a chronic nasal infection; these children should be distinguished from those with an acute URTI.

Algorithm for Management of Upper Respiratory Tract Infection

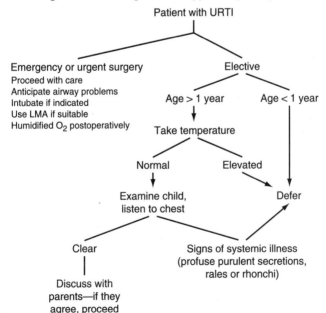

Several studies have suggested that patients with an uncomplicated URTI who are otherwise well do not have a higher incidence of serious perioperative problems after *minor* surgery performed under general anesthesia. They may have an increased incidence of intraoperative desaturation, which is usually easily treated, and desaturation may occur more rapidly in patients with URTI if they become apneic. Infants younger than 1 year of age with a URTI may have more serious complications (especially airway problems) during and after anesthesia. Pulmonary complications in patients having *major* surgery may be more common if there is a recent (within 2 weeks) history of URTI. This may result from the fact that viral infections alter the reactivity of the airway for such a period and may also predispose to other infections.

The following plan of action is suggested:

1. **Emergency or urgent surgery:** These patients must be accepted for general anesthesia for the needed procedure. No special modifications to the anesthesia technique should be made (e.g., endotracheal intubation should be performed for the usual indications), but make sure that gases are warmed and humidified. Sevoflurane has been found to be an acceptable agent in children with mild URTI. Airway problems and laryngospasm must be anticipated, and all necessities for their treatment should be immediately at hand. When suitable, the laryngeal mask airway (LMA) should be used as an alternative to intubation; it may result in fewer airway complications. The patient should be carefully observed postoperatively.

2. **Elective surgery**

   a. The patient should be carefully assessed. A history of the URTI should be obtained along with a detailed history of any other illnesses. A careful physical examination should be performed, looking particularly for any evidence of systemic illness, purulent nasal secretions, or lower respiratory tract disease.

   b. Patients with mild URTI but without pyrexia or any other evidence of disease may be accepted for needed minor surgical procedures, because studies indicate little increased risk of complications. (However, surgery for infants younger than 1 year of age should be deferred if possible.) The decision to proceed should be discussed with the parents, and due consideration should be given to their feelings in the matter. Be prepared to deal rapidly and effectively with any airway problems or desaturation that occurs.

   c. Surgery for patients with URTI who have pyrexia or evidence of lower respiratory tract disease or other disease and those having major surgery should be deferred for 3–4 weeks if possible.

   d. Patients who are in the recovery phase of a URTI, especially if there was also lower respiratory tract involvement (e.g., cough, wheezing) should have major surgery deferred for 2–3 weeks if possible.

Suggested Additional Reading

Cohen MM and Cameron CB: Should you cancel the operation when the child has an upper respiratory tract infection? Anesth Analg 72:282–288, 1991.

Kinouchi K, Tanigami H, Tashiro C, et al.: Duration of apnea in anesthetised infants and children required for desaturation of hemoglobin to 95%: the influence of upper respiratory infection. Anesthesiology 77:1105–1107, 1992.

Liu LMP, Ryan JF, Cote CJ, and Goudsouzian NG: Influence of upper respiratory infections on critical incidents in children during anesthesia. Abstracts of the 9th World Congress of Anaesthesia, 1988, p A0786.

Mcleod ME and Roy L: Anaesthesia and upper respiratory tract infection in the paediatric patient. Can Anaesth Soc J 30:S86, 1983.

Nandwani N, Raphael JH, and Langton JA: Effect of an upper respiratory infection on upper airway reactivity. Br J Anaesth 78:352–355, 1997.

Rieger A, Schroter G, Philippi W, et al.: A comparison of sevoflurane with halothane in outpatient adenotomy in children with mild upper respiratory tract infections. J Clin Anesth 8:188–197, 1996.

Rolf N and Cote CJ: Frequency and severity of desaturation events during general anesthesia in children with and without upper respiratory infections. J Clin Anesth 4:200–203, 1992.

Tait AR, Pandit UA, Voepel-Lewis T, et al.: Cancellation of pediatric outpatient surgery: Economic and emotional implications for patients and their families. J Clin Anesthesia 9:213–219, 1997.

Tait AR, Pandit UA, Voepel-Lewis T, et al.: Use of the laryngeal mask airway in children with upper respiratory tract infections: a comparison with endotracheal intubation. Anesth Analg 86:706–711, 1998.

ASTHMA

Asthma affects 4%–13% of the pediatric population in various parts of North America. The disease is characterized by variable cough, wheezing, and breathlessness and is episodic and seasonal in many patients. The symptoms result from bronchoconstriction, mucosal edema, and tenacious secretions in the small airways. Severe attacks may occur throughout childhood and may be life-threatening. Acute exacerbations may be associated with URTIs, allergens, irritants, exercise, or emotional stress. The usual treatment is with inhaled β-adrenergics for bronchodilation and to improve mucociliary clearance, and inhaled corticosteroids to control the inflammatory aspects of the disease. Theophylline is sometimes used to prevent nocturnal bronchospasm. Severe asthmatic attacks may require systemic corticosteroid therapy. The disease often improves as the child grows older.

When a child with asthma presents for elective surgery, it is most important to determine whether the child's current status is optimal. The following are important considerations.

1. If possible, surgery should be delayed for at least 1 month after the last acute attack; during this period, airway reactivity may be increased and residual mucosal edema and secretions may impair pulmonary function.
2. Elective surgery should be deferred if there is any evidence of an active viral URTI. A URTI can be predicted to precipitate an exacerbation of symptoms.
3. How often does the child have attacks, and what symptoms are there between attacks? Has admission to an intensive care unit or

ventilator therapy ever been needed? If so, repeat severe attacks are likely.

4. What medications is the child taking, and are they controlling the child's symptoms? Have systemic corticosteroids been necessary? If so, in what dose? If the child is receiving theophylline therapy, the blood level of the drug should be measured preoperatively.
5. Physical examination of the chest is important to detect bronchospasm and exclude any other current pulmonary pathology. If wheezing is present, elective surgery should be deferred.
6. The results of recent pulmonary function tests and especially any response to bronchodilator therapy should be noted.
7. A chest radiograph should be ordered for any child with significant symptoms. If there is any concern that the child is in other than optimal condition, discussion with the surgeon and pediatrician should be directed toward delaying elective surgery and improving the patient's status.

Anesthesia Management

Preoperative

1. Ensure that the child receives routine medications up to the time of surgery. Oral medications can be taken with a sip of water; inhalations may be repeated, if necessary, just before transfer to the operating room.
2. Order appropriate steroid therapy for those with a history of extensive or recent steroid therapy. An intravenous infusion of hydrocortisone may be commenced 1 hour before surgery.
3. Order appropriate sedation to calm the child. Oral midazolam is preferred, but some have advocated the use of promethazine in asthmatics. Atropine, if considered necessary, may be given orally or intravenously at induction; it decreases secretions and causes some bronchodilation.

Perioperative

1. For intravenous induction, thiopental is reported to release histamine and possibly to cause bronchoconstriction; propofol is a better choice. Alternatively, ketamine may be used; ketamine is a bronchodilator and may protect against bronchospasm.
2. Inhalation induction with sevoflurane is preferred. Halothane may be used, but beware of arrhythmias in patients receiving theophylline therapy.
3. Avoid agents known to release histamine and cause bronchospasm (e.g., atracurium, mivacurium, rapacuronium, morphine). Nitrous oxide, halothane, sevoflurane, isoflurane, fentanyl, pancuronium, and vecuronium are considered the drugs of choice.
4. Intubation, if necessary, should be performed gently while the patient is deeply anesthetized; otherwise, the procedure may trigger bronchospasm. Alternatively, lidocaine 1.5 mg/kg IV may be

administered 3–4 minutes before intubation. If possible, avoid intubation for minor or short procedures. The LMA may be a very useful alternative.
5. Anesthetic gases should be warmed and humidified.
6. Intraoperative wheezing may be treated by deepening the anesthesia and by giving bronchodilator aerosols via the endotracheal tube (e.g., albuterol). Be careful to exclude nonasthmatic causes for wheezing (e.g., a partially obstructed endotracheal tube).
7. At the end of the operation, atropine and neostigmine may be administered to reverse relaxant drugs as necessary. Neostigmine may increase bronchomotor tone, but this effect is counteracted by the atropine. Extubation is preferably performed with the patient still anesthetized to minimize the risk of precipitating bronchospasm. If awake extubation is indicated, intravenous lidocaine should be administered beforehand.

Postoperative

1. Humidified oxygen should be administered.
2. When practical, regional analgesia is ideal for pain relief; for major surgery, continuous regional analgesia may be planned. Otherwise, use intravenous fentanyl or meperidine in repeated doses or via patient-controlled analgesia (PCA) (*see* page 194).
3. Postoperative wheezing may call for additional doses of an aerosol bronchodilator and appropriate adjustment of other medications.

If a child with severe symptoms of asthma requires emergency surgery, every effort should be made to improve the bronchospasm before inducing anesthesia. The anesthesia technique should then be designed to serve the surgery and also to provide therapy for the chest. Ketamine, pancuronium, and halothane are the preferred agents. Obtain a preoperative chest radiograph, and beware of the possibility of pneumothorax or atelectasis.

Suggested Additional Reading

Kingston HGG and Hirshman CA: Perioperative management of the patient with asthma. Anesth Analg 63:844–855, 1984.

Lerman J: Allergic diseases. In Katz J and Steward DJ (eds.): Anesthesia and Uncommon Pediatric Diseases, 2nd ed. WB Saunders, Philadelphia, 1993, pp 613–628.

Pizov R, Brown RH, Weiss YS, et al.: Wheezing during induction of general anesthesia in patients with and without asthma. Anesthesiology 82:1111–1116, 1995.

CYSTIC FIBROSIS

Cystic fibrosis (CF) is a heritable disorder of unknown pathogenesis. It affects many body systems, including the lungs. Respiratory failure develops by the second or third decade of life. Even if they appear fairly well, all of these patients have severe pulmonary ventilation-perfusion ($\dot{V}/\dot{Q}$) inequality.

Surgery for children with this condition is most commonly nasal polypectomy (in many cases repeated), antral lavage, or bronchoscopy for removal of retained secretions and treatment of atelectasis. Some children with advanced disease may present for lung transplantation. Transplanted lungs do not appear to be affected by this otherwise generalized disease.

Special Anesthesia Problems

1. Copious, extremely viscous secretions are present in the respiratory tract. Violent coughing may occur during induction.
2. Because of the $\dot{V}/\dot{Q}$ disturbances:
   a. Hypoxia may develop rapidly during anesthesia.
   b. Induction of anesthesia with inhalational agents is prolonged.
   c. There is reduced lung compliance. In severe late cases, very high airway pressure may be required to provide adequate ventilation and prevent hypoxemia. Therefore, a cuffed endotracheal tube should be used.
4. Malnutrition and underweight for age is a result of malabsorption and chronic infection. Drug dosages should be carefully reduced accordingly.
5. Many children with advanced CF become severely emotionally upset. All of them require very careful and considerate handling and much reassurance.

Anesthesia Management

Preoperative

1. Assess the patient's condition carefully; ensure that the pulmonary status is optimized before surgery by means of physiotherapy, inhalations, and so on.
2. Pulmonary function is usually at its worst first thing in the morning. If possible, arrange for the surgery to be scheduled at a time that allows for chest physiotherapy and clearing of secretions preoperatively.
3. Do not give narcotic premedication. Give midazolam if indicated to counter anxiety.
4. Ensure optimal hydration; fluids must not be withheld for long periods. The patient should be offered clear fluids until 2 hours preoperatively.

Perioperative

N.B. Whenever possible, use local or regional analgesia.

1. Establish an intravenous line for hydration and emergency drug administration.

If general anesthesia is required:

2. Give 100% O_2 by mask for at least 5 minutes; then induce anesthesia intravenously with thiopental and a relaxant drug.
3. Intubate the patient using a cuffed endotracheal tube.
4. Suction the trachea and remove secretions as often as necessary.
5. Use humidified gases with sufficient oxygen added (100% O_2 may be necessary for patients with severe disease).
6. Do not give long-acting agents; use a technique that ensures the patient's early awakening postoperatively.

Postoperative

1. Give fluids intravenously until the patient is drinking well.
2. Nurse the patient with humidified oxygen.
3. Provide optimal analgesia. Use regional analgesia for postoperative pain whenever possible.
4. Encourage early chest physiotherapy.

Suggested Additional Reading

Di Sant'Agnese PA and Talamo RC: Pathogenesis and physiopathology of cystic fibrosis of the pancreas: fibrocystic disease of the pancreas (mucoviscidosis). N Engl J Med 277:1287, 1344, 1399, 1967.

Lamberty JM and Rubin BK: The management of anaesthesia for patients with cystic fibrosis. Anaesthesia 40:448, 1985.

Robinson DA and Branthwaite MA: Pleural surgery in patients with cystic fibrosis. Anaesthesia 39:655–659, 1984.

HEMATOLOGIC DISORDERS

Anemia

Children requiring surgery may be anemic. Remember that the hemoglobin (Hb) level, normally 18–20 g/dl at birth, falls to a low of about 10–11 g/dl by 3 months of age and thereafter climbs gradually to 14 g/dl by 6 years of age (Table 6–1).

In the preterm infant, the Hb often falls to lower levels because of a low red blood cell mass at birth, short survival time of fetal red blood

Table 6–1. Normal Average Hemoglobin Levels in Infants and Children

Age	Hemoglobin (g/dl)	Hematocrit
Newborn	19.5	0.54
1 week	18.3	0.52
1 mo	14.0	0.42
3 mo	12.0	0.36
1 yr	11.2	0.35
3 yr	12.5	0.36
10 yr	12.9	0.37

cells, and poor erythropoietin response. Frequent blood sampling compounds this anemia. In children, Hb levels below normal for age are most frequently caused by poor diet. Anemia discovered before elective surgery should be fully investigated and adequately treated before the operation is scheduled. Traditionally, elective surgery has been postponed if the Hb is less than 10 g/dl, but in each case the whole clinical situation must be fully considered before the decision is made. Many children with a Hb level of 8 or 9 g/dl can be safely anesthetized provided no further blood loss takes place. If, however, the Hb is lower than 7 g/dl, the physiologic consequences of anemia may significantly compromise the margin of safety during anesthesia. Anemic preterm infants are at greater risk for perioperative apnea.

The following considerations are relevant for patients with anemia:

1. Transport of oxygen to the tissues can be maintained only by increased cardiac output or increased oxygen extraction from the blood. The major compensation is the increase in cardiac output; shift of the $Hb-O_2$ dissociation curve, caused by increased 2,3-diphosphoglycerate (2,3-DPG), contributes relatively little. At an Hb level less than about 8 g/dl, the cardiac output must increase to compensate for the decreased oxygen-carrying capacity of the blood.
2. Coronary sinus blood is normally very desaturated; therefore, in anemia, oxygen transport to the heart muscle can be maintained only by increased coronary blood flow. At Hb levels lower than 5 g/dl, the ability of the myocardium to meet its own needs is compromised and congestive cardiac failure may occur.
3. Anemic patients may be at increased risk for cardiac arrest during anesthesia. The factual data to support this hypothesis are scant, but it seems reasonable to suppose that patients with severe anemia have a reduced margin of safety.
4. Patients with significant cardiac or respiratory disease require a higher Hb level than normal children: 14 g/dl should be considered the minimum acceptable, and some patients need higher levels (*see* page 118).
5. Preterm infants who are anemic are more prone to apnea.

The following plan of action is suggested for routine elective surgery:

1. If a significant anemia is discovered, delay surgery until the anemia has been diagnosed and treated. In patients with iron-deficiency anemia, the Hb level increases significantly after 3–4 weeks of oral iron therapy.
2. If surgery should not be delayed, a decision must be made whether to proceed despite the anemic state or to transfuse packed cells to correct severe anemia. This decision depends on many factors, such as the age and health of the child, the expected surgical blood loss, and so on.
3. For the anemic patient, use an anesthetic technique that is optimal for the anemic state:
   a. Avoid excessive preoperative sedation.
   b. Oxygenate the patient before induction.

   c. Use high concentrations of inspired oxygen during anesthesia.
   d. Always use an endotracheal tube.
   e. Use controlled ventilation and maintain normocapnia.
   f. Be cautious with myocardial depressant drugs, although halothane has been suggested to be advantageous because it also decreases myocardial oxygen demand.
   g. Carefully replace fluids to maintain the intravascular volume; hypovolemia must be avoided if the cardiac output is to be maintained.
   h. Do not extubate until the patient is fully awake.
   i. Give additional oxygen continuously during transportation to and in the postanesthesia care unit (PACU).
   j. Keep the patient warm throughout!

Suggested Additional Reading

Allen JB and Allen RB: The minimum acceptable level of hemoglobin. Int Anesth Clin 20:1–22, 1982.

Barrera M, Miletich DJ, Albrecht RF, and Hoffman WE: Hemodynamic consequences of halothane anesthesia during chronic anemia. Anesthesiology 61:36–42, 1984.

Blanchette VS and Zipursky A: Assessment of anemia in newborn infants. Clin Perinatol 11:489–510, 1984.

Cropp G: Cardiovascular function in children with severe anemia. Circulation 39:775, 1969.

Gillies IDS: Anaemia and anaesthesia. Br J Anaesth 46:589, 1974.

Herbert W and Hammond D: Preoperative evaluation of the anemic child. Am Surg 29:660–666, 1963.

Strauss RG: Current issues in neonatal transfusions. Vox Sang 51:1–9, 1986.

Sickle Cell States

In sickle cell conditions, an abnormal Hb is present. Sickle cell hemoglobin (HbS) forms a gel when deoxygenated, distorting the erythrocytes; these then occlude vessels, causing infarction. In addition, the erythrocyte life span is reduced and there is increased hemolysis with consequent anemia and increased bilirubin level. The course of the disease is one of many crises: sickling, hemolytic, or aplastic. Sickling crises result in ischemic pain, hemolytic crises result in further anemia, and aplastic crises may cause death. The disease is mainly confined to persons of African descent. The anesthesiologist may meet these patients when they require a surgical procedure or when they are experiencing a painful crisis and require analgesia.

Sickle cell disease may become evident during infancy as HbS replaces fetal hemoglobin (HbF); the latter offers some protection against sickling.

The severity of the disease depends on the percentage of HbS present and the presence or absence of other abnormal forms of Hb.

1. Sickle cell trait (mild form): low concentration of HbS (less than 50%). Sickling is unlikely to occur without very severe hypoxemia.

This form is unlikely to give rise to serious problems during anesthesia. The incidence of sickle cell trait is approximately 8% in the black population.

2. Sickle cell disease (severe form): high concentration of HbS (more than 75%). This may cause serious complications during anesthesia and surgery. Sickle cell disease occurs in 0.16%–1.3% of the black population.

3. The presence of another abnormal Hb may modify the disease. For example, HbC, the second most common abnormal Hb, may result in a greater tendency to sickling. Patients with HbSC can have a normal Hb level but be at great risk of sickling. On the other hand, HbF, if it is present (e.g., in thalassemia), may protect by reducing hemolysis and sickling. It is therefore most important to know the results of Hb electrophoresis.

4. Neonates who have a high percentage of HbF are not usually anemic or considered at risk of sickling. However, sickle cell crises have been reported in severely stressed neonates. Usually, the clinical signs appear by the time the child is a few months old.

5. Splenic function is impaired, serious infections may occur, and prophylactic antibiotics are indicated. Later autosplenectomy may occur as a result of vaso-occlusive events.

6. Renal impairment (hyposthenuria) may occur in young children, leading to increased obligatory urine output and consequent increased risk of dehydration.

7. Acute chest syndrome, consisting of chest pain, respiratory distress, fever, and multilobe lung infiltrates, is common in children with sickle cell (SS) disease and may lead to severe hypoxemia. Therapy includes antibiotics, fluid therapy, transfusion, and pain control (PCA, nonsteroidal anti-inflammatory drugs, and possibly epidural analgesia).

8. In later life, pulmonary infarction leads to pulmonary hypertension and cor pulmonale.

Special Anesthesia Problems

1. A sickling crisis may be precipitated by general or local hypoxemia.

2. Sickling is more likely if the patient is anemic, acidotic, hypotensive, dehydrated, and/or hypothermic or if the patient's blood contains another abnormal Hb.

3. If the patient has sickle cell disease, previous vascular occlusive crises may have permanently impaired cardiac, hepatic, and/or renal function.

4. Serum cholinesterase activity may be low.

Anesthesia Management

Perioperative management of the sickle cell diseases is evolving as more experience with these conditions is gained. The assistance of a hematologist may be helpful in deciding which measures are appropriate for each patient. Do not be surprised if some previously held concepts change!

Preoperative

1. All black patients who require anesthesia must be screened for sickle cells:
   a. Sickle cell preparation (microscopy for "sickled" cells) takes 2 hours to complete.
   b. Results of solubility tests (Sickledex, Sickleprep) are available in 5 minutes but do not differentiate disease from trait.
   c. Screening tests are unreliable in infants younger than 6 months of age because HbF masks the results; electrophoresis provides accurate diagnosis.
   d. Some authorities recommend that all patients at risk should have Hb electrophoresis to establish the exact diagnosis.
2. In general, a severe form of the disease is less likely if anemia is absent, but Hb electrophoresis is still essential to exclude any other abnormal Hb and to assess the severity of the condition (Table 6–2). Patients with HbSC disease may have a normal Hb level but are still at a risk of sickling.
3. If the patient has sickle cell trait (less than 50% HbS):
   a. Avoid preoperative dehydration; encourage clear fluid until 2 hours before surgery if appropriate, or start intravenous fluids during the fasting period.
   b. Avoid excessive preoperative sedation.
4. If the patient has sickle cell disease (70%–90% HbS):
   a. Assess the patient carefully, particularly for sequelae of previous sickling crises (e.g., cardiac or renal infarction).
   b. Preoperative transfusions may be given. One of two approaches may be taken:
      i. **Traditional approach:** Infusions of packed cells are given over several days; this suppresses erythropoiesis, as evidenced by a fall in the reticulocyte count. The HbS level may then be reduced to less than 40%, which has been considered safe for most operations.
      ii. **Conservative approach:** A blood transfusion is given as necessary to increase the Hb level to 10 g/dl or higher. This has been demonstrated to be as effective as the traditional approach in preventing complications and is more conservative in the use (and hence the dangers) of transfusion.

Table 6–2. Hemoglobin Electrophoresis in Older Children

Syndrome	HbA (%)	HbS (%)	HbF (%)	HbC (%)
Sickle cell anemia	0	80–95	2–20	0
Sickle C disease	0	45–50	1–5	45–50
Sickle β-Thalassemia	0–30	65–90	2–15	0
Sickle cell trait	50–60	35–45	1–2	0
Normal	95–98	0	1–2	0

   c. Those patients who require cardiopulmonary bypass with hypothermia should have packed cell infusions or exchange transfusion to reduce the HbS level to less than 5%.

   d. In an acute emergency, exchange transfusion may be performed.

Perioperative

1. Use high concentrations of inspired oxygen (at least 50%) to maintain 100% saturation and control ventilation.
2. Monitor acid-base status carefully and avoid acidosis.
3. Ensure maintenance of normal body temperature.
4. Maintain fluid balance carefully to avoid dehydration or excessive fluid administration.
5. Beware of regional ischemia:
   a. Do not use a tourniquet unless it is essential. If one is used, exsanguinate the limb well and use the tourniquet for a minimal time.
   b. Check the blood pressure cuff and other equipment frequently to see that no locally constricting effects are produced.

Postoperative

1. The patient must be awake before extubation.
2. Give additional oxygen continuously during transport to and in the PACU.
3. Hydration and warmth must be maintained.
4. Be alert for the possibility of pulmonary complications; they are common in patients with sickle cell disease.

Suggested Additional Reading

Esseltine DW, Baxter MRN, and Bevan JC: Sickle cell states and the anaesthetist. Can J Anaesth 35:385–403, 1988.

Lane PA: Sickle cell disease. Pediatr Clin North Am 43:639–664, 1996.

Riethmuller R, Grundy EM, and Radley-Smith R: Open heart surgery in a patient with homozygous sickle-cell states: a review. Anaesthesia 37:324, 1982.

Vichinsky EP and Styles L: Pulmonary complications. Hematol Oncol Clin North Am 10:1275–1287, 1996.

Vichinsky EP, Haberkern CM, Neumayr L, et al.: A comparison of conservative and aggressive transfusion regimens in the perioperative management of sickle cell disease. N Engl J Med 333:206–213, 1995.

Hemophilia

Factor VIII Deficiency (Classic Hemophilia Type A)

Classic hemophilia is inherited as an X-linked recessive disorder and is characterized by episodes of bleeding, either spontaneous or after minimal injury. The presenting sign may be bleeding from the umbilical cord in neonates or after circumcision in infants. The diagnosis can be confirmed by factor VIII assay. During childhood, many sites may be involved, hemarthrosis is common, and retroperitoneal bleeding may occur. Hemophilic children require special care during any operation, including (most frequently) dental extractions.

Owing to the use of factor VIII concentrates from multiple donors, a high percentage of children with hemophilia have become infected with human immunodeficiency virus (HIV). Recombinant factor VIII is now available; it is as effective as that obtained from blood, and should ensure viral safety.

Surgical Management

Patients with hemophilia should undergo elective surgery only in hospitals with full facilities to care for this condition. Team care by a hematologist, a surgeon, and an anesthesiologist is essential. If an emergency operation is essential but the facilities of a hematology department are not available, give fresh-frozen plasma (20 ml/kg) preoperatively.

Preoperative

1. If there is any doubt about the diagnosis, the patient's blood must be tested. Preoperative investigation should include screening for factor VIII inhibitors (found in 5%–10% of patients), even if the patient has never previously had inhibitors.
2. One hour before surgery, an infusion of factor VIII concentrate (25–50 units/kg) should be given, followed by an assay for plasma factor VIII activity. Surgery can proceed if factor VIII activity is greater than 50%.

Perioperative

1. Exercise great care during instrumentation of the airway. Avoid trauma that might provoke submucosal hemorrhage.
2. A continuous infusion of factor VIII (3–4 units/kg/hr) may be advisable during major surgery.

Postoperative

1. Depending on the nature of the surgery, the factor VIII levels in the blood should be maintained at 50% for several days. This is achieved by giving factor VIII, as dictated by repeated assay, preferably by continuous infusion.
2. After dental extraction, ϵ-aminocaproic acid (Amicar) may help to inhibit fibrinolysis of formed blood clot.

N.B. When factor VIII inhibitors are present, therapy presents a major challenge. Various methods have been used, including very high doses of factor VIII combined with immunosuppressive therapy, porcine factor VIII, and recombinant factor VIIa.

Factor IX Deficiency (Christmas Disease, Hemophilia Type B)

Patients with factor IX deficiency are treated as for factor XIII deficiency except that factor IX levels are assayed and factor IX infusions are given.

Suggested Additional Reading

Hedner U and Glazer S: Management of hemophilia patients with inhibitors. Hematol Oncol Clin North Am 6:1035–1046, 1992.

Lusher JM and Warrier I: Hemophilia A. Hematol Oncol Clin North Am 6:1021–1033, 1992.

Von Willebrand's Disease

Von Willebrand's disease is the most common congenital bleeding disorder; it may affect 1% of children. There are many forms of the disease, both congenital and acquired, and its incidence varies widely among different ethnic groups. It may occur secondary to another disease (e.g., Wilms tumor) and may resolve with treatment of that disease. The basic defect present in von Willebrand's disease is the lack of a plasma cofactor that protects factor VIII and is necessary for normal platelet function. There are three general types of the disease:

Type 1: Common (90% of cases) and mild—the bleeding time is prolonged, but the prothrombin time (PT) and partial thromboplastin time (PTT) are often normal.

Type 2: (a) With normal platelet count and (b) with thrombocytopenia.

Type 3: Most severe form (fewer than 1% of cases)—von Willebrand's factor and factor VIII are undetectable.

The clinical manifestations depend on the severity of the disease. Cutaneous and mucous membrane bleeding are common, but deep tissue bleeding may also occur. A history of easy bleeding or failure to clot after dental extraction should alert the anesthesiologist. In type 1 and type 2a disease, 1-deamino-8-D-arginine vasopressin (DDAVP) is effective, but it may exacerbate type 2b and is ineffective in type 3 disease. The latter must be treated with cryoprecipitate or fresh-frozen plasma.

If the type of disease is unknown preoperatively, it may be appropriate to assess the effect on coagulation studies of an infusion of DDAVP. If the bleeding time is shortened, DDAVP may be useful perioperatively. If not, blood products will be necessary.

Suggested Additional Reading

Cameron CB and Kobrinsky N: Perioperative management of patients with Von Willebrand's disease. Can J Anaesth 37:341–347, 1990.

Werner EJ: Von Willebrand disease in children and adolescents. Pediatr Clin North Am 43:683–707, 1996.

ATYPICAL PLASMA CHOLINESTERASES

The genetically determined abnormal cholinesterases may result in prolonged apnea after the administration of muscle relaxants (e.g., succinylcholine, mivacurium). In the homozygous state (about 1 in 2,500 children), recovery of muscle power may be delayed for hours; in the heterozygous state, the delay is usually 15–25 minutes (Table 6–3).

Table 6–3. Plasma Cholinesterases: Variation in Response to Succinylcholine

Genotype	Incidence	Response to Succinylcholine	Dubucaine No.	Fluoride No.
Homozygous				
$E1^uE1^u$		Normal	70	50
$E1^aE1^a$	1:2,800	Grossly prolonged	15–25	20–25
$E1^sE1^s$	1:140,000	Grossly prolonged	—	—
$E1^fE1^f$	1:300,000	Moderately prolonged	60–70	30–40
Heterozygous				
$E1^uE1^a$	1:25	Almost normal	50–70	40–50
$E1^uE1^f$	1:280	Almost normal	70–80	50–55
$E1^uE1^s$	1:190	Almost normal	70	50
$E1^aE1^f$	1:29,000	Grossly prolonged	45–50	30–40
$E1^aE1^a$	1:20,000	Grossly prolonged	15–25	20–25
$E1^fE1^s$	1:200,000	Grossly prolonged	60–70	30–35

Management of Prolonged Apnea

If muscle activity fails to recover after administration of succinylcholine or mivacurium:

1. Continue to ventilate the patient and continue anesthesia.
2. Confirm persistence of the neuromuscular block, using a nerve stimulator.
3. Allow the child to recover completely before ventilation is discontinued (this may take up to 3–6 hours).

N.B. Prolonged apnea after succinylcholine due to an atypical cholinesterase is not serious provided the above steps are followed. Do not attempt to modify the neuromuscular block by giving drugs, infusing fresh blood, and so on, because further complications may arise. Ventilate the child well, and be patient!

Blood samples for cholinesterase studies also should be obtained:

1. Cholinesterase activity (normal range is 60–200 units but varies with the individual laboratory)
2. Dibucaine number (DN; normal range, 75–85)
3. Fluoride number (FN; normal range, 55–65)

Characteristically, patients with the atypical enzyme have a low DN (0–20) and a low FN (15–25) (see Table 6–3). Those heterozygous for the condition have intermediate values (DN, 40–60; FN, 40–50). The results of these tests may not be available for some days and hence are of no value in the immediate management of the patient.

Other Considerations

When the diagnosis is confirmed, the patient's family should have blood tests and be informed of their status. Those having homozygous atypical states should be advised to carry a warning card or wear a Medic Alert bracelet.

Suggested Additional Reading

Woelfel SK, Brandom BW, McGowan FX, and Cook DR: Plasma cholinesterase activity and response to mivacurium in infants. Anesthesiology 76:A966, 1992.

DIABETES MELLITUS

Diabetes mellitus is the most common endocrine disorder of childhood. Children with symptomatic diabetes are all insulin dependent; type 2 diabetes can occur in children and adolescents, but it is asymptomatic and usually is undiagnosed.

Young children typically present with weight loss, polydipsia, and polyuria. However, the onset may be abrupt, and the child may present with ketoacidosis; this may be accompanied by abdominal pain and leukocytosis, mimicking appendicitis. Vascular complications seldom occur in diabetic children, so the renal, cardiac or peripheral vascular effects of the disease are not seen.

The current approach to juvenile diabetes is to maintain blood glucose levels as close to normal as possible throughout the day by the use of twice- or thrice-daily insulin doses; some children may be using an insulin infusion pump. In some cases control is difficult, and childhood diabetes is often unstable; the anesthesiologist should cooperate closely with the medical team in planning the management of these cases.

Anesthesia Management

Perioperative management must be designed to achieve as close control of the blood glucose level as is possible.

Preoperative

1. Close monitoring of blood glucose should be instituted several days before elective major surgery to permit stabilization of the diabetes.
2. Minor elective surgery for the child with well-controlled diabetes may be planned on an outpatient basis.
3. Severe hyperglycemia and ketosis should be treated with appropriate insulin adjustments before surgery is scheduled. Defer emergency surgery, if possible, until the diabetic ketoacidosis is corrected.
4. **Short procedures** (less than 1 hour):
   a. Schedule as early as possible in the morning.
   b. Determine the preoperative blood glucose level.
   c. Give one-half to two-thirds the usual dose of insulin as intermediate-acting insulin only (NPH or Lente). No short-acting insulin should be given.
   d. Start an intravenous infusion of 5% glucose-containing solution and infuse at a maintenance rate (3–4 ml/kg/hr) unless the blood glucose is less than 5.5 mmol/L (100 mg/dl), in which case the rate should be increased and the blood glucose rechecked.
   e. Determine the blood glucose concentration every hour during surgery and immediately after the procedure, using a handheld glucometer.
5. **Long procedures** (more than 1 hour): The preferred technique is to give an infusion of insulin plus an infusion of dextrose and monitor blood glucose levels frequently (every 30–60 minutes) using a glucometer.
   a. Add 50 units of regular insulin to 500 ml of isotonic saline. (Each milliliter contains 0.1 unit of regular insulin.) Saturate the insulin-binding sites of the intravenous tubing by allowing 50–100 ml of the solution to run through.
   b. Use a Y-tube or piggyback connection to the maintenance intravenous line, and control the rate with an infusion pump.
   c. Infuse 1 ml/kg/hr, to deliver 0.1 units of insulin per kilogram per hour.

   d. Infuse a 5% glucose solution at a rate to maintain blood glucose at 8.5–14 mmol/L (150–250 mg/dl).

   e. Blood glucose levels should be determined every half hour during the surgery.

   f. Postoperatively, the insulin infusion may be continued as long as necessary, depending on the circumstances. The child's pediatrician should control the rate and amount of the infusion based on the blood glucose concentration.

Postoperative

1. **Short procedures:**
   a. If the patient is receiving subcutaneous insulin, give appropriate doses of short-acting insulin as required based on blood glucose levels. Continue intravenous hydration until the child is taking fluids orally.
   b. The child's usual insulin regimen can be resumed the next day if the patient is able to tolerate fluids or food.
2. **Long procedures:**
   a. Change to subcutaneous insulin when the child's condition allows (e.g., when the child is taking fluids orally and intravenous hydration has been discontinued).
   b. Pediatricians should follow up and manage the patient's diabetes.

Emergency Surgery

Diabetic ketoacidosis may result from the physiologic stresses of the surgical disease, but remember also that the symptoms of ketoacidosis may mimic those of the acute abdomen.

1. Attempt to stabilize the patient before proceeding to the operating room (OR). Stabilization should be done in cooperation with the medical team.
2. Insert monitoring lines for central venous pressure (CVP) and arterial pressure to assist in correcting hypovolemia and hyperglycemia.
3. Infuse warmed fluids to correct hypovolemia; normal saline 10–20 ml/kg over 1 hour may be required, as indicated by CVP.
4. Intravenous regular insulin will be required. A bolus dose of 0.1 unit/kg followed by an infusion of 0.1 unit/kg/hr may be used.
5. Monitor blood glucose frequently; the objective is to decrease the level by a maximum of 100 mg/dl each hour. More rapid declines may result in detrimental osmotic shifts.
6. When the blood glucose level is less than 300 mg/dl, continue rehydration with 0.45% saline and 5% dextrose solution.
7. Monitor serum electrolytes frequently; hypokalemia is to be expected. Potassium must be added to the infusion provided that renal function is satisfactory.
8. Metabolic acidosis corrects spontaneously as hypovolemia is corrected and insulin administered. Ketones are metabolized, and

their production is halted. Sodium bicarbonate is unnecessary and may be deleterious except when very severe acidosis (pH less than 7.0) is present.
9. Subclinical brain swelling occurs during the treatment of diabetic ketoacidosis and, rarely, dangerous cerebral edema may develop. It is recommended that patients be closely monitored and that total fluid administration be limited to 4 $L/m^2/24$ hr.

Suggested Additional Reading

Gavin LA: Perioperative treatment of the diabetic patient. Endocrinol Metab Clin North Am 21:457, 1992.
Krane EJ, Rockoff MA, Wallman JK, and Wolfsdorf JI: Subclinical brain swelling in children during the treatment of diabetic ketoacidosis. N Engl J Med 312:1147, 1985.

MALIGNANT DISEASES

The anesthesiologist frequently has to care for children with malignant disease. Special problems may arise depending on the site and type of the disease, but all of these children require special attention to their emotional status. Extreme care must be taken to ensure a minimum of discomfort and upset for both child and parents.

Children require special care during painful diagnostic and therapeutic procedures (e.g., lumbar puncture, bone marrow aspiration), and these should be carefully planned.

1. The child and parents should be thoroughly informed and prepared before each procedure.
2. The procedure should be performed in a comfortable and pleasant room. Suitable oral premedication can be given (e.g., midazolam).
3. Optimal sedation, analgesia, or general anesthesia should be provided; propofol infusion is very satisfactory (*see* page 52).
4. A highly skilled operator should perform each procedure. This is no place for the intern to learn.

Special Anesthesia Problems

The child with a malignancy may present special problems:

1. Abnormal anatomy, including the airway, may cause problems. Be especially aware of the child with enlarged hilar lymph nodes.
2. Hematologic disease may result in anemia, coagulopathy, and immune deficiency. Check laboratory results. Coagulopathy may lead to intraoperative pulmonary hemorrhage and difficulty with ventilation. Urgent bronchoscopy is required in such cases to remove clots.
3. Increased susceptibility to infection means that care in asepsis is vital to these children.

4. A history of long-term steroid therapy necessitates consideration of preoperative corticosteroids.
5. Nausea and vomiting may complicate radiotherapy and/or drug therapy and lead to dehydration and electrolyte disturbance. Check the biochemistry levels.
6. Cardiomyopathy may follow total body irradiation and cyclophosphamide therapy or the use of doxorubicin or daunomycin *(see below)*.
7. Hypercalcemia may accompany malignant tumors of bone.
8. Nephropathy may lead to impaired renal function.
9. Raised intracranial pressure may occur with involvement of the central nervous system.
10. Peripheral neuropathy may occur.
11. Muscle weakness and hypotonia occur in advanced malignant disease.
12. Toxic effects of chemotherapy may be present *(see below)*.

Adverse Effects of Commonly Used Drugs

All antineoplastic drugs can cause the following effects:

1. Bone marrow suppression, with anemia, leukopenia, and thrombocytopenia
2. Anorexia, nausea, and vomiting
3. Stomatitis and alopecia
4. Decreased resistance to infection

Some of these agents produce additional adverse effects:

1. Hepatotoxicity (e.g., methotrexate, cyclophosphamide), so the indices of liver function should be checked.
2. Renal toxic effects (e.g., cisplatin, ifosfamide), which may be increased by the use of aminoglycoside antibiotics or diuretics (furosemide).

Furthermore, specific drugs have effects of special importance to anesthesiologists:

1. **Cardiotoxic effects**
   a. Both *daunomycin,* used in leukemia therapy, and *doxorubicin* (Adriamycin), used in therapy for solid tumors and leukemias, affect the heart, causing
      i. Nonspecific electrocardiographic (ECG) changes, with any dose
      ii. Disturbances of conduction, including supraventricular tachycardia, atrial and ventricular extrasystoles, and ventricular fibrillation
      iii. Drug-induced cardiomyopathy in 1%–2% of patients, leading to congestive heart failure
      iv. The cardiac effects of doxorubicin are dose-related. A total cumulative dose of 250 mg/m^2, or 150 mg/m^2 if combined with mediastinal radiation, must alert the anesthesiologist and

is an indication for a full cardiologic assessment. Patients with a history of congestive heart failure are particularly likely to experience perioperative complications.

    v. Myocardial depressant drugs (e.g., halothane) should be avoided and cardiac parameters should be closely monitored.

    vi. Propranolol and calcium channel-blocking drugs may dangerously increase the cardiotoxic effects and should be avoided.

  b. *Mitoxantrone* may cause cardiotoxicity, especially if given after previous anthracycline therapy and with cumulative doses greater than 120 mg/m².

  c. *Cyclophosphamide, cisplatin, 5-fluorouracil, amsacrine, mithramycin, mitomycin, vincristine,* and *actinomycin D* may all be cardiotoxic or contribute to cardiotoxicity at high doses.

  d. Assessment of cardiac status: ECG changes are nonspecific, but prolongation of the Q-T interval is suggestive of toxicity. The echocardiogram is the most useful index of cardiac function, and recent studies should be reviewed before anesthesia.

2. **Pulmonary toxicity**

  a. *Bleomycin,* used in therapy for testicular tumors and Hodgkin's disease, causes pulmonary fibrosis in approximately 10% of patients and may result in death (1%). The effects on the lung are accelerated by hyperoxia, and oxygen therapy should be carefully controlled at all times. Fluid overload may further compromise lung function.

  b. *Busulfan, carmustine, methotrexate,* and *mitomycin* may cause pulmonary fibrosis with high doses.

  c. *Cytosine arabinoside, vinblastine,* and *mitomycin* have been associated with noncardiac pulmonary edema.

3. **Anticholinesterase inhibition**

  a. *Cyclophosphamide* and other alkylating agents—used for lymphomas, Hodgkin's disease, leukemias—inhibit serum cholinesterase; prolonged apnea with succinylcholine or mivacurium may occur.

Suggested Additional Reading

Azizkhan RG, Dudgeon DL, Buck JR, et al.: Life-threatening airway obstruction as a complication to the management of mediastinal masses in children. J Pediatr Surg 20:816–822, 1985.

Burrows FA, Hickey PR, and Kolin S: Complications of anesthesia in Adriamycin treated pediatric patients. Anesthesiology 59:A434, 1983.

Keon TP: Death on induction of anesthesia for cervical node biopsy. Anesthesiology 55:471–472, 1981.

Klein DS and Wilds PR: Pulmonary toxicity of antineoplastic agents: anaesthetic and postoperative implications. Can Anaesth Soc J 30:399, 1983.

McQuillan PJ, Morgan BA, and Ramwell J: Adriamycin cardiomyopathy. Anaesthesia 43:301–304, 1988.

Sanderson PM and Hartsilver E: Acute airway obstruction in a child with acute lymphoblastic leukaemia during central venous catheterization. Paediatr Anaesth 8:516–519, 1998.

Tobias JD: Special considerations for the pediatric oncology patient. In Berry FA and Steward DJ (eds.): Pediatrics for the Anesthesiologist. Churchill Livingstone, New York, 1993, pp. 287–303.

DOWN SYNDROME

Down syndrome (trisomy 21; T21) is common (1.5 cases per 1,000 live births). Mental retardation is invariably present but varies in severity from patient to patient; many children with this syndrome are very alert and cooperative.

Associated Conditions

1. Congenital heart disease occurs in up to 60% of patients, particularly atrioventricular canal, ventricular septal defect, patent ductus arteriosus, and tetralogy of Fallot.
2. Respiratory infections are common. This may be related to the genetic anomaly, an immune deficiency, and/or the social and institutional implications of the syndrome.
3. Atlantoaxial joint instability occurs in 12% of patients and may lead to cervical spinal cord injury. The neck is particularly unstable in the flexed position, but caution should be exercised to minimize any excessive motion.
4. Congenital subglottic stenosis is common. Ensure that the endotracheal tube selected is not too large and that there is an adequate leak around it when airway pressure is applied.
5. Obstructive sleep apnea is common.
6. Thyroid hypofunction is common as the child grows older.
7. Polycythemia is a frequent finding in neonates and may necessitate phlebotomy to relieve circulatory failure.
8. Duodenal atresia of the newborn is common in patients with Down syndrome.

Special Anesthesia Problems

1. Airway: The large tongue and small nasopharynx predispose to respiratory obstruction, particularly during mask anesthesia and recovery stages. Have an oropharyngeal airway ready. Congenital subglottic stenosis predisposes to postoperative stridor.
2. Lungs: Is there any acute infection present that requires therapy before surgery? Is there a history suggestive of obstructive sleep apnea?
3. Problems of associated cardiac disease: antibiotic prophylaxis is needed against subacute bacterial endocarditis.
4. Atlantoaxial joint instability may predispose to injury during intubation. Any excessive neck movement should be avoided (especially flexion). Screening for atlantoaxial subluxation should be obtained whenever possible in all children older than 4 years of age.

5. Retarded children are more difficult to manage during induction of anesthesia. Often the parents can be of great help.

N.B. Children with Down syndrome have been reported to be especially sensitive to the effects of atropine. This is not true; in practice, we have used the same dosage schedule for these as for other patients without any problems.

Suggested Additional Reading

Kobel M, Creighton RE, and Steward DJ: Anaesthetic considerations in Down's syndrome: experience with 100 patients and a review of the literature. Can Anaesth Soc J 29:593, 1982.

Moore RA, McNicholas KW, and Warran SP: Atlantoaxial subluxation with symptomatic spinal cord compression in a child with Down's syndrome. Anesth Analg 66:89–90, 1987.

Morray JP, MacGillivray R, and Duker G: Increased perioperative risk following repair of congenital heart disease in Down's syndrome. Anesthesiology 65:221–224, 1986.

Williams JP, Somerville GM, Miner ME, and Reilly D: Atlanto-axial subluxation and trisomy-21: Another perioperative complication. Anesthesiology 67:253–254, 1987.

MALIGNANT HYPERTHERMIA

Malignant hyperthermia (MH), a potentially fatal abnormal response to anesthetic agents, is genetically determined. It is characterized by a rapid rise in body temperature and profound biochemical changes usually accompanied by generalized muscular rigidity. Any of the commonly used volatile anesthetic agents may trigger the condition, as may succinylcholine.

MH is a rare condition, probably occurring in fewer than 1 in 100,000 cases in which general anesthetics are given. Children and young adults have most frequently been affected, and it has been reported in a patient as young as 2 months of age. Increased awareness of MH, leading to earlier diagnosis and prompt institution of treatment, plus the availability of a specific therapy (dantrolene), has reduced the mortality rate from more than 70% to less than 10% in reported surveys.

Knowledge of the pathophysiology of MH has progressively increased. It is now clear that the disease process is associated with altered calcium homeostasis in skeletal muscle. Malignant hyperthermia-susceptible (MHS) patients demonstrate an elevated calcium ion concentration in skeletal muscle, and studies in MHS swine show a marked increase in the intracellular calcium level on exposure to triggering agents. This increased calcium level has been linked with a potential defect in the "calcium-induced calcium release" mechanism within the cell, now further linked with a defect in the calcium release channel of the sarcoplasmic reticulum. The mechanism of the disease process in the cell produces a sustained contracture of skeletal muscle with associated heat production. The further manifestations of the acute syndrome are secondary to the acceleration of metabolic processes within skeletal muscle, which is accompanied by large increases in oxygen consumption and carbon dioxide production. If the acute condition persists, cellular energy substrates become depleted, with consequent failure of cellular functions, including those regulating the intracellular and extracellular chemical composition. Substances released by damaged cells trigger the continuing manifestations of the acute crisis, including coagulopathy and renal failure.

Detection of Susceptibility

There are still no simple, reliable screening tests to identify MHS individuals preoperatively. Creatine phosphokinase (CPK) levels are usually increased, but this test is very nonspecific and many other causes of elevated CPK exist. Many MHS patients do have local or generalized muscular disease; however, most patients with a muscle disease are not MHS. Although a positive family anesthetic history of MH is the most reliable clue, its absence does not guarantee an individual's nonsusceptibility to triggering agents. Even uneventful previous anesthesia does not absolutely preclude an MH crisis during a subsequent anesthesia.

At present, MHS patients can be identified with reasonable certainty only by in vitro study of fresh living muscle tissue obtained at biopsy. Caffeine- and halothane-induced contracture of the biopsy specimen is usually diagnostic; this is presently the "gold standard." Up to the present time a relatively large biopsy specimen has been required, so the test is not usually recommended for small children (younger than 10 years of age). In recent years, much progress has been made toward standardizing contracture testing for MHS and establishing uniform criteria for a positive diagnosis to be made.

Less invasive tests to determine MH susceptibility have been disappointing so far. Magnetic resonance imaging has been used to seek abnormalities of skeletal muscle energy substrates in MHS subjects, but a reliable, specific marker for the disease has not been identified. The possible identification of an MH gene located on chromosome 19 also raised hopes for new methods to diagnose the trait, but these have not yet been demonstrated to be reliable. Therefore, at the present time, there are no noninvasive methods to diagnose the MH trait with certainty.

Clinical Manifestations

Nonspecific early signs are

1. Elevation of the end-tidal carbon dioxide, unexplained tachycardia, tachypnea (or attempts to breathe against the ventilator), sweating, cyanosis, and overheating of the soda lime
2. Hypertonus of the skeletal muscle
   a. It may occur immediately after the administration of succinylcholine.

      i. Failure of skeletal muscle to relax. This is an indication to postpone surgery and reevaluate.

     ii. Abnormally severe muscle fasciculations or intense masseter spasm. This should arouse suspicion.

  b. It may also occur later during anesthesia, after the use of potent agents, commonly halothane.

3. A rapid rise in body temperature (more than 1°C) is a later sign.

The prognosis is much more favorable if the syndrome is recognized before a severe pyretic reaction develops.

Confirmatory evidence of an impending MH crisis consists of biochemical changes: severe metabolic acidosis (base deficit greater than 25 meq/L) and severe respiratory acidosis (partial pressure of carbon dioxide [PCO_2] greater than 60 mmHg). Serum potassium *may* be elevated. Generalized muscle rigidity, ventricular arrhythmias, cyanosis, and increasing body temperature are highly predictive of an impending MH crisis.

Therapeutic Regimen*

1. Discontinue all inhalational agents; inform the surgeon of the diagnosis; insist that the surgery must be urgently terminated. **Send for help!**

2. Hyperventilate with 100% O_2 using a high flow. A T-piece type circuit (e.g., Bain) may not provide adequate ventilation for large patients even at high flows; therefore, change to a new circle absorber system as soon as possible.

3. Immediately give the following:

  a. *Dantrolene:* The initial dose is 2.5 mg/kg IV. If necessary, continue to infuse intravenously at 1 mg/kg/min until the heart rate begins to slow and become regular, decreased muscle tone becomes evident, and the patient's temperature starts to fall. Then withhold the dantrolene and observe the heart rate, muscle tone, and temperature. If these deteriorate again, the infusion can be repeated at intervals of not less than 15 minutes until clinical improvement is apparent.

  b. If an intravenous preparation of dantrolene is not available or if arrhythmias persist, infuse *procainamide* intravenously (1 mg/kg/min, up to a maximum of 15 mg/kg) and monitor the results with the ECG. This infusion may relieve muscle contracture promptly and prevent further increase in body temperature.

  c. *Sodium bicarbonate (7.5%):* 4 ml/kg IV immediately; repeat in accordance with blood gas analyses.

  d. *Mannitol:* 0.5 g/kg; some mannitol is present in the dantrolene mixture (150 mg for each mg of dantrolene), but

---

*Further advice can be obtained in North America from the MHAUS hotline telephone number: 209-634-4917.

      supplementation may be needed to maintain an adequate urine output (more than 1 ml/kg/hr).

4. Commence active cooling. Place the patient on a rubber sheet, apply ice bags and ice water, and use fans. Intragastric cooling and cold enemas may also be necessary. Infuse refrigerated saline solution intravenously at 10 ml/kg/hr as necessary.

5. Change to a vapor-free anesthetic machine and a vapor-free circuit (e.g., disposable plastic circuit) as soon as possible.

6. Continue monitoring the patient closely:
   a. Monitor by stethoscope, pulse oximeter, and ECG.
   b. If an arterial line is not already present, insert one to measure pressure and obtain samples.
   c. Insert a CVP line to monitor volume status.
   d. Insert a urinary catheter and monitor urine output.
   e. Attach a multichannel thermometer (rectal, esophageal, skin, and muscle leads). Beware of overtreatment leading to hypothermia.

7. Obtain frequent arterial blood samples for the following studies:
   a. Blood gas and acid/base determinations (repeat every 10 minutes)
   b. Serum electrolytes (Na, K, Cl, Ca, inorganic phosphate)
   c. CPK
   d. Serum enzymes: serum glutamic oxaloacetic transaminase (SGOT), lactate dehydrogenase (LDH), creatine kinase (CK), 3-hydroxybutyrate dehydrogenase (3-HBDH).
   e. Coagulation studies

8. Correct any electrolyte imbalance on the basis of biochemical indices. To treat hyperkalemia, give 0.15 units/kg of regular insulin with 0.5 g/kg of glucose.

9. Continue to measure urine output, and maintain it at 1 ml/kg/hr or greater, using diuretics as necessary.

10. Coagulopathy must be expected and may necessitate therapy on the basis of demonstrated factor deficiencies.

11. Avoid the administration of drugs that might complicate matters: calcium, digitalis, and adrenergic agents have previously been considered contraindicated. In fact they may not cause further problems, but they are probably best avoided unless definitely indicated. *Calcium channel-blocking agents are considered contraindicated; they may interact with dantrolene to produce profound myocardial depression and do not have a therapeutic role in MH.*

12. Monitor the patient in the intensive care unit; MH may recur within the first 24 hours. Sequelae of the episode may also demand aggressive therapy. For example:
    a. Cerebral edema may appear due to hypoxic insult.
    b. Pulmonary edema may present due to fluid overload or myocardial dysfunction.
    c. Coagulopathy and renal failure may require continued care.
    d. Oral dantrolene, 1 mg/kg every 6 hours, should be administered for the next 48 hours.

Anesthesia Regimen for Patients with Known Susceptibility to Malignant Hyperthermia

All personnel who may be concerned in the care of an MHS patient in the OR and PACU must be fully acquainted with a suitable protocol that describes the location of drugs, equipment, etc., and the procedures to be implemented if MH develops.

Patients at Risk

1. Survivors of an MH crisis
2. Patients with a positive muscle biopsy
3. A first-degree relative of anyone known to be MHS (i.e., positive muscle biopsy or survivor of an MH crisis)
4. Those with muscle abnormalities and/or an elevated serum CPK level, in whom MH may be suspected
5. Patients with central core disease

In the management of children, the clinician must frequently assume possible MH susceptibility on questionable evidence (e.g., a family history of anesthetic difficulties but no positive muscle biopsy in the family). The simple course then is to provide a trigger-free anesthetic.

Preoperative Investigation

A preoperative investigation should be done for patients with a positive or strongly suggestive family or personal history.

1. Review the family and personal history carefully, noting especially muscle disease, cardiac abnormality, and drug- or anesthesia-induced reactions.
2. Order laboratory investigations: serum enzymes (SGOT, LDH, CK, 3-HBDH) and coagulation indices.
3. Order an ECG and an echocardiogram.
4. If the findings indicate a strong possibility of MH susceptibility and the child is older than 12 years of age, it may be advisable to arrange for muscle biopsy at a suitably equipped center. Younger children and infants must be presumed to be at risk for MH and treated accordingly until they are old enough for testing (or until an improved, less invasive diagnostic test becomes available).

Preoperative Preparation

1. If major surgery is planned, the patient should be admitted to hospital 24 hours preoperatively (bed rest helps to alleviate anxiety and reduce muscle cramps). Minor surgery may be planned on an outpatient basis with appropriate additional precautions as outlined below.
2. Routine dantrolene pretreatment for all MHS patients is not recommended. It may be advantageous to administer dantrolene,

2–4 mg/kg IV, preoperatively to the very high risk MHS patient and to emergency or trauma patients known to be MHS.
3. If diagnostic muscle biopsy is to be performed, dantrolene must not be given (it affects the test results).

Anesthesia Management

Preoperative

1. Order a suitable barbiturate or diazepam to be given the evening before surgery.
2. Order oral midazolam (0.5–0.75 mg/kg) 30 minutes preoperatively.
3. Ensure that all necessary drugs and equipment have been prepared:
   a. Drugs for anesthesia—All intravenous induction agents, nondepolarizing relaxants, narcotic analgesics, nitrous oxide, ketamine, atropine, and anticholinesterases are safe.
   b. Drugs for emergency use if MH develops, including refrigerated lactated Ringer's solution, normal saline, 7.5% sodium bicarbonate, warmed 20% mannitol and 50% glucose solutions, dantrolene, procainamide, hydrocortisone, furosemide, potassium chloride, soluble insulin, heparin, chlorpromazine, and propranolol.
   c. Equipment: vapor-free anesthetic machine, plastic disposable circuit and reservoir bag, ventilator, hypothermia blankets, multichannel thermometer and probes. Ice and ice bags should be available to the OR suite.
4. Remove all triggering agents from the room (to avoid any possibility of accidental use).

Preoperative

1. Induce and maintain anesthesia using only nontriggering agents; these include thiopental, propofol, nitrous oxide, all narcotic analgesics, all benzodiazepines, all nondepolarizing muscle relaxants, and all local analgesics.
2. For all major procedures, insert arterial and CVP lines and monitor urine output.
3. Monitor closely for early signs of an MH crisis.

Postoperative (After Uneventful Anesthesia)

1. Transfer the patient to the PACU, with monitoring equipment, intravenous cannulas, and catheter in place.
2. Ensure that *all* PACU staff are aware of the possibility of a delayed MH reaction and know what to do if one occurs.
3. Vital signs are recorded at 5-minute intervals initially.
4. Do not transfer the patient to the ward or home until vital signs have been stable for 4 hours and the results of any laboratory tests are satisfactory.
5. After the patient is returned to the ward, vital signs are recorded hourly for 4 hours and then every 4 hours for 1 day.

6. Dantrolene should be administered to any patient who exhibits any untoward signs (e.g., persistent tachycardia or dysrhythmia, temperature rise).

Suggested Additional Reading

Cunliffe M, Lerman J, and Britt BA: Is prophylactic dantrolene indicated for MHS patients undergoing elective surgery? Anesth Analg 66:S35, 1987.

Hackl W, Mauritz W, Schemper M, et al.: Prediction of malignant hyperthermia susceptibility—statistical evaluation of clinical signs. Br J Anaesth 64:425–429, 1990.

Larach MG: Standardization of the caffeine halothane muscle contracture test. Anesth Analg 69:511–515, 1989.

Lerman J and Relton JES: Anesthesia for malignant hyperthermia susceptible patients. In Britt BA (ed.): Malignant Hyperthermia. Martinus Nijhoff, Boston, 1987, pp 369–392.

Levitt RC, Meyers D, Fletcher JE, and Rosenberg H: Molecular genetics and malignant hyperthermia. Anesthesiology 75:1–3, 1991.

Rosenberg H: Clinical presentation of malignant hyperthermia. Br J Anaesth 60:268–273, 1988.

Yentis SM, Levine MF, and Hartley EJ: Should all children with suspected or confirmed malignant hyperthermia susceptibility be admitted after surgery? A 10 year review. Anesth Analg 75:345–350, 1992.

Neuroleptic Malignant Syndrome

Neuroleptic malignant syndrome is a disorder characterized by fever, muscle rigidity, tachycardia, and autonomic instability that occurs in patients receiving antipsychotic medication. It is rare but has been reported in children, in whom the diagnosis may be missed or may be confused with MH. The disease can progress to hepatic and renal failure. Treatment is by withdrawal of the antipsychotic medication. The likelihood that this syndrome is associated closely with MH susceptibility is considered remote.

Suggested Additional Reading

Levine MF and Lerman J: Neuroleptic malignant syndrome in a child. Paediatr Anaesth 3:47–50, 1993.

Masseter Spasm

Masseter spasm may sometimes be observed when succinylcholine is administered intravenously to a patient who is anesthetized with halothane. This phenomenon has caused much confusion in the past, and it has been suggested that this form of masseter spasm might commonly be associated with MH trait. It is now recognized that many children respond with transient increased masseter tone if the "halothane followed by succinylcholine" sequence is used. This is probably a normal response that varies in intensity. We suggest that the whole problem can be avoided by not routinely giving succinylcholine to a patient who is anesthetized with halothane!

If masseter spasm does occur, various courses of action have been suggested, ranging from discontinuing the anesthesia and recommending a muscle biopsy to continuing the anesthesia with known MH-triggering agents. We suggest that a conservative approach is to continue with anesthesia, monitor the patient carefully, and avoid known triggering agents.

Masseter spasm after the thiopental plus succinylcholine sequence is very rare and must be considered a possible early sign of MH trait *(see above).*

Suggested Additional Reading

Lazzell VA, Carr AS, Lerman J: The incidence of masseter muscle rigidity after succinylcholine in infants and children. Can J Anaesth 41:475–479, 1994.

O'Flynn RP, Shutack JG, Rosenberg H, and Fletcher JE: Masseter muscle rigidity and malignant hyperthermia susceptibility in pediatric patients: an update on management and diagnosis. Anesthesiology 80:1228–1233, 1994.

Vanderspek AF: Triggering agents continued after masseter spasm: there is proof in this pudding. Anesth Analg 73:364–365, 1991.

Vanderspek AF, Fang WB, Ashton-Miller JA, et al.: Increased masticatory muscle stiffness during limb muscle flaccidity associated with succinylcholine administration. Anesthesiology 69:11–16, 1988.

LATEX ALLERGY

Latex allergy can cause a severe, life-threatening intraoperative immunoglobulin E-mediated anaphylactic reaction. Urticaria, bronchospasm, and/or circulatory collapse may occur. A history of repeated exposure to latex (e.g., frequent catheterization for neurogenic bladder, repeated surgery) and/or reactions to rubber balloons may be elicited. Up to 40% of patients with spina bifida have latex allergy. The risk of developing allergy may be related to the number of operations and the presence of atopy; hence, older patients are more likely to have developed allergy. Cross-reactivity to bananas, avocado, kiwi fruit, and chestnuts may be found. Skin-prick testing or radioallergosorbent testing (RAST) to latex may confirm the allergy, though there is some controversy as to the use of such tests.

Latex allergy should be considered if signs of an anaphylactic reaction occur during surgery and cannot be related to drug administration. The initial signs are increased airway pressure, decreased oxygen saturation, hypotension and tachycardia, and possibly urticaria.

The condition demands rapid, aggressive therapy including ventilation with oxygen, rapid infusion of warmed intravenous fluids to expand the blood volume, and epinephrine 1–5 µg/kg IV bolus followed by an infusion of 0.1–0.3 µg/kg/min. Other drugs that should be used include antihistamines (diphenhydramine, 1 mg/kg); histamine$_2$ (H_2) receptor-blocking drugs (cimetidine, 4 µg/kg); methylxanthines (aminophylline, 3–5 mg/kg); and corticosteroids (methylprednisolone, 25 mg/kg).

Patients at risk should be carefully reviewed; those with a history suggestive of latex allergy should be skin tested if possible. Those who are positive or with a history suggestive of latex allergy may be pretreated before surgery to minimize the risk of an anaphylactic reaction. A regi-

Table 6–4. Anesthesia Equipment That May Contain Latex

Plastic syringes	Catheters	Airway or bite block
Vials	Tourniquets	Ventilator bellows
Intravenous bag	Face mask	Blood pressure cuff
IV set (ports)	Endotracheal tube	Gloves
Adhesive tape	Anesthesia circuit and bag	

men of corticosteroids (prednisone, 1 mg/kg) and H_1- and H_2-blocking drugs (diphenhydramine, 1 mg/kg, and cimetidine, 5 mg/kg) has been suggested. The patient may then be anesthetized and carefully monitored. It is most important that all members of the surgical team use nonlatex (e.g., neoprene) gloves and that all latex materials be excluded from the surgical and anesthesia equipment (Table 6–4).

It is practical and important to eliminate latex from all items that may come into close contact with the patient (e.g., syringes, masks). It may be less practical and less important to change remote items (e.g., ventilator bellows). All items of equipment that are latex free should be clearly labeled as such in the storage area. All items containing latex should be clearly marked with a warning label.

It is strongly recommended that all patients at risk for development of latex allergy (e.g. those with myelomeningocele) should be treated in a latex-free environment from the outset.

In summary:

1. All patients should be questioned about a history of allergy.
2. Patients in high-risk groups should be identified and offered skin tests.
3. All equipment should be clearly labeled as to its latex content.
4. All procedures on patients who have a positive history or are at high risk for development of latex allergy should be performed in a latex-free environment.

Suggested Additional Reading

Kam PCA, Lee MSM, and Thompson JF: Latex allergy: an emerging clinical and occupational health problem. Anaesthesia 52:570–575, 1997.

McKinstry LJ, Fenton WJ, and Barrett P: Anaesthesia and the patient with latex allergy. Can J Anaesth 39:587–589, 1992.

Swartz J, Braude BM, Gilmour RF, et al: Intraoperative anaphylaxis to latex. Can J Anaesth 37:589–592, 1990.

Task Force on Allergic Reactions to Latex: Committee report. J Allergy Clin Immunol 92:16–18, 1993.

THE CHILD WITH A TRANSPLANT

There are now numerous children living with transplanted organs; these patients require special considerations.

1. These patients and their families have survived extensive medical and surgical interventions; they require very considerate emotional care.

2. All of these patients will be on a regimen of antirejection drugs, which may have important side effects.

   a. All of the antirejection drugs cause reduced resistance to infection. *Take extreme care with aseptic technique.* Insert only those intravenous and monitoring lines that are really needed, and have them removed as soon as possible.

   b. Cyclosporine can cause hypertension, hyperkalemia, and nephrotoxicity; therefore, check renal function tests. In addition, it may interact with and potentiate barbiturates, fentanyl, and muscle relaxants, especially vecuronium and atracurium.

   c. Azathioprine can cause bone marrow depression and hepatotoxicity; check liver function. It also has anticholinesterase effects and may prolong the action of succinylcholine and antagonize nondepolarizing relaxants.

   d. Prolonged steroid therapy demands the usual considerations and appropriate supplementation.

   e. OKT3, usually used to treat rejection crises, can cause anaphylaxis as well as acute pulmonary edema, especially if fluid overload is present. It may also cause psychiatric disturbances.

3. Children have a relatively high rate of noncompliance with their antirejection therapy. This may lead to problems with graft rejection.

Special Considerations for the Patient with a Transplanted Heart

Patients with a denervated transplanted heart have altered cardiac function.

1. Effects normally mediated via the autonomic nervous system are absent (e.g., vagal slowing, baroreceptor responses to blood pressure changes). Changes in heart rate as an index of light anesthesia or hypovolemia are unreliable.

2. Indirect drug effects that depend on autonomic pathways are absent (e.g., the chronotropic effects of atropine, pancuronium, or opioids).

3. Compensation for changes in blood volume and cardiac filling pressure is limited and delayed.

4. Coronary atherosclerosis is accelerated in transplanted hearts and may occur in children. In the denervated heart, ischemia may occur without pain and coronary angiography is required for diagnosis. Careful intraoperative ECG monitoring is essential.

The following are considerations for anesthesia in the child with a heart transplant:

1. The child should be carefully screened for signs of rejection, which if present may increase the risks of anesthesia and surgery. Signs include

   a. Poor appetite, irritability, fluid retention

   b. Decreased cardiac function on echocardiogram

   c. Low-voltage ECG

2. Practice meticulous asepsis. Avoid unnecessary cannulation; use only essential invasive monitoring lines.
3. Maintain normovolemia; ensure adequate fluid replacement.
4. Avoid high doses of drugs that have a direct cardiac depressant effect (e.g., halothane, lidocaine).
5. Maintain afterload; avoid agents and techniques that cause rapid changes in vascular tone.
6. If cardiotonic drugs are indicated, use direct-acting agents (e.g., isoproterenol, dopamine).

Most patients have been successfully managed using a narcotic- and relaxant-based anesthetic technique. Despite theoretic considerations of interaction between muscle relaxants and immunosuppressive therapy, the usual doses are often required (but neuromuscular blockade must be monitored).

Special Considerations for the Patient with a Transplanted Lung

Heart and lung transplantation may be performed for patients with cardiac disease complicated by pulmonary hypertension. Lung transplantation is performed in children with end-stage CF, primary pulmonary hypertension, or idiopathic pulmonary fibrosis. The transplanted lungs are prone to infection and also to obliterative bronchiolitis that progresses to respiratory failure.

Regular bronchial alveolar lavage with transbronchial biopsy is performed to monitor for infection or signs of rejection. General anesthesia usually is required. A technique using a propofol infusion and *cis*-atracurium with controlled ventilation has been found to be most satisfactory. The largest endotracheal tube that can easily be passed should be used. Many of these patients experience considerable dyspnea on emergence from anesthesia and are more comfortable if placed in a sitting position as they awaken. Secretions may also be troublesome.

Special Considerations for the Patient with a Transplanted Liver

After a successful liver transplantation, children can be expected to have normal metabolic functions and drug metabolism. Therefore any suitable anesthesia regimen can be used, and no agents are contraindicated. However, these children are prone to infections, particularly by viral agents (cytomegalovirus, Epstein-Barr virus, hepatitis virus), and require very careful aseptic precautions.

Those patients who have abnormal liver function can be expected to have abnormal drug distribution, protein binding, metabolism, and clearance. In addition they may have a coagulopathy. The PT is considered one of the most useful tests of hepatic function because it becomes prolonged before most other tests are abnormal. In these patients, anesthesia regimens should be carefully chosen; volatile agents may be used cautiously, but the response to opioids can be unpredictable. *Cis*-atracurium is the relaxant of choice.

Suggested Additional Reading

Cheng DCH and Ong DD: Anesthesia for non-cardiac surgery in heart transplanted patients. Can J Anaesth 40:981–986, 1993.

Black AE: Anesthesia for pediatric patients who have had a transplant. Int Anesthesiol Clin 33:107–123, 1995.

Chapter **7**

Postoperative Care and Pain Management

THE POSTANESTHESIA CARE UNIT

General Management

All patients must be placed in a lateral position for transport to the postanesthesia care unit (PACU); the anesthesiologist walks behind the cart or bed, in a good position to observe the child continuously. During transfer to the PACU there is a danger of respiratory obstruction, so be alert to this possibility. If the airway is in doubt, do not leave the operating room (OR). On route to the PACU, if the airway becomes precarious, apply digital pressure behind the pinna to sublux the temporomandibular joint (TMJ) and open the airway. All patients—other than absolutely healthy children having minor surgery—should have oxygen administered during transport. There is evidence from monitoring of oxygen saturation during transport that many children sustain a decrease in hemoglobin oxygen saturation at this time. A clear airway and good ventilation must be ensured. In the PACU, the anesthesiologist

1. Transfers the patient to the care of the nurses (*see below*) and explains the operative procedure as well as any complications of surgery or anesthesia.
2. Completes the anesthesia record.
3. Writes postoperative orders, including those for analgesics, intravenous fluids, and respiratory therapy.
4. Confirms the patient's vital signs on arrival as recorded by the receiving nurse.

In the PACU, every patient is given humidified oxygen via a face mask. The anesthesiologist should not hand over care of a patient until there is no doubt that the patient has a good airway, is ventilating well, and no longer needs a laryngeal mask airway or oropharyngeal airway. *A patient who still requires an oropharyngeal airway may still need an anesthesiologist.*

Remember that small infants (younger than 3 months of age) may not rapidly convert to mouth-breathing if the nasal passages are blocked (e.g., after cleft lip repair). If such obstruction occurs, insertion of an oropharyngeal airway or orogastric tube permits ventilation until the patient is fully awake.

The progress of recovery should be documented with the use of a postanesthesia scoring system along with regular recording of the vital signs. All patients should receive oxygen initially until they awaken and maintain an adequate saturation in room air. Oxygen saturation should be continuously monitored until the patient is fully awake and ready for discharge.

As soon as the child begins to waken, with stable vital signs and good pain control ensured, the parents should be allowed to come to the bedside. This decreases the child's anxiety in the PACU, reduces crying, and reduces the need for sedation.

After ketamine anesthesia, recovery should take place in a quiet area with minimal tactile and auditory stimulation. If, despite these precautions, hallucinations develop, give midazolam 0.05–0.1 mg/kg IV or diazepam (0.2–0.4 mg/kg IV).

Complications in the Postanesthesia Care Unit

Laryngospasm

Laryngospasm may occur and is more likely in those patients with blood or secretions in the pharynx. It should be managed by bag-and-mask ventilation with oxygen, maintaining slight positive pressure, and subluxation of the TMJ. Be ready to reintubate the trachea if necessary, and do not delay that procedure too long if desaturation progresses. Pulmonary edema may follow immediately on relief of severe laryngospasm. If it occurs, it should be treated with continued positive pressure ventilation.

Postoperative Stridor

Postoperative stridor, caused by subglottic edema, may occur, especially after endoscopy or after the unwise use of too large an endotracheal tube. Stridor is also more common in patients with Down syndrome and after surgery during which head movement occurred. Stridor usually appears within 30–60 minutes after extubation. The use of humidified oxygen and intravenous administration of dexamethasone (Decadron) may reduce subglottic edema. If stridor persists, administer racemic epinephrine by intermittent positive-pressure breathing for 15 minutes; this is usually efficacious. Very rarely, it may be necessary to reintubate a patient in the PACU for persistent severe stridor. In such cases a smaller-diameter tube may be appropriate.

Shivering and Rigidity

Shivering and rigidity are common during recovery from anesthesia; they greatly increase the metabolic rate and oxygen requirement. Shivering is often severe after halothane; if it causes concern (e.g., in an orthopaedic patient with a recently reduced fracture), an intravenous injection of methylphenidate HCl (Ritalin, 0.15–0.4 mg/kg) will abolish the symptoms.

Nausea and Vomiting

Postoperative nausea and vomiting may be troublesome in the recovery period; it is a leading cause of delayed discharge from the PACU or, more rarely, of unplanned admission of the day surgery patient. The incidence of postoperative nausea and vomiting can be significantly reduced by some general measures:

1. Avoid the indiscriminate use of narcotic analgesics; use other analgesic drugs (e.g., nonsteroidal anti-inflammatory drugs [NSAIDs]) or regional analgesia whenever possible.
2. Do not "push" fluids postoperatively; wait until the patient asks for them or is obviously thirsty.
3. Do not rush to mobilize the patient, especially after eye surgery.

When nausea and vomiting can be anticipated (e.g., eye surgery, tonsillectomy), the incidence can be reduced by the choice of anesthesia regimen (e.g., propofol) or by the prophylactic use of antiemetics. In those patients with unexpected nausea and vomiting, rescue medication with an antiemetic drug is necessary (Table 7–1).

Dimenhydrinate and metoclopramide have both been shown to be

Table 7–1. Antiemetic Drugs and Intravenous Doses

Drug	Dose
Dimenhydrinate	0.5 mg/kg
Metoclopramide	0.15 mg/kg
Droperidol	0.075 mg/kg
Ondansetron	0.1 mg/kg
Granisetron	10–20 µg/kg
Dexamethasone	0.15 mg/kg (maximum, 8 mg)

moderately effective and cause little sedation. Droperidol in doses adequate to combat nausea and vomiting may cause sedation, with delayed recovery and discharge. Ondansetron and granisetron are probably the most effective agents for postoperative nausea and vomiting, but they are expensive. Dexamethasone is reported to be very effective, particularly in patients undergoing tonsillectomy and adenoidectomy.

Duration of Stay in the Postanesthesia Care Unit

Patients are kept in the PACU until they are fully awake and have recovered from the effects of anesthesia. As a general rule a minimum stay of 30 minutes or two sets of vital signs is required. Infants weighing less than 5 kg are usually kept in the PACU for a longer period or transferred to a monitored bed. Be alert for possible postoperative complications (e.g., stridor after surgery of or near the airway or after endoscopy; bleeding after a kidney or liver biopsy), and specify a longer stay in the PACU for such patients.

Patients staying longer than 1 hour must have deep-breathing and coughing exercises and be turned hourly. Each patient should be signed out of the PACU by an anesthesiologist.

Suggested Additional Reading

Fujii Y, Toyooka H, and Tanaka H: Effective dose of granisetron for preventing postoperative emesis in children. Can J Anaesth 43:660–667, 1996.

Hamid SK, Selby IR, Sikich N, and Lerman J: Vomiting after adenotonsillectomy in children: a comparison of ondansetron, dimenhydrinate, and placebo. Anesth Analg 86:496–500, 1998.

Larson PC: Laryngospasm—the best treatment. Anesthesiology 89:1293–1294, 1998.

Lee KWT and Downes JJ: Pulmonary edema secondary to laryngospasm in children. Anesthesiology 59:347–349, 1983.

Roy WL and Lerman J: Laryngospasm in paediatric anaesthesia. Can J Anaesth 35:93–98, 1988.

Schreiner MS, Nicholson SC, Martin T, and Whitney L: Should children drink before discharge from day surgery? Anesthesiology 76:528–533, 1992.

Splinter WM and Roberts DJ: Dexamethasone decreases vomiting by children after tonsillectomy. Anesth Analg 83:913–916, 1996.

Steward DJ: A simplified scoring system for the post-operative recovery room. Can Anaesth Soc J 22:111–113, 1975.

MANAGEMENT OF PAIN

The ability of infants and children to feel pain was misunderstood in the past, and this led to undertreatment of pain. It is now recognized that the biochemical and nervous components of the pain perception pathways are completely formed during fetal life and that even the preterm infant can feel pain. Furthermore, the adverse effects of unmodified pain have been documented even in very young infants. Studies suggest that inadequate treatment of pain in infants may lead to increased sensitivity to pain later in life.

There are many reasons why pediatric pain was undertreated in the past and why even today inadequate therapy is often applied:

1. Infants cannot tell us when they are in pain, and it is sometimes difficult to tell whether they are crying because they are in pain or for another reason.
2. The older child's response to pain differs from that of the adult; often these children are quiet and withdrawn, failing to announce their extreme discomfort.
3. In the days when intramuscular injection of a narcotic was the standard therapy for postoperative pain, children often feared the injection more than the pain and preferred to suffer in silence. This tended to perpetuate the myth that children do not feel pain as much as adults.
4. Physicians have been uncertain of the safety of the analgesic drugs given to infants. It was stated that infants are "exquisitely sensitive" to the respiratory depressant effects of morphine; this led to an ultraconservative approach in prescribing.
5. Many physicians, and especially those junior staff to whom the responsibility for pain management was customarily delegated, have been unsure of the correct dosage of analgesics for pediatric patients.
6. Nurses have tended to underestimate pain as well, but they have also overestimated the danger of the child's becoming addicted to potent analgesic drugs.

More recently a much greater understanding of childhood pain has been acquired. We know that all pediatric patients can experience pain, we are better equipped to assess pain levels, and we have better means to control pain. Postoperative pain management should be planned when the preoperative evaluation is performed, and it should be discussed with the patient and parents.

Assessment of Pain

The first essential in the optimal management of pediatric pain is to establish regular, objective pain level assessments that are recorded on the patient's medical record. In infants, the level of pain may be assessed by either physiologic or behavioral indices. Physiologic indices include tachycardia, tachypnea, increased blood pressure, and sweating. Of the behavioral indices, facial expression may be most reliable, but cry characteristics and body movement (especially flexion of the limbs) are also useful. The opinion of the parent and of the child's nurse in interpretation of these behavioral signs may be very useful. These indices are incorporated into a numeric scale that can be scored and recorded; an example is shown in Table 7–2.

Older children may be asked to report their pain level using one of a variety of visual analog scales, such as the Wong-Baker FACES Pain Rating Scale. They may also be asked to rate their pain on a color scale or to report it by coloring their pain on a body outline.

Table 7–2. A Pain Scale for Preverbal and Nonverbal Infants (FLACC Scale)

Category	Score		
	0	1	2
Face	No particular expression or smile	Occasional grimace or frown, withdrawn, disinterested	Frequent to constant quivering chin, clenched jaw
Legs	Normal position or relaxed	Uneasy, restless, tense	Kicking or legs drawn up
Activity	Lying quietly, normal position, moves easily	Squirming, shifting back and forth, tense	Arched, rigid or jerking
Cry	No cry (awake or asleep)	Moans or whimpers, occasional complaint.	Crying steadily, screams or sobs, frequent complaints
Consolability	Content, relaxed	Reassured by occasional touching, hugging, or being talked to; distractable	Difficult to console or comfort

Reproduced with permission of Merkel SI, et al: The FLACC: A behavioral scale for scoring postoperative pain in young children. Pediatr Nurs 23:392, 1997.

Wong-Baker FACES Pain Rating Scale

0	1	2	3	4	5
No Hurt	Hurts Little Bit	Hurts Little More	Hurts Even More	Hurts Whole Lot	Hurts Worst

Alternate coding					
0	2	4	6	8	10

Adolescents can be assessed with the use of standard adult self-report scales. Note, however, that at this age psychological and emotional factors may influence the response much than in younger children. *When treating pain at any age, it is essential to monitor the response to therapy with an objective scoring system.*

Suggested Additional Reading

Abu-Saad HH, Bours GJJW, Stevens B, and Hamers JPH: Assessment of pain in the neonate. Semin Neonatol 22:402–416, 1998.

Anand KJS and Hickey PR: Pain in the fetus and neonate. N Engl J Med 317:1321–1329, 1987.

Beyer JE and Wells N: The assessment of pain in children. Pediatr Clin North Am 36:837–854, 1989.

Merkel SI, Voepel-Lewis T, Shayevitz JR, and Malviya S: The FLACC: a behavioral scale for scoring postoperative pain in young children. Pediatric Nursing 23:293–297, 1997.

Schechter NL: The undertreatment of pain in children: an overview. Pediatr Clin North Am 36:781–794, 1989.

Taddio A, Katz J, Ilersich AL, and Koren G: Effect of neonatal circumcision on pain response during subsequent routine vaccination. Lancet 349:599–603, 1997.

POSTOPERATIVE PAIN

The provision of optimal postoperative analgesia for every infant and child should be the objective: postoperative pain hurts and may have adverse physiologic and psychological effects. Good pain relief minimizes the metabolic rate for oxygen, reduces cardiorespiratory demands, promotes early ambulation, and speeds recovery. In addition, it has been shown that postoperative emotional disturbance is reduced if pain is well controlled. There is now a variety of means to combat postoperative pain, and most can be applied to pediatric patients. Plan for optimal postoperative pain control when the patient is first seen preoperatively; some of the methods that might be chosen require advance planning. Discuss the plans for postoperative pain management with the parents and with those children who are old enough to understand.

Systemic Analgesic Drugs

After minor procedures, when no regional or local analgesia regimen is possible, the use of a systemic analgesic is indicated. Dosages in common use are listed in Table 7–3.

The appropriate drug should be chosen for the magnitude of the pain, and a satisfactory effect should be confirmed. It is preferable to administer the first dose of the analgesic drug before the patient emerges from general anesthesia—for example, for tonsillectomy give 1.5 mg/kg of meperidine IM, and for minor superficial surgery give 30–40 mg/kg acetaminophen PR after induction of anesthesia. Avoid ordering intramuscular injections for awake patients; give analgesics by the intravenous, rectal, or oral route.

Acetaminophen

Acetaminophen is a mild analgesic and antipyretic drug, but it provides good analgesia after minor procedures, especially if given before the surgery. It is considered safe in neonates, but metabolism and elimination are delayed in neonates compared with adults, so repeat doses should be given at 6- rather than 4-hour intervals. Excessive doses can cause hepatic failure; the total dose should not exceed 100 mg/kg/day. Make sure that clear instructions are given to parents about dosage after the child goes home. Hepatic damage has also been reported at lower dose levels when acetaminophen was given to debilitated children; it is wise to avoid the drug in such cases. After major surgery, acetaminophen combined with narcotics reduces the need for the latter, thereby reducing the risk of respiratory depression. Acetaminophen does not affect coagulation of the blood.

Codeine

Codeine has been used to treat moderate pain. It may be given intramuscularly or orally, but it must not be given intravenously, because apnea and severe hypotension may occur. Codeine has been considered a safe drug for infants and children, but respiratory depression similar to that associated with morphine use may occur, especially after repeated doses.

Table 7–3. Common Dosages for Systemic Analgesic Drugs

For minor procedures
    Acetaminophen, 10–20 mg/kg PO or 30–40 mg/kg PR
    Codeine, 1–1.5 mg/kg IM or PO q4h
    Ibuprofen, 5–10 mg/kg PO
    Ketorolac, 1 mg/kg IM
For more major procedures
    Meperidine, 1 mg/kg IM q4h or 0.2 mg/kg IV q2h
    Morphine, 0.1–0.2 mg/kg IM q4h

A dose of 1–1.5 mg/kg IM or PO (maximum, 60 mg) is usually recommended.

Ibuprofen

Ibuprofen, an NSAID, may be given by the oral or rectal route. It has been found effective in reducing the child's requirements for narcotic analgesics postoperatively. However, ibuprofen can cause gastrointestinal upset (nausea, vomiting, diarrhea), and it also affects platelet aggregation, which could result in increased bleeding.

Ketorolac

Ketorolac is another NSAID; its potent analgesic effects may rival those of morphine without the respiratory depressant effects of the latter. When given before surgery, ketorolac 1 mg/kg IV appears to provide postoperative analgesia comparable to 0.1 mg/kg of morphine. In common with other NSAIDs, ketorolac inhibits platelet aggregation and is not recommended where bleeding may be a problem. Other serious although uncommon potential side effects include gastrointestinal hemorrhage, interstitial nephritis, and acute renal failure.

Continuous Narcotic Infusions

Morphine by continuous infusion, using a dilute solution and a syringe pump, provides for even levels of analgesia with good sedation and is appropriate for many patients after major surgery. The patient must have close nursing supervision and be monitored by pulse oximeter when this technique is used. The dose administered should be frequently titrated against the observed pain level.

Recommended doses:

Children older than 1 year:	Loading dose, 0.1 mg/kg IV
	Infusion,* 10–30 μg/kg/hr
Infants younger than 1 year:	Loading dose, 0.05 mg/kg
	Infusion, 5–15 μg/kg/hr

Lower rates of infusion may be adequate after cardiac surgery, when the clearance rates for morphine have been demonstrated to be lower.

Infants receiving a morphine infusion should be carefully monitored during the infusion and for 24 hours after the infusion is discontinued to detect any depression of ventilation.

Suggested Additional Reading

Anderson BJ: What we don't know about paracetamol in children. Paediatr Anaesth 8:451–460, 1998.

---

*An infusion can be prepared by adding 1 mg of morphine for each kilogram body weight to 100 ml of fluid. This solution, infused at 1 ml/hr, will equal 10 μg/kg/hr. For some patients, the loading dose may have to be repeated to establish an initial satisfactory level of analgesia.

Chay PCW, Duffy BJ, and Walker JS: Pharmacokinetic-pharmacodynamic relationships of morphine in neonates. Clin Pharmacol Ther 51:334–342, 1992.

Esmail Z, Montgomery C, Court C, et al.: Efficacy and complications of morphine infusions in postoperative paediatric patients. Paediatr Anaesth 9:321–328, 1999.

Gaudreault P, Guay J, Nicol O, et al.: Pharmacokinetics and clinical efficacy of intrarectal solution of acetaminophen. Can J Anaesth 35:149–152, 1988.

Heubi JE, Barbacci MB, and Zimmerman HJ: Therapeutic misadventures with acetaminophen: Hepatotoxicity after multiple doses in children. J Pediatr 132:22–27, 1998.

Koren G, Butt W, Chinyanga H, et al.: Postoperative morphine infusion in new-born infants: assessment of disposition characteristics and safety. J Pediatr 107:963–967, 1985.

Lynn AM, Opheim KE, and Tyler DC: Morphine infusion after pediatric cardiac surgery. Crit Care Med 12:863–866, 1984.

Maunuksela EL, Ryhanen P, and Janhunen L: Efficacy of rectal ibuprofen in controlling postoperative pain in children. Can J Anaesth 39:226–230, 1992.

Miller RP, Roberts RJ, and Fischer LJ: Acetaminophen elimination kinetics in neonates, children, and adults. Clin Pharmacol Ther 19:284–294, 1976.

Watcha MF, Jones MB, Lagueruela RG, et al.: Comparison of ketorolac and morphine as adjuvants during pediatric surgery. Anesthesiology 76:368–372, 1992.

Patient-Controlled Analgesia

Pediatric patients older than 5 years of age are able to manage a patient-controlled analgesia (PCA) system and so obtain good pain relief. Children may especially benefit from PCA; they do not have to ask for pain relief and can be "in control." Most children are familiar with computer games and have no problem mastering the principles of PCA. It is important that a safe regimen be established and that both child and parents be reassured that the system has an appropriate lockout time and total dosage safeguards. The parents should be warned not to trigger the system for the child. All children should have a loading dose of opioids. Whether a background infusion is required to supplement boluses has been controversial, but in children a slow continuous infusion with PCA supplements may give the best results, in terms of both pain control and sleep pattern.

The regimen used should be modified for the type of surgery; patients who have had orthopaedic operations have higher morphine requirements than those who have had general surgery, and those who have had spinal surgery require even higher doses. It is convenient to adjust the background infusion rate to suit the type of surgery (Table 7–4).

Side effects of PCA include the following:

1. *Nausea and vomiting:* This may be troublesome and may require reduction of dosage and administration of promethazine (0.25–0.5 mg/kg). Be aware that promethazine may produce increased sedation.

2. *Excessive sedation:* Monitor patients carefully and have naloxone ready for administration in the treatment unit. Be alert to the possibility that someone who is unaware that the patient is receiving PCA may order a "stat dose" of another analgesic drug and thereby produce

Table 7–4. Suitable Regimens for Patient-Controlled Analgesia

Initial bolus doses	0.1–0.2 mg/kg IV until settled
PCA bolus dose	10 μg/kg
Lockout period	10 min
Background infusion	
For general surgery	20 μg/kg/hr
For orthopaedic surgery	25 μg/kg/hr
For spinal surgery	40 μg/kg/hr
Maximum hourly dose	100 μg/kg

depression. Write specific orders on the charts of PCA patients that they are to have no additional drugs without the knowledge of the PCA team.

Suggested Additional Reading

Gillespie JA and Morton NS: Patient controlled analgesia for children: a review. Paediatr Anaesth 2:51–59, 1992.

Peters JWB, Bandell Hoekstra IENG, Huijer Abu-Saad H, et al.: Patient controlled analgesia in children and adolescents: a randomized controlled trial. Paediatr Anaesth 9:235–241, 1999.

Regional Analgesia for Postoperative Pain

The pain that occurs after many pediatric procedures can be effectively treated by regional analgesic techniques, and these should be used whenever possible. Frequently, no other or only mild analgesics (e.g., acetaminophen) will be required. In this manner the side effects of narcotics are avoided and the child rapidly returns to full activity after minor surgery. Provision should be made, however, for transition to systemic analgesics after the block wears off. Studies have shown that significant pain may occur at this time, especially in outpatients. The parent should be carefully instructed to administer an analgesic drug (e.g., acetaminophen) in anticipation of this need.

After major surgery, appropriate nerve blocks (e.g., intercostal nerve block) using local analgesic drugs may permit a reduction of the narcotic dosage and earlier mobilization of the patient.

The possibility that a regional block established before the surgery (preemptive analgesia) may modulate total postoperative pain by preventing biochemical changes ("windup") within the central nervous system is appealing, but the results of well-designed studies have been disappointing. Regional block performed before the commencement of surgery does provide some intraoperative analgesia and therefore reduces the need for general anesthetic drugs. It also ensures that the block is well established before the patient emerges from anesthesia.

Peripheral Nerve Block or Local Infiltration

The following blocks are commonly used in pediatric patients; for details of technique, see pages 129–147 and the articles listed at the end of this section. Bupivacaine or ropivacaine to a maximum of 3 mg/kg is commonly used. More prolonged analgesia may be obtained if dextran 40 is mixed with the local anesthetic (e.g., equal volumes of 0.5% bupivacaine and dextran 40). In children, peripheral nerve block has been shown to have the lowest incidence of complications compared with other techniques for regional analgesia.

1. For thoracotomy or flank incisions (e.g., renal), block the appropriate intercostal nerves using 1–2 ml of 0.25% bupivacaine. Use equal volumes of dextran 40 and 0.5% bupivacaine to produce a more prolonged block.
2. For inguinal surgery, block the ilioinguinal and iliohypogastric nerves just medial to the anterior superior iliac spine. This block has been shown to be as effective as caudal analgesia for such procedures.
3. For umbilical surgery, block the tenth intercostal nerve bilaterally.
4. For circumcision, perform a penile nerve block or use topical lidocaine gel, which may also be effective.
5. Local infiltration of the incision site before surgery, using 0.125% bupivacaine, may provide pain relief when there is no suitable nerve to block. Preincisional infiltration of the tonsils with 0.25% bupivacaine with epinephrine reduces postoperative pain and discomfort on swallowing.

Caudal Analgesia

Caudal analgesia is useful for many abdominal, perineal, and lower limb procedures. Insertion of a catheter provides for continued pain relief (*see* page 133).

Thoracic or Lumbar Epidural Analgesia

Continuous epidural analgesia has been used to provide pain relief after thoracic, abdominal, perineal, and lower limb surgery. Bupivacaine is commonly used and may be delivered by continuous infusion via an epidural catheter or by intermittent top-up doses. Lower infusion rates should be used for infants, because they metabolize bupivacaine less rapidly (Table 7–5); it has been suggested that intermittent top-up doses may be safer in small infants.

All patients must have constant nursing observation. The level of analgesia should be monitored and the patient should be observed for early signs of toxicity (e.g., restlessness, twitching, tinnitus, lightheadedness).

Suggested Additional Reading

Dalens B and Hasnaoui A: Caudal anesthesia in pediatric surgery: success rate and adverse effects in 750 consecutive patients. Anesth Analg 68:83–89, 1989.

Dalens B, Tanguy A, and Haberer JP: Lumbar epidural anesthesia for operative and postoperative pain relief in infants and young children. Anesth Analg 65:1069–1073, 1986.

Table 7–5. Suggested Dosages for Epidural Analgesics

Bupivacaine	
Loading dose (0.25%)	0.5 ml/kg
Infusion (0.125%)	0.1–0.3 ml/kg/hr (children)
	0.05–0.1 ml/kg/hr (infants)
Morphine	
Single-shot lumbar or caudal injection	0.05–0.1 mg/kg of preservative-free morphine in up to 15 ml preservative-free saline
Fentanyl	
Infusion	0.5–2.0 µg/kg/hr
PCA doses	0.5–1.0 µg/kg (lockout period, 15 min)

Desparmet J, Meistelman C, Barre J, and Saint-Maurice C: Continuous epidural infusion of bupivacaine for postoperative pain relief in children. Anesthesiology 67:108–110, 1987.

Giaufre E, Dalens B, and Gombert A: Epidemiology and morbidity of regional anesthesia in children: a one-year prospective survey of the French Language Society of Pediatric Anesthesiologists. Anesth Analg 83:904–912, 1996.

Rice LJ, Pudimat MA, and Hannalah RS: Timing of caudal block placement in relation to surgery does not affect duration of postoperative analgesia in paediatric ambulatory patients. Can J Anaesth 37:429–431, 1990.

Shelley MP: Intercostal nerve block for children. Anaesthesia 42:591–592, 1987.

Tree-Trakarn T and Pirayavaraporn S: Postoperative pain relief for circumcision in children: comparison among morphine, nerve block and topical analgesia. Anesthesiology 62:519–522, 1985.

Uemura A and Yamashita M: A formula for determining the distance from the skin to the lumbar epidural space in infants and children. Pediatr Anaesth 2:305–307, 1992.

Wolf A, Valley RD, Fear DW, et al.: The minimum effective concentration of bupivacaine for caudal analgesia after surgery in pediatrics. Anesthesiology 67:A509, 1987.

Epidural Narcotics

Epidural narcotic analgesics by the lumbar or the caudal route have been shown to be effective after major cardiac, general, urologic, or orthopaedic surgery in children. Some investigators claim that more effective pain relief may be obtained if the narcotic is administered before surgery. A single dose of morphine provides analgesia for up to 18 hours, at which time the dose can be repeated if necessary.

The complications seen are similar to those observed in adults, with pruritus, urinary retention, and nausea being the most common. Ventilatory depression may occur, and the ventilatory response to carbon dioxide is depressed for up to 24 hours.

Fentanyl administered by the lumbar or caudal epidural route may be less likely to cause respiratory depression because it has increased fat solubility and consequently more limited distribution and decreased rostral spread. Fentanyl may be added to continuous infusions of bupivacaine or given alone by epidural infusion, which may be by PCA in older children (see Table 7–5).

All patients should receive appropriate nursing observation and should be monitored by a cardiorespiratory monitor and pulse oximeter. Nurses should be instructed to check the patient's level of consciousness frequently; increased somnolence is the most reliable early sign of impending respiratory depression. The patient should be observed for at least 24 hours after the last administration of an epidural narcotic.

Common complications include the following:

1. *Pruritus:* This may be controlled without loss of analgesia by the use of small bolus doses of naloxone (1–2 μg/kg) or by a naloxone infusion (1–2 μg/kg/hr). A very small dose of propofol has also been reported to relieve pruritus.
2. *Urinary retention:* This may require catheterization; for this reason, epidural narcotics may be contraindicated if it is necessary to avoid catheterization.
3. *Nausea and vomiting:* This may be improved by the use of antiemetics, metoclopramide, naloxone, or a scopolamine patch.
4. *Respiratory depression:* This effect is more rare and may occur later (up to 24 hours). It is particularly a danger if systemic narcotics are concurrently administered. It may be reversed by the administration of naloxone.

Suggested Additional Reading

Irving GA, Butt AD, and Van Der Veen B: A comparison of caudal morphine given pre or post surgery for postoperative analgesia in children. Pediatr Anaesth 3:217–221, 1993.

Krane EJ, Jacobson LE, Lynn AM, et al.: Caudal morphine for postoperative analgesia in children. Anesth Analg 66:647–653, 1987.

Rose JB, Francis MC, and Kettrick RG: Continuous naloxone infusion in paediatric patients with pruritus associated with epidural morphine. Pediatr Anaesth 3:255–258, 1993.

Tyler DC and Krane EJ: Epidural opioids in children. J Pediatr Surg 24:469–473, 1989.

Anesthesia for Specific Procedures

Chapter **8**

Neurosurgery and Invasive Neuroradiology

GENERAL PRINCIPLES

1. Perioperative management must be planned to minimize the possibility of increasing the intracranial pressure (ICP) and to ensure optimal operating conditions for the neurosurgeon.
2. Light general anesthesia is adequate for neurosurgical operations. Additional techniques may be required to prevent or treat increased ICP. All anesthetic drugs used should be short-acting, capable of being rapidly eliminated. This ensures that the patient speedily emerges from anesthesia, permitting accurate, continuous postoperative neurosurgical assessment.
3. Prior infiltration of the scalp incision site with bupivacaine with epinephrine by the surgeon reduces blood loss, blunts any response to the initial incision, reduces the need for general anesthetic drugs, and possibly minimizes postoperative pain.
4. Postoperative pain after intracranial surgery must be effectively treated, but respiratory depression must be avoided. For major procedures, a morphine infusion may be titrated to achieve satisfactory analgesia. For minor procedures, codeine (oral or intramuscular) or acetaminophen may suffice.
5. Some patients may benefit from a period of postoperative controlled ventilation after major intracranial surgery.

Intracranial Physiology and Pathophysiology

1. Normally, autoregulation of the caliber of the cerebral vessels ensures maintenance of constant blood flow during alterations in mean arterial blood pressure (BP). This system operates throughout a wide range of systemic BPs (65–180 mmHg in adults, and even as low as 40–50 mmHg in the supine infant).
2. Cerebral blood flow (CBF) is higher in infants and children (90–100 ml per 100 g per minute) than in adults (50–60 ml per 100 g per minute). CBF varies directly with changes in arterial carbon dioxide tension ($PaCO_2$) while the latter is between 20 and 80 mmHg. A 1-mm change in $PaCO_2$ leads to a 4% change in CBF.
3. Vasodilation of normal reactive cerebral vessels reduces blood flow in low-resistance vessels—for example, arteriovenous (AV) malformations and vascular tumors—and in areas that have lost autoregulation—for example, infection and trauma (intracerebral steal).
4. Vasoconstriction of normal reactive cerebral vessels has the opposite effect (inverse intracerebral steal).
5. The total volume of the intracranial contents cannot alter. However, any of its three constituents—blood, cerebrospinal fluid (CSF), and brain tissue—can increase or decrease if compensated by an equal and opposite change in the volumes of the others (revised Munro-Kelly hypothesis).
6. The effect of a space-occupying lesion on ICP depends on its volume and rate of expansion. Initially, the lesion displaces CSF and/or

venous blood from the skull, and ICP increases slowly if at all. As expansion continues, compensation is no longer possible, and small increases in volume result in progressively larger increases in ICP. With a rapidly expanding lesion (e.g., intracranial bleeding), pressure increases rapidly from the outset.

7. Infants have a less rigid skull than adults; an increase in the contents may be accommodated by expansion of the fontanels and separation of the suture lines. The ICP may be estimated by palpation of the fontanel.

Effects of Specific Anesthetic Drugs on Intracranial Physiology

1. All inhalation agents may increase CBF and ICP:
   a. Nitrous oxide (N_2O) may cause a very small increase in CBF but has been used successfully for neurosurgery for many years. It may increase ICP if air is present within the cranium and in these circumstances is contraindicated.
   b. Sevoflurane increases CBF less than isoflurane, which in turn has less effect than halothane. Desflurane is a more potent cerebral vasodilator than the other volatile agents.
   c. Cerebral autoregulation during changes in arterial BP is lost with higher concentrations of volatile agents, but the response to changes in carbon dioxide tension (PCO_2) is retained. Therefore hyperventilation tends to reverse the effect of the agent on CBF. Autoregulation appears to be preserved at 1 minimum alveolar concentration (1 MAC) of isoflurane or sevoflurane anesthesia.
   d. Hypocarbia tends to modify or reverse the effects of agents that increase CBF (e.g., halothane, isoflurane, sevoflurane). Prior induction of hypocapnia minimizes the increase in ICP with halothane. Isoflurane (1 MAC) increases CBF less than halothane, and during isoflurane anesthesia the CBF returns to control levels more rapidly with hyperventilation. Sevoflurane has the least effect on CBF and ICP.
   e. The cerebral metabolic rate for oxygen ($CMRO_2$) is reduced by halothane, isoflurane, and sevoflurane. Isoflurane and sevoflurane at higher concentrations may provide some cerebral protection.
2. Intravenous anesthetic agents (with the notable exception of ketamine) either have no effect on CBF or decrease it, but hypercarbia tends to modify or reverse these effects:
   a. Thiopental reduces ICP and therefore is an ideal induction agent in neurosurgery. It does not prevent an increase in BP and ICP during laryngoscopy and intubation; these may, however, be attenuated by prior administration of lidocaine 1–1.5 mg/kg IV.
   b. Propofol reduces CBF and $CMRO_2$, preserves autoregulation, and may offer some cerebral protection. Induction doses may cause some hypotension but also blunt the responses to laryngoscopy and intubation.

   c. The narcotic analgesics fentanyl and sufentanil have little effect
      on CBF provided that ventilation is maintained. Autoregulation
      and the cerebrovascular response to $PaCO_2$ are also maintained.
      Alfentanil has been demonstrated to increase CSF pressure in
      patients with cerebral tumors.

   d. Ketamine increases CBF and $CMRO_2$; CSF pressure is increased.
      This drug should not be used in neurosurgical patients with
      raised ICP.

   e. Midazolam and diazepam decrease CBF, $CMRO_2$, and ICP and
      may control seizures. Flumazenil, which antagonizes
      benzodiazepines, also antagonizes their effects on CBF and ICP.
      Therefore, it should be used with caution.

3. Nondepolarizing muscle relaxants have no direct effect on CBF.
   (Vasodilation resulting from histamine release due to *d*-tubocurarine,
   atracurium, or rapacurium is a possible exception.)

4. Succinylcholine may very slightly elevate CBF and ICP in patients
   with a space-occupying lesion; this response may be attenuated by
   prior administration of a small dose of a nondepolarizing relaxant
   drug. Hyperkalemia may occur if succinylcholine is given to patients
   with cerebral trauma and some other central nervous system
   diseases, including paraplegia, encephalitis, and subarachnoid
   hemorrhage.

5. Sodium nitroprusside, nitroglycerin, adenosine, and the calcium
   channel-blocking drugs impair cerebral autoregulation and may
   increase CBF and ICP.

6. Dexamethasone (0.15 mg/kg IV to a maximum of 10 mg) may
   decrease focal cerebral edema in response to surgical trauma of
   brain tissue.

7. If an independent vasodilator effect is absent, drugs that depress
   neuronal function decrease CBF.

8. Drugs that enhance neuronal function increase CBF.

9. Somatosensory evoked potentials (SSEPs), which may be used to
   monitor brain or spinal cord function, are depressed by volatile
   anesthetic agents if these agents are given in more than minimal
   concentration. Fentanyl and sufentanil have little effect on SSEPs.

ANESTHESIA MANAGEMENT

Premedication

Patients with increased ICP should not receive any drug that can depress
respiration, prolong recovery, or hamper postoperative assessment.
Therefore, with one exception *(see below)*, do not give heavy sedative
premedication to patients undergoing craniotomy. Some patients may
benefit from a small dose of midazolam to calm them before surgery,
but they should be closely observed. Patients with normal ICP who are
undergoing elective or noncranial surgery (e.g., laminectomy) may be
given the usual dose of oral midazolam before anesthesia.

   Exception. Patients with a vascular aneurysm or AV malformation,
especially if there is a history of hemorrhage, should have sedative

premedication. Midazolam may be given intravenously by the anesthesiologist in the ward or in the intensive care unit. The patient is then closely observed and the dose is repeated if necessary before the patient is brought to the operating room (OR).

EMLA cream or amethocaine gel (Ametop) should be applied to the area over a selected vein for intravenous access.

Induction of Anesthesia

Management during induction of anesthesia should be planned to minimize changes in ICP caused by hypoxia or hypercapnia, the effects of anesthetic drugs, or instrumentation of the airway.

Gentle preoxygenation preceding intravenous induction, using thiopental or propofol, and followed by a muscle relaxant to facilitate intubation and ensure optimal ventilation, is preferred. Lidocaine (1–1.5 mg/ kg IV) may be given 3 minutes before intubation to minimize changes in ICP associated with this procedure.

Patients with vascular anomalies should be induced with thiopental or propofol; anesthesia should then be deepened with an inhalation agent, using gentle controlled ventilation to avoid hypercapnia. A generous dose of a suitable relaxant and lidocaine 1.5 mg/kg IV are given before intubation. The blood pressure is carefully monitored during induction to watch for hypertension, which should be treated.

Some patients undergoing emergency surgery have a full stomach and should have a rapid sequence induction using succinylcholine with all precautions to avoid aspiration.

For surgery in the prone position, for small infants, and for any procedures that entail changes in position, use a nasotracheal tube. (An orotracheal tube may kink in the prone patient or become dislodged if saliva loosens the adhesive tape; a nasotracheal tube is easier to secure firmly and accurately in the infant.) For surgery on older children in the supine or lateral position, use an armored orotracheal tube; throat packing placed in the mouth limits the flow of saliva from the mouth.

N.B. Sudden preoperative apnea may occur in neurosurgical patients awaiting operation and may indicate acutely raised ICP. If this occurs, hyperventilate the patient with oxygen and advise the surgeon so that a CSF tap can be performed immediately.

Maintenance

Volatile anesthetic agents may increase CBF; therefore, they should be used in the lowest concentration compatible with adequate anesthesia and should be accompanied by muscle relaxant drugs and moderate hyperventilation. Otherwise, N_2O together with short-acting narcotics (e.g., fentanyl, sufentanil), which ensure rapid postoperative recovery, may be preferred. Deep anesthesia is unnecessary. Propofol infusions may be a useful alternative in some patients, particularly toward the end of a long procedure when other agents have been discontinued to provide for rapid emergence.

Ventilation

Controlled hyperventilation is used to decrease brain bulk and ICP during intracranial surgery and to improve the quality of cerebral arteriograms during neuroradiology. A $PaCO_2$ of 27–30 mmHg is preferred during controlled ventilation.

Patient Monitoring

The patient should be monitored as follows:

1. Esophageal stethoscope, pulse oximeter, automated BP cuff
2. Continuous recording of body temperature (esophageal or rectal)
3. Electrocardiogram (ECG)
4. End-tidal carbon dioxide monitor; this is useful both as a guide to the adequacy of ventilation and as a means of detecting air embolism.
5. For major neurosurgery, an arterial line should be inserted.
6. Measurement of urinary output via catheter, during all major neurosurgery and if diuretics may be given
7. A precordial Doppler flowmeter should be used for operations when air embolism is a danger. This includes those performed with the patient in the sitting or head-up position and all major cranial reconstructions (including cranioplasty for craniosynostosis). The Doppler probe should be placed over the right atrium (second right interspace adjacent to the sternum).
8. A central venous catheter may be inserted both to monitor central venous pressure (CVP) and to attempt to aspirate air should embolism occur.

INTRAVENOUS THERAPY AND CONTROL OF INTRACRANIAL PRESSURE

A very reliable intravenous cannula is essential for pediatric neurosurgical patients; a 22-gauge cannula is used for infants, an 18-gauge cannula for older children.

General Rules for Intravenous Therapy

1. Avoid giving hypoosmolar fluids, because they increase brain edema; use normal saline.
2. Avoid dextrose-containing solutions except for documented hypoglycemia. Dextrose administration may increase the risk of neurologic damage secondary to local ischemia, including that caused by surgical retraction. If there is concern that hypoglycemia might result (e.g., in infants), regular blood glucose determinations should be performed.
3. Maintain the intravascular volume but avoid excessive fluid administration; third-space losses are very small in neurosurgical

patients. Use isotonic fluids; normal saline is preferred because it maintains the osmolarity of the intravascular compartment and minimizes cerebral edema formation. In addition, the syndrome of inappropriate antidiuretic hormone secretion (SIADH) may follow neurosurgical procedures and may result in hyponatremia; the use of hypotonic solutions adds to this danger.

4. Blood losses are difficult to measure; therefore, replace volumes, using cardiovascular indices (heart rate, BP, and CVP) as a guide. Give normal saline as necessary to replace fluid deficits and maintain intravascular volume. Colloid solutions or blood may be required for extensive losses *(see below)*.

Control of ICP and Reduction of Brain Volume

Most important in the conduct of neuroanesthesia is to ensure that the surgeon has absolutely optimal intracranial operating conditions. This can be ensured as follows:

1. Avoid any episodes of underventilation or hypoxemia during the induction process.
2. Provide a clear, unobstructed airway at all times. The largest endotracheal tube that will pass easily should be used. It should be positioned so that there is no possibility of kinking or compression. Reinforced tubes should be used where applicable.
3. Provide hyperventilation to a $PaCO_2$ of ± 30 mmHg.
4. A slight head-up tilt is preferred (15°); veins in the neck should be totally unobstructed.
5. Provide furosemide 0.5 mg/kg IV followed by mannitol 20% (0.5–1 g/kg) infused over 20–30 minutes as the skull is being opened.

After a diuretic is used, the schedule of fluid therapy depends also on the urine output. When urine volume equals 10% of the estimated blood volume (EBV), further urine losses are replaced (volume for volume) with normal saline. Subsequently, serum electrolyte determinations should be made to exclude abnormalities and guide replacements.

Blood Replacement

Because blood loss during neurosurgery cannot be measured accurately, it must be gauged clinically from observation of the amount of bleeding and measurement of the patient's cardiovascular indices. The systolic BP must be monitored carefully; fluid replacements should maintain it at 60 mmHg in infants and 70–80 mmHg in larger children. (**Note:** The latter may lose up to 20% of EBV without a fall in BP.) When surgery is complete but before the dura is closed, enough fluid is given to return the arterial pressure to the preloss level. During closure, a fluid volume equal to 10% of the EBV is given. The decision to transfuse blood may be based on determination of the hematocrit or clinical judgment of the losses that are occurring in relation to the allowable blood loss.

If major blood transfusion has been necessary, particularly in small infants, serum Ca^{++} may fall. Hypotension unresponsive to further volume replacement should be treated with calcium gluconate.

Hypotensive Techniques

A safe range of systolic BP in the supine position is 50–65 mmHg in children up to 10 years of age and 70–75 mmHg in older children. If the patient is tilted head-up, position the transducer at the level of the head.

Drugs to Induce Hypotension

1. *Isoflurane.* The inspired concentration can be increased progressively until the desired pressure is obtained. This method is easy to apply and results in very stable BP levels.
2. *Sodium nitroprusside.* It has been widely used to induce hypotension but may result in tachyphylaxis, often results in wide swings in pressure, and in large doses may cause toxic effects. Because sodium nitroprusside (SNP) interferes with cerebral autoregulation and may increase ICP, its infusion should not be commenced until the skull is opened.

Air Embolism

Air embolism is a particular hazard when surgery is performed with the patient in the sitting position, but it may also occur when the patient is prone or supine if the head is at all elevated. It is relatively common during craniosynostosis repair and has also occurred during laminectomy. Air may be drawn in rapidly if a venous sinus is entered, or it may trickle in through veins within the bone. Air embolism detected by Doppler ultrasonography has a similar incidence in children and in adults but is more likely to produce cardiovascular instability in children.

Embolism usually occurs during opening of the skull. The signs, in order of decreasing sensitivity, include the following:

1. Changes in Doppler ultrasound over the precordium/appearance on transesophageal echocardiogram
2. Sudden decrease in end-tidal carbon dioxide level (or increase in end-tidal nitrogen level)
3. Hypotension
4. Change in heart sounds

Early diagnosis and rapid therapy are required to prevent a serious outcome.

1. Inform the surgeon, who will compress and/or flood the wound to prevent the entrainment of further air.
2. Lower the head; this increases the venous pressure at the wound and augments venous return from the legs.
3. Compress the jugular veins in the neck.

4. Ventilate with 100% O_2; discontinue N_2O to prevent further expansion of air emboli within the bloodstream.
5. Attempt to aspirate air via the central catheter; this is successful in fewer than 60% of cases.
6. Apply cardiopulmonary resuscitation and other measures (e.g., inotropes) as required.

Postoperative Considerations

All patients should be fully recovered from the effects of anesthetic drugs and awake at completion of the procedure. Extubation should be smooth, without coughing or bucking; this can be facilitated by giving lidocaine 1.5 mg/kg IV. If the patient remains unresponsive or any ventilatory depression is present, the endotracheal tube should be left in and controlled ventilation continued until the cause is determined. In some instances after major neurosurgery, it may be preferable to continue with controlled ventilation into the postoperative period and extubate the patient later.

Postoperative nursing care should include routine monitoring of neurologic signs. The fluid status should be carefully monitored, because regulatory mechanisms (e.g., antidiuretic hormone levels) may be altered after craniotomy.

Suggested Additional Reading

Cucchiara RF and Bowers B: Air embolism in children undergoing suboccipital craniotomy. Anesthesiology 57:338–339, 1982.

Faberowski LW, Black S, and Mickle JP: Incidence of venous air embolism during craniectomy for craniosynostosis repair. Anesthesiology 92:20–23, 2000.

Hammer GB and Krane EJ: Perioperative care of the neurosurgical pediatric patient. Int Anesthesiol Clin 34:55–71, 1996.

Lam AM and Gelb AW: Cardiovascular effects of isoflurane-induced hypotension for cerebral aneurysm surgery. Anesth Analg 62:742, 1983.

Meridy HW, Creighton RE, and Humphreys RP: Complications during neurosurgery in the prone position in children. Can Anaesth Soc J 21:445, 1974.

Hydrocephalus

Hydrocephalus may be caused by a congenital defect (e.g., Arnold-Chiari malformation, aqueduct stenosis) or by acquired disease (e.g., hemorrhage, infection, tumor). In the newborn, hydrocephalus may be secondary to the Arnold-Chiari malformation. (In many cases it is accompanied by meningomyelocele; this combined defect is present in 1–3 of every 1,000 live births.)

Surgical Procedures: Creation of Cerebrospinal Fluid Shunts

For noncommunicating hydrocephalus, the following procedures are performed:

1. Ventriculoperitoneal shunt (lateral ventricle to peritoneum)—most common and preferred, because it allows the most room for growth
2. Ventriculoatrial shunt (lateral ventricle to right atrium)—still used occasionally but may lead to long-term complications, especially pulmonary thromboembolism and cor pulmonale
3. Ventriculopleural shunt (lateral ventricle to pleural cavity)—rare
4. Fourth ventriculostomy

For communicating hydrocephalus, a lumboperitoneal shunt (lumbar subarachnoid space to peritoneum) is performed.

Endoscopic instruments are now commonly used to position shunts in the lateral ventricles and for fourth ventriculostomy. Very occasionally, these endoscopic procedures may be accompanied by considerable bleeding. Alternatively, shunts may be positioned under ultrasound guidance.

Special Anesthesia Problems

1. Increased ICP may occur and is sometimes severe. In such cases the patient may have been vomiting and may have had a poor fluid intake preoperatively; check fluid and electrolyte status. Occasionally, acute symptoms of raised ICP demand immediate surgery.
2. Many patients have had repeated anesthesia for shunt revisions.
3. Blood loss is usually minimal, but very occasionally bleeding occurs from a large vessel. Always be prepared with a good intravenous route.
4. The patient should be fully awake at the end of procedure to permit neurologic assessment.

Anesthesia Management

Preoperative

1. Exercise special care if the ICP is increased. The patient should be monitored carefully until surgery can be arranged, because the patient's condition can deteriorate suddenly, necessitating immediate ventricular tap or lumbar puncture (depending on whether the hydrocephalus is noncommunicating or communicating).
2. If the patient becomes apneic, intubate, hyperventilate, and arrange for an immediate ventricular tap.
3. Assess fluid status. Intravenous fluids should be given to correct hydration in those with inadequate oral intake.

Perioperative

1. Exercise special care during induction of anesthesia to prevent hypoventilation, hypoxia, or systemic hypertension.
   a. An intravenous induction with propofol or thiopental plus a muscle relaxant is preferred, so that the airway can be secured rapidly and excellent ventilation ensured.
   b. Lidocaine 1.5 mg/kg IV may be given to attenuate the hypertensive response to laryngoscopy and intubation.

2. During surgery, maintain anesthesia with N_2O and low concentrations of isoflurane or halothane. Addition of a nondepolarizing relaxant drug (*cis*-atracurium preferred for short cases) permits the use of minimal volatile agent, with rapid recovery on reversal. Controlled ventilation is preferred for all patients.

3. Pay special attention to the following situations:
   a. Hypotension at the time of CSF tap. If the arterial BP was elevated secondary to increased ICP and if excessive inhalation agents have been given, the BP may fall precipitously as the ICP returns to normal (at the time of CSF tap). Withdraw all anesthetic agents and ventilate with 100% O_2 until the arterial BP returns to a normal level.
   b. Bradycardia and other arrhythmias. These may occur after placement of the intraventricular catheter, probably as a result of shifts in intracranial contents.
   c. Ventriculoatrial shunts. Apply controlled positive-pressure ventilation to prevent air embolism while the vein is open for insertion of the cardiac end of the ventriculoatrial shunt. The ECG may be used as a guide for positioning the atrial end of the shunt. Fill the shunt tubing with hypertonic saline and attach it by an extension wire to the left-arm ECG lead. Switch the ECG to lead III. Advance the tubing; as the tip approaches the right atrium the P waves grow higher, and when it reaches its correct position in the atrium they become small and biphasic (Fig. 8–1).

4. Blood loss is usually minimal, requiring no replacement, but a reliable, adequate-bore intravenous line should always be placed.

5. Discontinue potent anesthetic agents before the end of surgery, so that the patient is wide awake and responsive before leaving the OR.

Postoperative

1. Order routine postcraniotomy nursing care.
2. Order analgesics as required, but avoid excessive doses of narcotic analgesics; intramuscular codeine is usually effective.

Craniosynostosis

Premature fusion of a suture between bones of the vault of the skull leads to deformity. Most frequently only the sagittal suture is involved, leading to cosmetic deformity. Fusion of more than one suture may lead to raised ICP and later to mental retardation and possibly optic atrophy. Early surgical repair (at less than 6 months of age) gives improved cosmetic results with less blood loss than repair at an older age.

Associated Conditions

1. Craniofacial abnormalities such as Crouzon's disease and Apert's syndrome

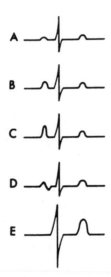

Figure 8–1. Drawing of ECG tracings obtained as a VA shunt catheter is advanced toward the heart. **(A)** When the catheter tip is in the SVC, P waves become large as the tip approaches the right atrium **(B, C)**, then smaller and biphasic as the atrium is entered **(D)**. If the catheter is advanced too far into the ventricle, the QRS complexes become very large **(E)**.

Surgical Procedure

1. Craniectomy—division of skull along suture lines

Special Anesthesia Problems

1. Possible increased ICP.
2. Sudden massive blood loss from damaged cerebral venous sinuses. Continued bleeding owing to the vascularity of the scalp and other membranes.
3. Difficult airway in patients with craniofacial syndromes.
4. Air embolism is definitely a potential intraoperative danger.

Anesthesia Management

Preoperative

1. Check that blood is available in the OR for transfusion.
2. Use caution with premedication if the ICP is increased.

Perioperative

1. Intravenous induction with thiopental and a relaxant is optimal to rapidly secure the airway and prevent hypoventilation. A

nasotracheal tube is preferred; otherwise, use an armored oral tube. (Choanal atresia is occasionally associated with craniosynostosis.)
2. Maintain anesthesia with N_2O/O_2, low concentrations of sevoflurane or isoflurane, and a relaxant; control ventilation.
3. Establish a reliable wide-bore intravenous line and have blood ready in the OR. Monitor blood loss carefully. An arterial line should be inserted if extensive surgery is planned.
4. Hyperventilation and possibly diuresis may be needed to ensure that the volume of the intracranial contents is not increased.
5. Position a precordial Doppler probe and monitor carefully for air embolism as the skull is opened.
6. Discontinue potent anesthetic agents before the end of surgery so that the patient is wide awake and responsive before leaving the OR.

Postoperative

1. Order routine postcraniotomy nursing care.
2. Exercise caution with narcotic analgesics.

Myelodysplasia: Meningomyelocele and Encephalocele

Meningomyelocele and encephalocele result from failure of the neural tube to fuse in the fetus. The incidence of meningomyelocele is approximately 1–4 per 1,000 live births, with a large geographic variation. Encephalocele is much less common. Early operation should be performed because of the risk of infection and to avoid further damage to nerve tissue. Extensive skin dissection to mobilize flaps may be needed in some cases, and this may result in considerable blood loss.

Associated Conditions

Hydrocephalus, in many cases with Arnold-Chiari malformation and aqueductal stenosis, occurs in 80% of infants with meningomyelocele or encephalocele.

Short trachea has been described in association with meningomyelocele.

Surgical Procedures

Excision of the sac and repair of the defect is usually performed as soon as possible after birth.

Special Anesthesia Problems

1. Potential difficulty in positioning the patient for intubation; be aware that patients with meningomyelocele may also have a short trachea. *Ensure that the endotracheal tube is not in an endobronchial location.*
2. Blood losses, which are difficult to measure and may be considerable.

3. Difficulty maintaining body temperature during surgery.
4. Possibility of postoperative ventilatory depression or apnea. Hydrocephalus and Arnold-Chiari syndrome are associated; apart from this, ventilatory control may be abnormal in infants with meningomyelocele.

> **N.B.** *Succinylcholine* does not *cause hyperkalemia in infants with myelome-ningocele.*

Anesthesia Management

Observe all special precautions for the neonate.

Preoperative

1. The lesion is kept covered with sterile dressing.
2. Ensure that cross-matched blood (250 ml) is available in the OR.
3. Ensure that the OR has been warmed to at least 24°C.

Perioperative

1. Use warming blankets under bolsters, a Bair hugger, radiant heat lamps, a heated humidifier, and a woolen cap on the patient's head.
2. Induce anesthesia and intubate. Laryngoscopy and intubation are easier if the patient is placed left side down, with an assistant applying forward pressure at the back of the head and backward pressure on the shoulders to prevent neck extension. If intubation cannot be performed in this position, place the infant supine, supported on a ring cushion to protect the defect. Check the position of the tube carefully.
3. Continue anesthesia with N_2O and isoflurane or sevoflurane, with controlled ventilation. An arterial line should be inserted if an extensive procedure is necessary.
4. For surgery, the patient is positioned prone on bolsters.
5. Do not give neuromuscular blocking agents until it has been ascertained whether the surgeon wishes to use a nerve stimulator to identify the nerve roots.
6. Blood loss cannot be measured accurately. Estimate the amount of bleeding and monitor the arterial systolic pressure and the hematocrit as a guide to replacement.

Postoperative

1. Return the patient to a warm incubator, to be nursed prone on a frame.
2. Instruct the nursing staff to observe closely for signs of raised ICP, especially in cases of encephalocele. Monitor ventilation carefully.
3. Do not give narcotic analgesics.
4. Check hemoglobin and hematocrit on arrival in the postanesthesia care unit.

Arnold-Chiari Malformation

The Arnold-Chiari malformation consists of an elongated cerebellar vermis that herniates through the foramen magnum with associated compression of the brain stem. Infants with this disease may present with difficulty swallowing, recurrent aspiration, stridor, and possible apneic episodes. The gag reflex may be depressed or absent.

Associated Conditions

Syringomyelia is often associated and leads to arm weakness and possible sensory deficit.

Surgical Procedure

The surgical procedure consists of decompression of the posterior fossa, enlargement of the foramen magnum with upper cervical laminectomy, opening of the dura, and lysis of adhesions. If syringomyelia is present, it is treated by drainage of the hydromyelia.

Special Anesthesia Problems

1. Control of ventilation is abnormal; preoperative ventilation may be required, and postoperative apnea may occur.
2. Recurrent aspiration frequently results in impaired pulmonary function, complicating the ventilatory status.
3. Stridor may occur and is not always improved immediately after surgery.
4. The patient must be positioned prone and with the neck flexed for surgery; a very carefully positioned nasotracheal tube is preferred.

Anesthesia Management

Anesthesia management is the same as for posterior fossa exploration. The patient should be very carefully monitored postoperatively. Rarely, the endotracheal tube must be left in place if the patient cannot maintain a safe airway; later, tracheostomy may be required.

Craniotomy for Tumors and Vascular Lesions

Intracerebral tumors are relatively common during childhood, with a peak incidence at the age of 5–8 years; about 60% are in the posterior fossa. Epileptogenic foci and benign vascular lesions may also be indications for craniotomy.

Surgical Procedures

1. Exploratory biopsy and/or excision of lesion.

Special Anesthesia Problems

1. Elevated ICP and/or hydrocephalus may be present and may result in nausea, vomiting, and electrolyte disturbance.

2. Anesthesia techniques must be designed to provide optimal intracranial conditions for surgery.
3. Blood losses are difficult to measure and may be massive.
4. Small infants with AV malformation may have associated high-output congestive heart failure. These patients have a low diastolic blood pressure and do not tolerate further reduction in blood pressure intraoperatively (cardiac arrest may occur). Anesthesia in older children with aneurysm or AV malformation must be very carefully managed to avoid intraoperative hypertension; controlled hypotension may be required to facilitate the surgery.
5. Postoperatively, the patient must be free of residual effects of anesthesia to permit accurate neurologic assessment and monitoring.
6. In a few cases it may be necessary to perform intraoperative neurophysiologic studies. During surgery for epilepsy, it may be necessary to record the electroencephalogram (EEG) directly from the brain tissue; in such cases it is preferable to avoid giving large doses of drugs known to suppress seizures (e.g., thiopental, diazepam). In others, it may be necessary to record cortical SSEPs intraoperatively. The use of 0.5% isoflurane in N_2O has been demonstrated to be satisfactory during such monitoring. Higher concentrations of volatile agents may interfere with the recording.
7. In very few cases, the patient is required to be awake and to cooperate during surgery (e.g., to map the speech area).

Anesthesia Management

Preoperative

1. Assess the patient carefully. Review and understand the pathology and the surgical procedures that will be required. Check hematology and biochemistry results.
2. Check that blood is available for transfusion (at least 1,000 ml for craniotomy and more for removal of vascular malformations).
3. Do not give narcotic sedative premedication except for patients with vascular lesions. Establish rapport with older children; reassure them, and explain the planned procedures.

Perioperative

1. Induce anesthesia, preferably using intravenous thiopental 5–7 mg/kg, lidocaine 1.5 mg/kg, and a full dose of a relaxant; this method permits the airway to be secured rapidly and prevents hypoventilation, hypoxia, coughing, or straining.
2. Intubate using the largest endotracheal tube that passes the larynx easily. A nasotracheal tube is preferred for small infants and for those in whom postoperative ventilation may be required.
3. Light general anesthesia is adequate for neurosurgery (e.g., N_2O and isoflurane 0.5%–0.75% plus a relaxant drug). A small dose of a potent narcotic (e.g., fentanyl 2 µg/kg) may be given at the start of the surgery; little analgesia is required once the skull is open. Controlled ventilation with *cis*-atracurium or vecuronium given

intermittently while the neuromuscular block is monitored is very satisfactory and can readily be reversed. Monitor the neuromuscular block with a nerve stimulator or by electromyography (EMG).
4. Insert an arterial line for all patients and also a CVP line in patients with vascular lesions. A urinary catheter should be inserted and urine output monitored.
5. Encourage the surgeon to infiltrate the area for the proposed scalp incision with 0.125% bupivacaine with epinephrine 1:200,000 (maximum volume, 2.0 ml/kg).
6. Give a diuretic to reduce the brain mass as the skull is being opened.
7. Give dexamethasone 0.15 mg/kg IV (maximum dose, 10 mg) to minimize focal cerebral edema).
8. If it is planned to extubate the patient, discontinue volatile anesthetic agents before the end of surgery so that the patient is wide awake and responsive before leaving the operating room.

Special Considerations: Anterior and Middle Fossa Surgery

1. Use an armored orotracheal tube or a nasotracheal tube.
2. Position patient with a 15° head-up tilt.
3. Maintain anesthesia and monitor as previously described.
4. Watch for arrhythmias or changes in BP, especially during dissections in the region of the pituitary gland and hypothalamus. If these occur, alert the surgeon to discontinue surgery until the situation resolves. Intravenous atropine may be required for bradycardia.

Special Considerations: Posterior Fossa Surgery (Prone Position)

1. Use a nasotracheal tube. It can be precisely secured at the nostril, it is less likely to kink than an oral tube, and its taping is unlikely to be loosened by saliva.
2. The patient should lie prone on a frame (e.g., Relton frame) or bolsters, with a 15° head-up tilt and with the thorax and abdomen hanging free.
3. Anesthetize as for anterior or middle fossa surgery *(see above)*. Monitor vital signs very carefully during manipulations in the region of the brain stem.

Special Considerations: Posterior Fossa Surgery (Sitting Position)

Many pediatric neurosurgeons use the prone or park-bench position, but unfortunately some still prefer to operate with the patient in the sitting position.

1. Air embolism is a prime concern; monitor carefully with a precordial Doppler probe and capnograph and place a CVP line at the junction of the superior vena cava and right atrium using ECG guidance. The CVP line can be used to aspirate air in case of embolism and also as a guide to fluid therapy.

2. Cardiovascular stability is the next problem; the lower limbs should be bandaged to promote venous return, and the patient positioned carefully while the blood pressure is monitored.

Postoperative

1. The patient must have recovered fully from the effects of anesthesia before leaving the OR.
2. Order routine postcraniotomy nursing monitoring and care.
3. Be very cautious with narcotic analgesics to avoid respiratory depression; a morphine infusion at an appropriately low rate is usually very effective. *N.B. The patient is often also given an antiseizure medication.*
4. Body temperature may rise; measures to restore normothermia may then be required.
5. SIADH may occur with resulting oliguria and electrolyte disturbance.

Craniopharyngioma

This most common of pituitary tumors in children may become very large and compress adjacent structures (e.g., the optic chiasma), may cause a considerable increase in ICP, and may result in significant endocrine disturbance. Even after aggressive removal of the tumor under microscopic guidance, recurrence is not uncommon (10%).

Special Problems

1. Children with this disease often have growth retardation due to growth hormone deficiency, and they tend to be obese. They may also have behavior disturbances.
2. Adrenal insufficiency must be anticipated postoperatively; corticosteroid replacement therapy should be commenced before operation.
3. Diabetes insipidus may be present preoperatively and almost certainly will appear intraoperatively or postoperatively. Monitor CVP, urine output, and serum electrolytes during the operation. Be prepared to replace excessive urine losses and to administer 1-deamino-8-D-arginine vasopressin (DDAVP) if necessary.
4. The surgical approach via a frontal craniotomy requires optimal reduction of brain mass (i.e., perfect neurosurgical anesthesia) if good access to the tumor is to be obtained.
5. The procedure may be prolonged; the patient must be very carefully positioned.
6. After excision of a craniopharyngioma, children require thyroid and growth hormone replacement therapy.

Aneurysm of the Vein of Galen

This uncommon disease, an AV malformation involving the great cerebral vein of Galen, is a considerable challenge to the pediatric neuroanesthesiologist. The disease may manifest in the neonate, evidenced by severe congestive cardiac failure and a cerebral bruit; the operative risk is highest in lesions that appear at this age. Current management usually is by initial transcatheter coil occlusion of the feeding vessels. When lesions of the vein of Galen manifest later in life, the course is more benign, and the lesion may be managed like other AV malformations.

Special Anesthesia Problems

1. Neonates and very young infants are likely to be in severe congestive cardiac failure preoperatively. This condition can sometimes be improved by embolization of some of the aberrant vessels. Staged closed embolization may represent the safest therapeutic approach to this disease.
2. The surgical mortality rate has been high, usually because of uncontrollable bleeding or intraoperative cardiac arrest. The use of profound hypothermia with circulatory arrest has been attempted, but the results were poor. Current management is by transcatheter embolization of feeding vessels in the neuroradiology suite, possibly followed by surgical excision. Careful intraoperative management of the cardiovascular parameters may improve the outlook.

Anesthesia Management

1. It is important that hypovolemia or hypotension be avoided before the vessels are clipped. The AV shunt through the lesion places a great stress on the heart; failure is common, and myocardial perfusion is threatened by the low diastolic pressure. If the diastolic pressure falls, myocardial perfusion will be inadequate and cardiac arrest will occur. Hypotensive techniques are contraindicated, and the blood pressure should be maintained until the aneurysm can be clipped or embolized. Aggressive cardiovascular monitoring is recommended for accurate monitoring of the intraoperative status and replacement of fluids as needed.
2. When the aneurysm is clipped, the ventricular afterload suddenly rises and decompensation may occur. Vasodilators and inotropic agents should be prepared to compensate for this development if necessary.
3. Use of N_2O should be avoided, because it may depress the myocardium and slightly elevate pulmonary vascular resistance. High-dose fentanyl anesthesia is recommended.
4. If general anesthesia is employed during closed embolization, careful attention to the volume of contrast medium used is essential; excessive doses may lead to further volume overload.

Suggested Additional Reading

McLeod EM, Creighton RE, and Humphreys RP: Anaesthetic management of arteriovenous malformations of the vein of Galen. Can Anaesth Soc J 29:307, 1982.

Rasch DK, Webster DE, Hutyra J, et al.: Anesthesia management of hemodynamic changes during vein of Galen clipping. Anesthesiology 69:993–995, 1988.

Electrocorticography and Operations for Epilepsy

Many older children (beyond 8 years of age) cooperate adequately during neuroleptanalgesia for electrocorticography and operations for epilepsy (e.g., temporal lobectomy).

Special Anesthesia Problems

1. Drugs that modify the EEG significantly (e.g., barbiturates) must not be given. Propofol may be used.
2. The patient must be awake and cooperative (including being able to speak).
3. Anesthesia techniques must be designed to provide optimal intracranial conditions for surgery.
4. Blood losses are difficult to measure and may be considerable.
5. Postoperatively, the patient must be free of residual effects of anesthesia, to permit accurate neurologic assessment and monitoring.

Anesthesia Management

Preoperative

1. At the preoperative visit, assess the child and judge the likelihood that the child will cooperate.
2. Explain to the patient the anesthetic technique proposed and the reasons for it. Encourage enthusiastic cooperation in the procedure (i.e., explain that in this procedure patients experience a dreamy state and feel no pain, but they themselves must help make the operation a success).
3. Do not give premedication.
4. Omit anticonvulsant drugs the morning of the surgery.
5. Check that blood is available for transfusion.

Perioperative

1. Ensure that equipment is at hand for emergency intubation and ventilation.
2. Start a large-bore intravenous infusion (use a local analgesic).
3. Give intravenous atropine followed by droperidol 0.1 mg/kg; titrate doses of fentanyl 2 µg/kg until the patient is comfortable but responsive. Hypnosis, as required, may be provided by a low-dose propofol infusion, but avoid producing excessive ventilatory depression. Low concentrations of N_2O may also be provided via a nasal catheter.
4. Allow surgeons to shave the patient's head and to insert a urinary catheter (ensure that lidocaine jelly is used).
5. Perform a scalp block on the side of surgery using 1% lidocaine with 0.25% bupivacaine, with 1:200,000 epinephrine.
6. Monitor the BP and arterial blood gases via an indwelling cannula.
7. During craniotomy, give increments of fentanyl (2 µg/kg) to

provide additional analgesia and give $O_2 \pm N_2O$ via nasal prongs. (One prong may be used to monitor end-tidal carbon dioxide.)
8. Talk with the patient and encourage regular deep breathing (to avoid hypoventilation).
9. While the skull is being opened, give mannitol 1–2 g/kg or furosemide 0.6 mg/kg and dexamethasone 0.2 mg/kg.
10. If excessive respiratory depression occurs, reverse it with levallorphan 0.05 mg/kg. Avoid the use of naloxone at this stage if possible; naloxone may result in excessive reversal of sedation and analgesia, and the patient may become very restless.

Postoperative

1. If the patient remains excessively drowsy, give a small dose of naloxone (0.5–5 µg/kg).
2. Order routine postcraniotomy nursing care.

Suggested Additional Reading

Soriano SG, Eldredge EA, Wang FK, et al.: The effect of propofol on intraoperative electrocorticography and cortical stimulation during awake craniotomies in children. Paediatr Anaesth 10:29–34, 2000.

Spinal Cord Tumors and Tethered Cord

Spinal cord tumors are less common in children than in adults, but they can occur at any site in the spinal cord.

Tethered cord causes bladder and bowel symptoms and weakness of one or both lower limbs. This syndrome is confirmed by myelography and computed tomography, which demonstrate a low conus, a thickened filum, and a transverse orientation of nerve roots.

Surgical Procedure

Surgical division of the filum terminale is the treatment.

Special Anesthesia Considerations

1. Muscle relaxants should not be used if the surgeon wishes to use nerve stimulation intraoperatively to identify peripheral nerves. Anorectal manometry or SSEPs from the pudendal nerve may also be used to monitor neurologic function intraoperatively.
2. The patient must be carefully positioned on a frame or bolsters to avoid pressure on the abdomen. Such pressure diverts blood from the abdominal veins to the vertebral venous plexus and increases bleeding at the surgical site.
3. General endotracheal anesthesia with N_2O, low concentrations of isoflurane, and small doses of fentanyl with controlled ventilation is very satisfactory.

Selective Posterior Rhizotomy for Spasticity

Some patients with spasticity secondary to cerebral palsy may benefit from rhizotomy of some of the fascicles of the posterior roots of L2 to S1 bilaterally. Intraoperative EMG monitoring is used to determine which fascicles demonstrate a normal response to stimulation (brief local contraction) and which give an abnormal response (a sustained or diffuse contracture). The latter are then divided. Many children benefit significantly, with a generalized reduction of spasticity, improved limb function, and even improved speech function. Sensation is not significantly affected.

Management of anesthesia should be as for tethered cord *(see above)*. Nondepolarizing muscle relaxants should not be administered, because the resulting neuromuscular block compromises interpretation of the EMG findings. Succinylcholine may be given for intubation if required; it is safe to use in the patient with cerebral palsy.

Suggested Additional Reading

Alfery DD, Shapiro HM, and Gagnon RL: Cardiac arrest following rapid drainage of CSF fluid in a patient with hydrocephalus. Anesthesiology 52:443, 1980.

Creighton RE, Relton JEW, and Meridy HW: Anaesthesia for occipital encephalocoele. Can Anaesth Soc J 21:403, 1974.

Dierdorf SF, McNiece WL, Rao CC, et al.: Failure of succinylcholine to alter plasma potassium in patients with myelomeningocele. Anesthesiology 64:272–273 1986.

Fitch W, Barker J, Jennett WB, and McDowall DG: The influence of neuroleptanalgesic drugs on cerebrospinal fluid pressure. Br J Anaesth 41:800, 1969.

Frost EAQ: Anesthesia for elective intracranial procedures. Anesth Rev 7:13, 1980.

Hellbusch LC and Nihsen BJ: Rectal sphincter pressure monitoring device. Neurosurgery 24:775–776, 1989.

Lassen NA and Christensen MS: Physiology of cerebral blood flow. Br J Anaesth 48:719, 1976.

McLeod EM, Creighton RE, and Humphreys RP: Anesthesia for cerebral arteriovenous malformations in children. Can Anaesth Soc J 29:299–306, 1982.

Peacock WJ, Arens LJ, and Berman B: Cerebral palsy spasticity: selective posterior rhizotomy. Pediatr Neurosci 13:61–66, 1987.

Robertson JT, Schick RW, Morgan F, and Matson DD: Accurate placement of ventriculo-atrial shunt for hydrocephalus under electrocardiographic control. J Neurosurg 18:255, 1961.

Rockoff MA: Anesthesia for children with hydrocephalus. Anesthesiol Rev 6:28–34, 1979.

Shapiro HM: Intracranial hypertension: therapeutic and anesthetic considerations. Anesthesiology 43:445, 1975.

Vandesteene A, Trempont V, Engelman E, et al: Effect of propofol on cerebral blood flow and metabolism in man. Anaesthesia 43(Suppl):43, 1988.

Wells TR and Jacobs RA: Incidence of short trachea in patients with myelomeningocele. Pediatr Neurol 6:109, 1990.

Wood CC, Spencer DD, Allison T, et al.: Localization of human sensorimotor cortex during surgery by cortical surface recording of somatosensory evoked potentials. J Neurosurg 68:99–111, 1988.

Anesthesia for Pediatric Invasive Neuroradiology

The development of microcatheters and occlusive materials that can be delivered via microcatheters has altered the management of pediatric neurovascular lesions. AV malformations and vein of Galen or other intracranial aneurysms are being treated by neuroradiologists using endovascular techniques. Therapeutic materials include particulate and nonparticulate embolic substances and microcoils.

Although morbidity after the use of these methods may be generally less than after open surgery, providing anesthesia to these patients in the radiology suite introduces some problems for the anesthesiologist.

Special Anesthesia Problems

1. The radiology suite may be at a distance from the OR and anesthesia support services; ensure that all equipment and supplies that might be needed are available before commencing anesthesia. Make sure that communications to the OR are readily available so that additional equipment or help can be obtained if needed.
2. General endotracheal anesthesia with neuromuscular block (using a nerve stimulator) is always required for infants and young children; it is crucial that patients do not move, especially during injections of embolizing materials.
3. Access to the patient may be limited by the radiologic equipment; check ventilation carefully after intubation, and secure the endotracheal tube firmly. A RAE tube* may be suitable for some cases, but usually a standard tube is preferred because it can be used if postoperative ventilation is required. Ensure that ventilator circuits and monitoring lines can be routed so that they are absolutely secure throughout the procedure.
4. Maintenance of normal body temperature may be difficult when the patient is on the x-ray table. Use humidified, warmed gases and forced-air warming mattresses. Keep the patient covered as much as possible.
5. SSEPs may be monitored to guide the procedure; for this reason, volatile agents must be limited to low concentrations. In some cases an amobarbital (Amytal) infusion may be used together with SSEPs to map cortical areas before embolization.
6. After the procedure the patient's neurologic status must be assessed and monitored. Therefore, a technique should be used that permits rapid and complete awakening.
7. Potential complications of the procedure include perforation of a vessel or aneurysm, accidental closure of normal vessels or draining veins, and adhesion of catheters. Some cases might need to proceed to craniotomy.

---

*RAE tube, Mallinckrodt, Inc., St. Louis, MO.

Anesthesia Management

1. No preoperative sedation is routinely administered, but it may be preferred for some patients with intracranial aneurysm or AV malformation.
2. Induction and intubation should be planned as for craniotomy to minimize changes in ICP dynamics.
3. N_2O with sevoflurane (up to 1%) may be used for maintenance and does not significantly affect SSEP monitoring. Small doses of narcotic analgesics (e.g., fentanyl 1–2 µg/kg) may be given and will also minimize postoperative headache and discomfort.
4. A nondepolarizing muscle relaxant should be used (vecuronium or rocuronium), and the degree of neuromuscular block should be carefully monitored.
5. The patient should be carefully positioned and padded to avoid pressure injuries. Means to maintain body temperature should be provided *(see above)*.

Postoperative Care

1. It is desirable for the patient to rest quietly but to not be obtunded, so that an accurate early postprocedure neurologic assessment can be made.
2. The catheterization sites and the distal circulation should be regularly checked.
3. Suitable sedation and gentle restraint may be necessary to prevent movement that might result in bleeding or hematoma at the catheterization sites.

Chapter 9

Ophthalmology

GENERAL PRINCIPLES

1. General anesthesia is almost always required, because children do not tolerate sedation for eye surgery.
2. Intraocular surgery and surgery of the nasolacrimal duct and eyelids require a bloodless field. Although induced hypotension is seldom indicated for these operations, all measures should be taken to ensure that the anesthetic does not increase bleeding. Smooth, general anesthesia—with optimal airway, good positioning of the patient, and quiet emergence without coughing or straining—is important.
3. The oculocardiac reflex is powerful in children but can readily be blocked by giving intravenous atropine in the usual dosage (0.01–0.02 mg/kg) at the time of induction. Do not rely on atropine given intramuscularly or on local anesthetic (retrobulbar) blocks to avoid this reflex. *Monitor the heart rate carefully during manipulation of the eyes.* In the rare event that atropine is contraindicated, remember that the oculocardiac reflex is more likely to be triggered by a sudden pull than by a gradually applied progressive traction on the extraocular muscles. The reflex usually fatigues rapidly; that is, a second pull does not elicit the same powerful effect.
4. Some children may be taking drugs that have significant side effects:
   a. Echothiophate iodide (Phospholine Iodide), a long-acting plasma cholinesterase inhibitor, is given as eye drops to children with glaucoma and to some patients with strabismus (esotropia).

Significant systemic absorption occurs and may result in toxic symptoms (nausea, vomiting, abdominal pain) and prolonged apnea after administration of succinylcholine or mivacurium.

b. Timolol maleate topical (a β-blocking agent) is also used as an antiglaucoma agent in children. It is absorbed from the conjunctiva and may cause bradycardia refractory to atropine and bronchospasm. Children with asthma may experience an exacerbation with this drug.

c. Acetazolamide (Diamox) may cause a metabolic acidosis, and depletion of sodium, potassium, and water. It may also rarely trigger anaphylaxis, Stevens-Johnson syndrome, and bone marrow depression.

5. Drugs applied to the conjunctiva or injected into the eye during surgery may cause systemic effects or have significant implications for the anesthesiologist.

a. Epinephrine and phenylephrine may cause hypertension and arrhythmias, effects that are potentially dangerous especially during halothane anesthesia. (Epinephrine eye drops are specifically contraindicated in patients with tetralogy of Fallot because they may precipitate a cyanotic "tet" spell.) Phenylephrine drops cause fewer problems, especially if the concentration is limited to 2.5%; but if instilled on a hyperemic conjunctiva they may cause severe hypertension. Monitor the heart rate and blood pressure carefully after drug instillation.

b. Cyclopentolate (Cyclogyl), a mydriatic, may cause ataxia, disorientation, psychosis, and convulsions, especially if a 2% solution is used. A 0.5% solution should be used for infants, and a 1% solution for children.

c. Tropicamide (Mydriacyl) may cause behavior disturbance, psychotic reactions, and, rarely, vasomotor collapse.

d. Scopolamine eye drops may cause excitation and disorientation, which may be treated with physostigmine 0.01 mg/kg IV.

e. Pilocarpine may cause hypertension, tachycardia, bronchospasm, nausea, vomiting, and diarrhea.

f. Intraocular injection of acetylcholine, to produce miosis after lens extraction, may cause increased secretions, salivation, bronchospasm, and bradycardia.

g. Sulfur hexafluoride gas or air may be injected to assist in retinal reattachment surgery. If so, discontinue nitrous oxide (N_2O) for 20 minutes beforehand, to avoid an increase in intraocular pressure (IOP) followed by an even more dangerous fall in IOP as the N_2O is withdrawn; this could damage the retinal reattachment.

6. The effects of anesthetic drugs and techniques on IOP must be remembered:

a. Atropine causes only a very slight increase in IOP when given intramuscularly, intravenously, or orally. Its use as a premedicant is not contraindicated in patients with glaucoma.

b. All potent inhalation anesthetic agents, intravenous agents (barbiturates, propofol, neuroleptics, and opioids) and nondepolarizing relaxants decrease IOP, and the effect may be dose related.

c. Intravenous succinylcholine may cause a transient increase in IOP that is not reliably prevented by pretreatment with a nondepolarizing relaxant drug. The increase in IOP occurs within 30 seconds after administration but abates quickly, returning to normal within 6 minutes. Succinylcholine is usually avoided in children undergoing intraocular surgery. The rise in IOP may be less in those patients with already increased IOP (glaucoma), but it seems prudent to omit succinylcholine in such patients, especially if measurement of IOP is part of the operation. The use of succinylcholine for patients with penetrating eye trauma has been controversial. Although it was originally thought to be contraindicated, it has been shown to be safe in at least one large series. When given after thiopental in a rapid sequence induction, succinylcholine causes no increase in IOP. However, With the introduction of new, rapid-acting nondepolarizing relaxants (e.g., rocuronium), there are alternatives to succinylcholine for rapid sequence induction in patients with penetrating eye injury.

d. Ketamine, originally thought to increase IOP, probably has little effect.

e. Diuretic drugs decrease IOP and may reduce the increase in IOP after succinylcholine administration.

Anesthesia Techniques and Intraocular Pressure

f. Laryngoscopy and endotracheal intubation may increase IOP; this effect can be modified by the administration of lidocaine 1 mg/kg IV, preferably 3 minutes before intubation. The insertion of a laryngeal mask airway (LMA) causes less increase in IOP, and its removal may be associated with less coughing and straining. Therefore, the LMA may be useful for patients undergoing eye surgery.

g. Coughing, bucking, crying, and straining all increase IOP markedly. Smooth extubation without coughing can be effected by administration of lidocaine 1–2 mg IV immediately before removal of the tube.

h. Hypercapnia increases IOP, and hypocapnia decreases it.

7. Succinylcholine causes contracture of the extraocular smooth muscles and interferes with forced duction testing that is performed within 15 minutes after its administration.

8. Anesthesia for ophthalmology must be deep enough to ensure that the eyes are immobile and fixed centrally; during light anesthesia, the eyes often "roll up." Ketamine is generally found to be unsatisfactory for ophthalmic surgery.

9. Postoperative pain may be troublesome after eye operations, but nonsteroidal anti-inflammatory drugs such as acetaminophen are often sufficient for pain management. Nausea and vomiting is common postoperatively. It may be reduced by the use of propofol

as the primary anesthetic, and it may be further reduced by the intraoperative administration of intravenous dimenhydrinate (0.5 mg/kg), ondansetron (0.1 mg/kg), or metoclopramide 0.15 mg/kg. Metoclopramide does not cause sedation and is appropriate if adjustable sutures are being used.

10. Be very cautious when using mask anesthesia for surgery of the eyelids and similar operations (e.g., chalazion excision). Do not allow high concentrations of oxygen to leak around the mask when the surgeon is using a cautery; serious facial burns may occur.

CORRECTION OF STRABISMUS

Correction of strabismus is the most common eye operation in children.

Associated Conditions

Malignant hyperpyrexia is very rare, but strabismus or ptosis may be associated conditions. Be constantly aware of this possibility.

Special Anesthesia Problems

1. Oculocardiac reflex—Severe bradycardia and even cardiac arrest can occur as a result of traction on the extraocular muscles (*see above*).
2. "Oculogastric reflex"—vomiting after eye muscle surgery is very common and should be prevented as outlined above. Vomiting may also be precipitated by "pushing" fluids postoperatively and by early ambulation.
3. Postoperative pain may be considerable in older children.
4. If adjustable sutures are used, the patient must be assessable postoperatively; excessive sedation should not be ordered. If a second anesthetic might be required to adjust the suture, an intravenous line or a heparin lock should be left in place to facilitate induction of a second anesthetic. Do not use droperidol in such patients, because they will then be too drowsy to cooperate; metoclopramide is preferred (*see below*).

Anesthesia Management

Preoperative

1. *Do not give heavy sedation.*
   a. The surgeon may wish to examine the patient immediately before the operation.
   b. Narcotics can increase the tendency to vomit postoperatively.
   c. Midazolam (0.75 mg/kg for children 1–6 years of age) is an effective premedication with rapid onset. Clonidine (4 μg/kg PO) is effective as a premedication in these patients, but it must be given 60–90 minutes before surgery. It may cause bradycardia and hypotension but does provide some postoperative analgesia.
2. Give atropine, preferably intravenously, at induction.

Perioperative

1. Induction is accomplished either intravenously (with thiopental or propofol plus atropine, followed by a relaxant) or by inhalation of halothane or sevoflurane.
2. If induction was by inhalation, give atropine intravenously before the start of surgery.
3. For orotracheal intubation, spray the larynx well with lidocaine and use an oral RAE tube. Alternatively, in suitable patients, use a well lubricated LMA.
4. Maintain anesthesia with N_2O/O_2/halothane or sevoflurane; allow spontaneous ventilation (provided the surgery is not excessively long).
5. From the start of surgery, listen to the patient's heart sounds continuously via a precordial stethoscope and monitor the electrocardiogram. If bradycardia occurs, ask the surgeon to discontinue manipulation until you have given a further dose of intravenous atropine.
6. Give dimenhydrinate (0.5 mg/kg) or ondansetron (0.1 mg/kg) intravenously before surgery starts to reduce postoperative vomiting, or metoclopramide (0.15 mg/kg) immediately after the operation.

Postoperative

1. To avoid subconjunctival hemorrhage, the trachea must be extubated or the LMA removed without causing coughing and straining by the patient. Extubate while the child is still deeply anesthetized, and allow the patient to awaken smoothly while supporting the airway and administering oxygen by mask. Intravenous lidocaine (1.5 mg/kg) administered before extubation reduces coughing.
2. Provide analgesics for pain (e.g., acetaminophen orally or per rectum or morphine (0.05 mg/kg IV) as required).
3. Intravenous rehydration during surgery should obviate the need for early oral ingestion in the postanesthesia care unit. Delaying ingestion of oral fluids decreases the incidence of poststrabismus vomiting.
4. If nausea and/or vomiting occurs, order additional antiemetic therapy and continue with intravenous fluids.

INTRAOCULAR SURGERY AND EXAMINATION UNDER ANESTHESIA FOR GLAUCOMA OR TUMOR

Children most commonly require general anesthesia for cataract or glaucoma surgery, treatment of detached retina, or examination under anesthesia (EUA) for glaucoma or tumor.

Special Anesthesia Problems

1. The oculocardiac reflex *(see above)*.

2. Intraocular pressure—may be affected by anesthesia drugs and techniques (*see above*).
3. Coughing and straining—*may elevate the intraocular pressure.* (Induction of and emergence from anesthesia should be as quiet and smooth as possible.)

Anesthesia Management

Preoperative

1. Give adequate sedation to avoid coughing and straining.
2. It is safe to give atropine to patients with congenital open-angle glaucoma.

Perioperative

1. Induce anesthesia as smoothly as possible, intravenously with thiopental or propofol or by inhalation of N_2O and halothane or sevoflurane.
2. *Do not give succinylcholine.*
3. Deepen anesthesia and spray the larynx with lidocaine before intubation, or insert a well-lubricated LMA. For longer surgical procedures (i.e., other than a short EUA), administer a nondepolarizing relaxant drug before intubation.
4. Maintain anesthesia with N_2O/O_2/halothane or sevoflurane. Allow spontaneous ventilation for very short EUA procedures; otherwise, control the ventilation to avoid hypercapnia. The alternative, the use of propofol by infusion to maintain anesthesia, may be advantageous in reducing postoperative vomiting.
5. Discontinue N_2O early if sulfur hexafluoride or air is to be injected into the eye.
6. At the end of surgery, suction the pharynx carefully and extubate the patient, or remove the LMA, while the child is still deeply anesthetized. Lidocaine 1.5 mg/kg mg IV, administered before extubation, decreases the risk of coughing or straining during emergence.
7. Reapply the mask, support the airway, and give oxygen only until the patient wakens.

Postoperative

1. Order adequate sedation and analgesics.
2. Order an antiemetic as required.

PROBING OF THE NASOLACRIMAL DUCT AND CHALAZION EXCISION

These minor procedures are performed on an outpatient basis and give rise to no special problems. Endotracheal intubation is usually unnecessary, and the procedure can often be carried out with an anesthesia mask in place. Beware of oxygen leaks under the mask if cautery is being used (*see above*). If it appears that the procedure may be more difficult and prolonged, intubation or use of an LMA is preferred.

PENETRATING EYE TRAUMA

Penetrating eye trauma is a relatively common injury in children.

Special Anesthesia Problems

1. Any increase in IOP may result in extrusion of anterior chamber structures and/or vitreous humor. Crying, coughing, and straining should be avoided as much as possible. Sedate the child as necessary. Short-acting, nondepolarizing relaxants such as rocuronium may be used to facilitate relaxation during a rapid sequence induction in children with penetrating eye injury. Intravenous lidocaine minimizes any increase in IOP caused by laryngoscopy.
2. It may be difficult to position a mask if the eye is covered with a dressing.
3. The patient may have a full stomach.

Anesthesia Management

Preoperative

1. Give light sedation and analgesics as required; avoid upsetting the child.
2. If indicated, as early as possible before induction, give metoclopramide (Reglan) 0.1 mg/kg IV to expedite gastric emptying.
3. Give intravenous atropine at induction. (**Note:** Atropine blocks the effect of metoclopramide and therefore should not be given earlier.)

Perioperative

1. Most children require a rapid sequence induction; give 100% O_2 by mask for 4 minutes before injection of lidocaine.
2. Inject intravenous lidocaine 1 mg/kg slowly, followed 3 minutes later by thiopental or propofol, with atropine, and rocuronium.
3. Have an assistant apply cricoid pressure.
4. Intubate the patient without prior lung inflation. Aspirate the stomach.
5. Control ventilation and maintain anesthesia with N_2O/O_2 and halothane, sevoflurane, or propofol infusion.

Postoperative

1. Administer intravenous lidocaine before extubation to decrease coughing.
2. Extubate when the patient is fully awake and in the lateral position.

ANESTHESIA FOR RADIOTHERAPY

Infants and children with retinoblastoma may require daily repeated radiotherapy for which they must remain absolutely still; hence, general anesthesia is required.

The problem is to give short-acting anesthetics and have the child return to normal activity and feeding as soon as possible. A lens-sparing radiotherapy technique may be used, which means that the head must be firmly and accurately restrained; this may compromise the airway. Various techniques have been used, including inhaled halothane, sevoflurane, or propofol with or without an LMA. This avoids repeated risk of laryngeal trauma and should maintain a good airway despite positioning of the head.

More recently, the use of the Head/Fix Immobilization Device,* which uses suction to a mold of the palate, firmly supports the head and also generally maintains a very good airway without further instrumentation. Hence, a propofol infusion can be used with some confidence.

An intravenous cannula may be placed at the administration of the first anesthetic and maintained in place with a heparin lock for use on subsequent occasions.

Photoradiation therapy using a hematoporphyrin derivative (HpD) to mark tumor cells for subsequent argon laser therapy is sometimes used. Patients undergoing HpD therapy must be kept in total darkness to prevent skin pigmentation and burns. General anesthesia in darkness is required; pulse oximetry is safe and reliable in the presence of HpD. It is suggested that, if necessary, intubation and other procedures can be performed with the use of a night vision scope.

Suggested Additional Reading

Apt L, Isenberg S, and Gaffney WL: The oculocardiac reflex in strabismus surgery. Am J Ophthalmol 76:533, 1973.

Arthur DS and Dewar KMS: Anaesthesia for eye surgery in children. Br J Anaesth 52:681, 1980.

Ausinsch B, Rayburn RL, Munson ES, and Levy NS: Ketamine and intraocular pressure in children. Anesth Analg 55:773, 1976.

Benjamin KW: The toxicity of ocular medications. Int Ophthalmol Clin 19:199, 1978.

Broadman LM, Cerruzi W, Patane PS, et al.: Metoclopramide reduces the incidence of vomiting following strabismus surgery in children. Anesthesiology 72:245–248, 1990.

Edmondson L, Lindsay SL, Lanigan LP, et al.: Intraocular pressure changes during rapid sequence induction of anaesthesia. Anaesthesia 43:1005–1010, 1988.

Eustis S, Lerman J, and Smith DR: Effect of droperidol pretreatment on post-anesthetic vomiting in children undergoing strabismus surgery: the minimum effective dose. J Pediatr Ophthalmol Strabismus 24:165–168, 1987.

France NK, France TD, Woodburn JD, and Burbank DP: Alteration of forced duction testing by succinylcholine. Anesthesiology 51:S326, 1979.

Fraunfelder FT and Scafidi AR: Possible adverse effects from topical ocular 10% phenylephrine. Am J Ophthalmol 85:447, 1978.

---

*Medical Intelligence, Schwabmunchen, Germany.

Lansche RK: Systemic reactions to topical epinephrine and phenylephrine. Am J Ophthalmol 61:95, 1966.

Lederman IR: Fire hazard during ophthalmic surgery. Ophthalmic Surg 16:577, 1985.

Libonati MM, Leahy JJ, and Ellison N: The use of succinylcholine in open eye surgery. Anesthesiology 62:637–640, 1985.

McGoldrick KE: Considerations for pediatric eye surgery. Int Anesthesiol Clin 28:72, 1990.

McGoldrick KE: Ocular drugs and anesthesia. Int Anesthesiol Clin 28:72–77, 1990.

Meyers EF, Krupin T, Johnson M, and Zink H: Failure of nondepolarizing neuromuscular blockers to inhibit succinylcholine-induced increased intraocular pressure: a controlled study. Anesthesiology 48:149, 1978.

Meyers EF and Tomeldan SA: Glycopyrrolate vs atropine in prevention of oculocardiac reflex during eye surgery. Anesthesiology 51:350, 1979.

Mikawa K, Nishin K, Maekawa N, et al.: Oral clonidine premedication reduces vomiting in children after strabismus surgery. Can J Anaesthesiol 42:977–981, 1995.

Murphy DF: Anesthesia and intraocular pressure. Anesth Analg 64:520–530, 1985.

Rose JB, Martin TM, Corddry DH, et al.: Ondansetron reduces the incidence and severity of poststrabismus repair vomiting in children. Anesth Analg 79:486–489, 1994.

Samuels SI and Maze M: Beta receptor blockade following the use of eye drops. Anesthesiology 52:369, 1980.

Schreiner MS, Nicolson SC, Martin T, and Whitney L: Should children drink before discharge from day surgery? Anesthesiology 76:528–533, 1992.

Taylor DH and Child CS: The laryngeal mask in pediatric radiotherapy. Anesthesiology 45:690, 1990.

Uchida U, Kinouchi K, and Tashiro C: A new photoradiation therapy and anesthesia. Anesth Analg 70:222–223, 1990.

Vener DF, Carr AS, Sikich N, et al.: Dimenhydrinate decreases vomiting after strabismus surgery in children. Anesth Analg 82:728–731, 1996.

Weir PM, Munro HM, Reynolds PI, et al.: Propofol infusion and the incidence of emesis in pediatric outpatient strabismus surgery. Anesth Analg 76:760–764, 1993.

Wellwood M and Goresky GV: Systemic hypertension associated with topical administration of 2.5% phenylephrine HCl. Am J Ophthalmol 93:369, 1982.

Chapter **10**

Otorhinolaryngology

GENERAL PRINCIPLES

Although much of it is simple and commonplace, ear, nose, and throat surgery has a disproportionately large potential for anesthetic and surgical complications. It demands meticulous attention to all aspects of the patient's perioperative care.

1. Because many of these operations involve the airway, the anesthesiologist must be prepared to provide good surgical access to that area while maintaining a safe ventilatory pathway for the patient.
2. The advent of the surgical microscope has permitted development of delicate and precise surgery for the middle ear. Anesthesia for such procedures must provide quiet operating conditions with minimal bleeding, smooth emergence from anesthesia, and minimal disturbance postoperatively.
3. After surgery involving the airway, skilled nursing care in the postanesthesia care unit is essential, so that signs of impending complications can be detected early and appropriate therapy instituted immediately.
4. The use of the laser to treat lesions of the larynx has created some additional potential problems of anesthesia management. In these patients, as in all others, the simplest techniques may be the safest.
5. When topical vasoconstrictors are used, the anesthesiologist must be aware of the drugs and dose that will be used, because significant systemic absorption may cause dangerous effects. A maximum initial dose of 20 μg/kg of phenylephrine has been recommended for children, but this seems to be considerably less than has been used in common practice. Monitor the child carefully when topical vasoconstrictors are applied. Topical phenylephrine may lead to hypertension, but usually it resolves rapidly and no treatment is necessary. Occasionally very severe hypertension may occur; it should be treated with the use of direct vasodilators (e.g., sodium nitroprusside) or α-adrenergic receptor antagonists (e.g., phentolamine). Do not use β-blockers or calcium channel blockers, because they may cause a disastrous fall in cardiac output and pulmonary edema may occur.

Suggested Additional Reading

Groudine SB, Hollinger I, Jones J, and Debouno BA: New York State guidelines on the topical use of phenylephrine in the operating room. Anesthesiology 92:859–864, 2000.

CHOANAL ATRESIA

If it is complete (as in 90% of cases), choanal atresia (membranous or bony occlusion of the posterior nares) causes respiratory distress immediately after birth. Because neonates are primarily nose-breathers, nasal obstruction must be relieved immediately by insertion of an oro-pharyngeal airway. The diagnosis can be confirmed by the inability to pass even a fine nasal catheter. Once the diagnosis is established, the passage of an orogastric tube not only maintains an oral airway but enables feeding of the infant. Definitive surgery is sometimes delayed until the infant is older, but endonasal puncture and stenting may be performed in the neonate. It is now recognized that even lesser degrees of choanal atresia may lead to chronic nasal problems; therefore, early repair is indicated.

Associated Conditions

The "CHARGE" association consists of coloboma, congenital heart disease, choanal atresia, growth and mental retardation, ear anomalies, and genitourinary abnormalities with genital hypoplasia.

Surgical Procedures

1. Transpalatal repair is usually performed at age 1–2 days in the healthy, full-term infant. Stents are left in for 3–6 months.
2. Transnasal puncture may be performed in preterm infants or in those with associated significant disease (e.g., the CHARGE association).

Special Anesthesia Problems

The primary problem is maintenance of the airway until completion of surgery.

Anesthesia Management

Preoperative

1. Adequate ventilation requires continued use of an oropharyngeal airway.
2. Do not order sedatives.

Perioperative

1. Observe all special precautions for neonates.
2. Leave the oropharyngeal airway in place: give 100% O_2 by mask.
3. Induce anesthesia by inhalation of sevoflurane or halothane. Confirm that manual ventilation via the mask and oropharyngeal airway is successful and, if so, administer a short acting muscle relaxant; intubate using an oral RAE tube.*
4. Maintain anesthesia with nitrous oxide (N_2O) and low concentrations of sevoflurane or halothane with controlled ventilation.
5. Suction the pharynx very carefully at the end of the operation and ensure that the stents are clean and patent.
6. Do not extubate until the patient is fully awake.

Postoperative

1. Order humidified oxygen. The stents must be regularly suctioned with a fine catheter to keep them clear.

---

*Mallinckrodt Inc., St. Louis, MO.

2. Constant observation is essential, because aspiration of feeding solution commonly occurs after repair of choanal atresia.
3. Subsequent repairs may be necessary during later childhood for restenosis, but these operations present no other special anesthetic problems.

NASOPHARYNGEAL TUMORS

Teratomas, dermoid cysts, nasal encephaloceles, and other tumors may occur in pediatric patients and require surgical excision. Juvenile nasal angiofibroma is a rare benign but very vascular tumor that may involve the nose. Biopsy of these tumors may result in extensive bleeding that is very difficult to control; therefore, diagnosis is usually made on the basis of imaging studies. Operation to remove the tumor may result in massive blood loss and should be prepared for accordingly. Postoperatively there may be persistent nasal obstruction and continued bleeding; the endotracheal tube should be left in place until the patient is fully awake.

SURGERY OF THE NOSE

The most common procedures for nasal surgery are reduction of nasal fractures, septoplasty, rhinoplasty, and excision of nasal polyps.

Special Anesthesia Problems

1. The nasal airway may be blocked. The surgeon may wish to pack the nose with gauze and a vasoconstrictor (e.g., cocaine) preoperatively.
2. Children with nasal polyps usually have cystic fibrosis.
3. Functional endoscopic sinus surgery (FESS) may precipitate special problems *(see below)*.

Anesthesia Management

Preoperative

1. Assess the nasal airway.
2. If the patient has cystic fibrosis, order appropriate preoperative care.

Perioperative

1. Induce anesthesia by inhalation or intravenously with thiopental or propofol, followed by a relaxant drug.
2. If the nose is blocked, insert an oropharyngeal airway before attempting mask ventilation.
3. Perform orotracheal intubation, with a cuffed tube.
4. Insert a throat pack to prevent blood pooling in the pharynx and esophagus.
5. Position the patient with a slight head-up tilt.
6. Extubate when the patient is fully awake; premature extubation may lead to laryngospasm or airway obstruction from other causes.

Postoperative

1. Order analgesics as required.
2. Administer humidified oxygen by mask.
3. Postoperative airway obstruction may occur and, if prolonged, may predispose to postobstructive pulmonary edema. This requires therapy with oxygen and, if severe, with reintubation and positive-pressure ventilation.

FUNCTIONAL ENDOSCOPIC SINUS SURGERY

FESS has become a standard surgical treatment for chronic sinus disease. Precise endoscopic resection of diseased tissue and relief of obstruction while preserving normal mucosa is the objective, in order to restore normal sinus function.

Special Anesthesia Problems

1. Many of the patients may have chronic diseases (e.g., cystic fibrosis).
2. The successful use of endoscopy requires extensive use of vasoconstrictors. Ensure that maximal permissible doses are not exceeded: 1 mg/kg of cocaine (2%) and epinephrine 1:200,000 solution; maximum, 10 μg/kg. If hypertension ensues, treat it by deepening anesthesia or using vasodilators; do not use β-blockers or calcium channel-blocking agents.
3. Bleeding may be considerable and may require that packing remain in place postoperatively. Because this is likely to cause complete nasal obstruction, have the patient fully awake before extubation.
4. Rarely, the surgery may encroach on the orbit or intracranial space. In the latter case intracranial bleeding may occur. There is also a danger of pneumoencephalos if positive pressure is applied via a face mask.

TONSILLECTOMY AND ADENOIDECTOMY

Chronic inflammation and hypertrophy of lymphoid tissues in the pharynx may necessitate surgery to relieve obstruction or to remove the focus of infection. Repeated middle ear infections may be improved by adenoidectomy. Rarely, acute infection of a tonsil may result in a peritonsillar abscess (quinsy).

Tonsillectomy and adenoidectomy surgery is now often performed in the day surgery unit; this demands special considerations in the selection of suitable patients and in their postoperative evaluation before discharge home. An efficient follow-up service must be provided to deal with unexpected complications. Some patients may not be suitable for outpatient tonsillectomy.

The following patients are recommended for admission after tonsillectomy:

1. Those younger than 3 years of age
2. Those with abnormal coagulation studies or a history suggestive of increased bleeding tendency
3. Those with evidence of significant obstructive sleep apnea *(see below)*
4. Those with other systemic diseases that place them at additional perioperative risk (e.g., congenital heart disease, endocrine or neuromuscular disease, chromosomal abnormalities, obesity)
5. Those with craniofacial or airway abnormalities, including Down syndrome
6. Those with a history of peritonsillar abscess
7. Those who live at an excessive distance from the medical facility or whose home, social, or parental situation might preclude safe postoperative care.

Tonsillectomy is still one of the most common procedures in children and should be very safe. However, tonsillectomy-related deaths do still occur: the usual cause is excessive sedation of children with airway compromise or mismanagement of postoperative bleeding.

Obstructive Sleep Apnea. Chronic obstruction due to lymphoid hyperplasia may result in obstructive sleep apnea, and this is now a most common indication for tonsillectomy. Affected children may be obese, show daytime somnolence and behavior problems, snore at night, and sweat profusely. The parents may report that the child has interrupted breathing when sleeping.

If such a history is obtained preoperatively, sleep studies (polysomnography) should be performed; if the results are significantly abnormal, admission after tonsillectomy is advised. Polysomnographic indications for admission after tonsillectomy for the child with a history of obstructive sleep apnea include

1. A baseline value for partial pressure of carbon dioxide (PCO_2) of 50 mmHg or higher
2. A baseline awake oxygen saturation value of 90% or less
3. Episodes of oxygen desaturation of 80% or less
4. More than 10 episodes of obstructive apnea or hypopnea per hour of sleep

Patients with mild obstructive sleep apnea are reported to have few complications after tonsillectomy.

The child with obstructive sleep apnea should be closely monitored before and after operation; heavy narcotic sedation should be avoided. Postoperative sleep studies show that 90% or more improve. Those who do not should be investigated for residual soft tissue obstruction and may need uvulopalatopharyngoplasty.

Cardiorespiratory Syndrome. In very rare instances, severe chronic airway obstruction by adenoidal tissue may lead to pulmonary hypertension and right-sided heart failure (cardiorespiratory syndrome). This condition usually occurs in boys and is more common in black children.

There is usually a history of symptoms lasting 1 year or longer. The child is usually febrile with tachycardia and tachypnea. Chest radiography reveals cardiomegaly, and the electrocardiogram indicates right ventricular enlargement. Children with cardiorespiratory syndrome may be critically ill and may require emergency intubation to relieve the obstruction. Once this is done and the heart failure is controlled with digitalis and diuretics, tonsillectomy and adenoidectomy should be performed.

Surgical Procedures

1. Tonsillectomy
2. Adenoidectomy
3. Incision of peritonsillar abscess (quinsy)

Special Anesthesia Problems

1. Sharing the airway with the surgeon
2. Difficult intubation when acute infection or extreme lymphoid hypertrophy is present
3. Danger of postoperative bleeding
4. A history of bleeding tendency or recent salicylate therapy. Salicylate ingestion during the days before operation has been demonstrated to increase blood loss at tonsillectomy. If such a history is obtained, a test of bleeding time should be performed; if the time is prolonged (more than 10 minutes), the operation should be deferred.
5. A history suggestive of sleep apnea; such patients may be at risk for perioperative apnea *(see above)*.

Anesthesia Management

Preoperative

1. Patients with acute infection (e.g., quinsy) should be closely observed for impending airway obstruction. Check the extent to which the mouth can be opened; significant trismus may be present.
2. Do not give sedation, particularly to patients with any degree of airway obstruction.

Perioperative

1. Induce anesthesia intravenously with thiopental and relaxant or by inhalation.
2. Perform endotracheal intubation; an RAE tube may be used and then placed under a slotted tongue blade of the mouth gag. In this case check the airway patency carefully after the gag is positioned. Check for bilateral ventilation, because the RAE tube has a tendency to pass into the bronchus, especially if the head is flexed.
3. Maintain anesthesia with N_2O and sevoflurane or isoflurane, and assist ventilation. Plan for postoperative analgesia; meperidine or codeine 1.5 mg/kg IM or fentanyl 2 µg/kg IV during anesthesia will provide for immediate postoperative analgesia. In addition, infiltration of the tonsil beds with bupivacaine *before* surgery is effective in reducing postoperative pain.

4. An intravenous infusion should be given to replace the calculated fasting deficit: replace half of this deficit in the first hour, and the other half over the next 2 hours. In addition, give 3 ml of intravenous fluid for every 1 ml of blood lost. Discontinue the intravenous infusion after 3 hours, provided that the patient is not bleeding or vomiting. It is particularly important to ensure that children undergoing tonsillectomy and adenoidectomy on an outpatient basis are well hydrated before discharge.
5. Measure and chart blood losses carefully.
6. Carefully suction the pharynx; the presence of small amounts of blood in the pharynx may lead to laryngospasm. Extubate when the patient is fully awake and airway reflexes are fully restored. Do not pass suction catheters through the nose, because doing so may make the adenoid area bleed.

Postoperative

1. Order an analgesic—but not salicylate, which may precipitate bleeding. Acetaminophen (Tylenol 10–20 mg/kg PO) or Tylenol with Codeine is often adequate if a narcotic has been given and/or bupivacaine has been infiltrated intraoperatively.
2. Order fluids by mouth as taken, not pushed (e.g., cola beverages, Popsicles) when the patient is awake. Nausea and vomiting are common after tonsillectomy, and antinausea therapy may be required. If the decision is made to use potent antinausea drugs (e.g., ondansetron), be aware that they might prevent the patient who is continuing to bleed from vomiting and thus conceal the hemorrhage.
3. Closely monitor those patients who have a possible history of sleep apnea; such children may become apneic with sedation and/or airway obstruction. Constant nursing attention should be provided (i.e., retain the patient in the postanesthesia care unit overnight or admit the patient to a special unit).
4. Be cautious in ordering narcotic analgesics for the restless child, especially if there is any evidence of airway compromise. Restlessness may be a symptom of hypoxia secondary to obstruction, and narcotics may produce apnea.
5. The outpatient should be evaluated directly by the surgeon and the anesthesiologist before discharge. It is a general recommendation that patients should be observed for not less than 4 hours before discharge.
6. A telephone consultation service should be provided for follow-up of outpatients on the evening after surgery.
7. Complaints of abdominal pain after tonsillectomy are suggestive of swallowed blood from continued bleeding.

Reoperation for Bleeding After Tonsillectomy

Special Anesthesia Problems

1. The stomach may contain blood, which may be regurgitated during induction of anesthesia.

2. Hypovolemia may be present and is easily underestimated. There may be little blood to be seen, but much may have been swallowed.
3. The child may have a bleeding disorder that has been missed.

Anesthesia Management

Preoperative

1. Ensure that sufficient fluids have been transfused to restore the blood volume, correct severe anemia, and produce normal cardiovascular indices. Bleeding is virtually never so rapid that complete restoration of blood volume cannot be achieved before operation.
2. Check that further blood is available in case of need.
3. Check coagulation indices.
4. In some instances, gentle restraint permits examination, insertion of packing, or ligation of bleeding vessels without the need for general anesthesia.

Perioperative

1. Prepare all equipment for a rapid sequence induction.
2. Check again that the child has been adequately transfused.
3. Give 100% O_2 by mask.
4. Rapidly inject thiopental with atropine added, followed immediately by succinylcholine.
5. Have an assistant immediately apply cricoid pressure.
6. Intubate the trachea as rapidly as possible.
7. Maintain anesthesia as for tonsillectomy *(see above)*.
8. Extubate when the patient is fully awake.

Postoperative

1. Check the patient's hemoglobin level to confirm adequacy of blood replacement.
2. Be alert to the possibility of further bleeding.
3. Order suitable doses of analgesic (not acetylsalicylic acid), but bear in mind that, if the surgeon has inserted a pack
   a. Oversedation could result in complete obstruction of the airway.
   b. Restlessness may indicate hypoxia rather than a need for sedation.

Peritonsillar Abscess

Special Considerations

1. Trismus and swollen tissues in the pharynx may make intubation difficult.
2. There is a danger that the abscess may burst and flood the pharynx with pus.

Anesthesia Management

1. Check that the patient can open the mouth. Ensure that good suction is available. Give atropine 0.02 mg/kg IV.
2. Induce anesthesia by inhalation of N_2O and sevoflurane or halothane. Maintain spontaneous ventilation. Position the patient with the head slightly down and turned to the affected side.
3. Do not give muscle relaxants. (Airway obstruction may occur.)
4. When the patient is deeply anesthetized, discontinue N_2O and continue with halothane/O_2; give 1 mg/kg lidocaine IV to reduce the risk of coughing or breath-holding during laryngoscopy and endotracheal intubation. Be careful not to rupture the abscess during instrumentation.
5. Maintenance is the same as for tonsillectomy *(see above)*.
6. Suction carefully and extubate the fully awake patient in a lateral position.

N.B. Sometimes the inflammatory swelling involves the supraglottic structures, and postextubation obstruction may occur. Close observation is essential.

Suggested Additional Reading

Brown OE and Cunningham MJ: Tonsillectomy and adenoidectomy. In Patient Guidelines: Recommendations of the AAO-HNS Pediatric Otolaryngology Committee. American Academy of Otolaryngology, Head and Neck Surgery Bulletin, September 1996, pp 13–15.

Esclamado RM, Glenn MG, McCulloch TM, and Cummings CW: Perioperative complications and risk factors in the surgical treatment of obstructive sleep apnea syndrome. Laryngoscope 99:1125–1129, 1989.

Gabalski EC, Mattucci KF, Setzen M, and Moleski P: Ambulatory tonsillectomy and adenoidectomy. Laryngoscope 106:77–80, 1996.

Mandel EM and Reynolds CF: Sleep disorders associated with upper airway obstruction in children. Pediatr Clin North Am 28:897–903, 1981.

Spaur RE: The cardiorespiratory syndrome: cor pulmonale secondary to chronic upper airway obstruction from hypertrophied tonsils and adenoids. Ear Nose Throat J 62:562–570, 1982.

Tate N: Deaths from tonsillectomy. Lancet 2:1090, 1963.

OTOLOGIC CONDITIONS

Special Anesthesia Problems

1. The child may have had repeated procedures and may be very apprehensive.
2. The child's hearing may be impaired, making communication difficult.
3. During middle ear procedures, even a small amount of bleeding may interfere with surgery. Position the child carefully and avoid anesthetic causes of bleeding. However, induced hypotension is not usually warranted for this type of surgery in children.
4. The surgeon may wish to use vasoconstrictor drugs (e.g.,

epinephrine, cocaine). In such cases, halothane should be avoided and sevoflurane or isoflurane substituted.

5. Otologic procedures can be lengthy; if this is the case, the patient's ventilation should be controlled and careful attention should be paid to positioning, padding, and maintenance of body temperature.
6. In rare cases, the patient's cooperation is required during surgery (*see* Neuroleptanalgesia).
7. Postoperative nausea secondary to labyrinthine disturbance is common. Prior therapy with antinauseants (e.g., ondansetron) may be useful.

Major Otologic Procedures

Anesthesia Management

Preoperative

1. Order adequate sedation, especially for children who have had surgery previously.

Perioperative

1. Induce anesthesia by inhalation or intravenously with thiopental or propofol, followed by a suitable relaxant.
2. Spray the larynx with lidocaine; then insert an orotracheal tube.
3. Maintain anesthesia with N_2O/O_2 and a potent volatile agent; anesthesia must be deep enough to prevent any possibility of bucking on the tube, which increases bleeding.
4. Position the patient with a 15° head-up tilt to minimize bleeding.
5. If epinephrine is to be infiltrated, avoid halothane for maintenance.
6. The patient may be nauseated postoperatively; therefore, give adequate intravenous maintenance fluids and consider antinausea therapy.
7. For tympanoplasty, while the graft is being positioned, delete N_2O from the inspired mixture. (N_2O bubbles might float the graft off the desired position.)
8. Smooth extubation, without coughing, is essential. Therefore, administer intravenous lidocaine and remove the tube while the patient is still anesthetized. Maintain the airway and allow the patient to awaken while administering oxygen by mask.

Postoperative

1. Order analgesics and antiemetics as required.

Minor Otologic Procedures

Minor otologic procedures are usually performed in the outpatient department. N_2O has been shown to pass into the middle ear cavity if air is present and may modify findings at operation, but in general its use is not contraindicated. N_2O does not increase the incidence of postoperative vomiting.

Special Anesthesia Problems

1. Some patients who require repeated minor otologic procedures have associated congenital deformities of the upper airway that predispose to their ear disease (e.g., cleft palate, Pierre Robin syndrome). Check carefully for potential airway problems during anesthesia.
2. Many of these children present for anesthesia with signs of an upper respiratory tract infection (URTI). In such instances, the decision to proceed must be based on the urgency of surgery (e.g., acute middle ear infection) compared with the severity of the URTI. If the child's temperature is normal and no abnormal signs are present in the chest, the decision usually is to proceed.

Anesthesia Management

Preoperative

1. Sedation is often unnecessary, but oral midazolam is useful for the very upset child, though it delays recovery after very brief surgery.

Perioperative

1. Induce anesthesia by inhalation or intravenously with thiopental or propofol.
2. Maintain anesthesia with N_2O and sevoflurane or halothane by mask.
3. Intubation is not required, but a laryngoscope and tubes should be at hand in case of unexpected difficulties.
4. Ensure that you can comfortably hold the patient's head very still during the procedure.

Postoperative

1. Analgesics are not usually required, but Tylenol may be given if ear pain ensues.

Neuroleptanalgesia for Ear Surgery

For certain operations (e.g., ossicular reconstruction), the surgeon may wish to assess hearing during the surgical procedure. Most older children cooperate well if such operations are performed under a combination of neuroleptic agent and local analgesia.

Anesthesia Management

Preoperative

1. Explain in detail what will happen during the operation and reassure the patient that there will be no pain.

2. Order midazolam, to be given orally, sufficient to ensure a degree of sedation preoperatively.

Perioperative

1. Establish an intravenous line using a local analgesic.
2. Give droperidol 0.1 mg/kg IV and wait until it is effective, then titrate small doses of fentanyl (1–2 µg/kg) until the patient is comfortable. Atropine in the usual dosage may reduce any tendency to intraoperative nausea.
3. Ensure that the patient is positioned comfortably, and warn the patient not to cough or move the head.
4. Supplement analgesia as required with increments of fentanyl 1–2 µg/kg. Talk with the patient periodically to assess the effects of the drugs, but allow the patient to sleep when cooperation is not required. A low-dose infusion of propofol may be used.
5. Monitor ventilation and, if necessary, remind the patient to breathe deeply periodically.

Postoperative

1. Smaller than usual doses of analgesics are effective in most cases.
2. The continuing antiemetic effect of the neuroleptic agent usually minimizes postoperative nausea.

ENDOSCOPY

Endoscopy is often indicated in infants and children for diagnosis (e.g., stridor) or for therapy (e.g., removal of a foreign body).

Procedures

1. Laryngoscopy
2. Bronchoscopy—alone and for bronchography
3. Esophagoscopy

Special Anesthesia Problems

1. Existing airway problem or tracheotomy
2. Difficulty maintaining optimal ventilation during endoscopy, particularly in a patient with a very small airway
3. Possibility of complete airway obstruction during some procedures (e.g., removal of foreign body)
4. Danger of postoperative reduction in airway lumen by subglottic edema

N.B. Many conditions for which endoscopy is performed can progress to complete obstruction under anesthesia. Always have a selection of laryngoscopes and endotracheal tubes prepared; from the start of anesthesia, ensure that the endoscopist is at hand in case tracheotomy becomes urgently necessary.

General Anesthesia Management

1. *Spontaneous ventilation* is usually preferred during endoscopy in children. It may be safer than controlled ventilation if there is airway compromise, and it allows the endoscopist to examine the anatomic structure of the airway under normal physiologic conditions. Airway compression or collapse may not be detected during controlled ventilation.
2. *Controlled ventilation* is necessary for patients who are in respiratory failure and for those who cannot maintain effective ventilation when anesthetized.

Laryngoscopy

Anesthesia Management

Preoperative

1. Do not give heavy sedation to patients with airway problems. Midazolam given orally is useful for some older children having repeated endoscopy, but beware of sedating any child with a dubious airway.

Perioperative

1. Apply monitors, including pulse oximeter, and induce anesthesia by inhalation of N_2O and O_2 with sevoflurane or halothane.
2. When the patient is asleep, discontinue the N_2O and continue with sevoflurane or halothane in O_2. When the patient is deeply anesthetized, perform laryngoscopy and spray the larynx and supraglottic structures with lidocaine (maximum dose, 5 mg/kg).
3. Replace the mask until the lidocaine becomes effective (2–3 minutes). During the surgical procedure, maintain anesthesia with a propofol infusion.
4. Monitor ventilation carefully using a stethoscope.

Postoperative

1. Observe the patient closely until patient wakens.
2. Order humidified oxygen postoperatively.
3. Order nothing by mouth until 2 hours after application of the lidocaine spray.

N.B. The above method of anesthesia, employing topical analgesia and a propofol infusion with spontaneous ventilation, is considered overall the safest and most satisfactory method. Endotracheal tubes get into the surgeon's field of vision, and all other methods are cumbersome and complicated and therefore may fail. "Jet ventilation" methods can be dangerous in children, especially if the high-pressure jet is allowed to migrate distal to an obstructing lesion. In such circumstances, fatal pneumothorax and pneumomediastinum may occur.

Special Considerations

Laryngomalacia. A common cause of inspiratory stridor in the newborn, laryngomalacia can be diagnosed during laryngoscopy while the infant is awake or is awakening from anesthesia. The stridor usually disappears during deeper levels of anesthesia. In this condition, there is incomplete maturation of the cartilages of the larynx and a tendency for the epiglottis or one of the arytenoid cartilages to prolapse into the glottis on inspiration, causing marked inspiratory stridor. The condition is self-limited and disappears as the child grows; no special therapy is required. However, laryngoscopy is indicated to rule out other causes of stridor (e.g., cysts).

Congenital Cysts. Congenital cysts may occur in the region of the epiglottis and aryepiglottic folds. There may be inspiratory and expiratory stridor and a poor cry. The diagnosis is usually confirmed by radiologic imaging. Therapy is by excision or marsupialization.

Subglottic Hemangioma. Subglottic hemangioma may manifest with crouplike symptoms and a barking cough. The child frequently has other visible hemangiomata. The symptoms persist or recur, and diagnosis is confirmed at endoscopy. Current therapy is by laser destruction of the tumor.

Laryngeal Papillomas. These rare lesions are caused by a virus, and the cauliflower-like papillomas can cause serious obstruction to ventilation. Various therapies have been tried, including cryoprobing, ultrasound, and immune sera. The presently preferred therapy is resection by laser. Children with this condition usually present at 2–4 years of age and return for repeated laryngoscopy and resection. Recurrences are almost certain until adolescence, when the lesions usually regress spontaneously. Increasing hoarseness and dyspnea are the usual indications for reoperation, and on each occasion the extent of regrowth is impossible to determine before laryngoscopy. Sometimes extensive papillomas completely obscure the glottis. A cautious approach is indicated in all cases. Provide humidified gases postoperatively.

Special Anesthesia Problems

1. Acute airway obstruction may occur during induction of anesthesia.
2. The glottic opening may be difficult to visualize. Therefore, barbiturates and relaxants are contraindicated.
3. Surgical therapy by laser demands an unobstructed view of the larynx and immobile vocal cords.
4. Instrumentation of the trachea below the glottis should be avoided, because it may "seed" papillomas into the lower airways. Therefore, endotracheal tubes should be avoided if possible, and tracheostomy is usually considered to be contraindicated.

Anesthesia Management for Laser Surgery

The safest plan is as outlined above: no premedication, careful inhalation induction followed by laryngoscopy, and lidocaine spray to the larynx. If obstruction develops during induction (which happens rarely but is not unknown), an endotracheal tube must be inserted to establish the airway. The tube can be removed when the patient is deeply anesthetized and most of the papillomas have been resected. Usually intubation is not necessary, and laser resection can proceed once topical analgesia has been applied. Maintain anesthesia with a propofol infusion.

Alternatively, a nonflammable endotracheal tube (flexometallic or foil-wrapped) may be inserted. In this case ventilation can be controlled, but the surgeon must work around the tube.

N.B. Jet ventilation can be very dangerous in cases of obstructing lesions of the airway. Laryngeal obstruction during jet ventilation may lead to pneumomediastinum and pneumothorax. If jet ventilation is used, extreme care must be taken to avoid barotrauma: the jet must not be advanced beyond the lumen of the laryngoscope, and distal airway pressure should be monitored whenever possible.

Special Precautions for Use of the Laser

1. Cover the patient's eyes.
2. Use reduced concentrations of O_2 (less than 30%, if such a level provides satisfactory oxygenation) to limit the conflagration at the lesion. N_2O also supports combustion and should be avoided. If the use of an endotracheal tube is essential, use a nonflammable tube (e.g., the laser shielding tube*). Alternatively, if these are not available, a plastic tube may be wrapped in aluminum foil or packed away from the line of the laser with damp gauze. If a tube should ignite, it must be immediately disconnected from the anesthetic circuit and withdrawn from the patient. Injury results both from the burn and from the products of tube combustion.
3. All personnel in the operating room (OR) should wear eyeglasses for protection in case the laser beam is accidentally reflected in their direction. Post a warning sign on the door that the laser is in use.

Bronchoscopy

Bronchoscopy may be performed for various indications (e.g., removal of foreign body, diagnosis of respiratory disease, removal of secretions, treatment of atelectasis). For bronchoscopy in patients with cystic fibrosis, refer to that section. General anesthesia is usually required.

Special Anesthesia Problems

1. Difficulty maintaining adequate ventilation during the procedure, when the airway must be shared with the endoscopist
2. Existing impairment of ventilation in some cases

---

*Phycon laser shielding tube, Fuji Systems Corp., Tokyo, Japan.

Anesthesia Management

Preoperative

1. Assess the airway and the respiratory status carefully.
2. Do not give heavy narcotic premedication if there is any doubt about the airway or ventilation.

Perioperative

Spontaneous ventilation is preferred for all patients except those with respiratory insufficiency.

1. Induce anesthesia by inhalation of N_2O and sevoflurane or halothane in O_2.
2. Discontinue the N_2O and deepen anesthesia with sevoflurane or halothane in O_2.
3. When the patient is adequately anesthetized, remove the mask and perform laryngoscopy. Spray the larynx, trachea, and bronchi with lidocaine (maximum, 5 mg/kg).
4. Replace the mask; continue anesthesia with O_2 and halothane or sevoflurane until the lidocaine takes effect (2–3 minutes), at which time the bronchoscope can be inserted.
5. Supply O_2 and sevoflurane or halothane to the side arm and allow spontaneous ventilation, but remember that when a telescope is in use through a small Storz bronchoscope (3.5 mm or smaller), the resistance to ventilation is high. At such times, ventilation should be assisted or controlled and the telescope may have to be removed periodically.
6. Monitor the ventilation and heartbeat through two stethoscopes: one is taped to the precordium; the other is moved over the lung fields. Monitor oxygenation continuously, using the pulse oximeter.
7. Be alert to the possibility of pneumothorax, a rare complication of pediatric bronchoscopy.
8. When controlled ventilation is essential, as for patients in respiratory failure, a Venturi device (e.g., Sanders injector) may be used, but remember that patients whose severe chronic respiratory disease has reduced lung compliance may not ventilate well with this method. For such patients, the anesthetic circuit may be connected to the side arm of the bronchoscope and controlled ventilation continued (Fig. 10–1).

Postoperative

1. Order nothing by mouth for at least 2 hours (after lidocaine spray).
2. Order humidified O_2.
3. Watch for signs of stridor.

Flexible Bronchoscopy

Small-diameter flexible fiberoptic bronchoscopes have become available that permit diagnostic bronchoscopy to be performed with the patient

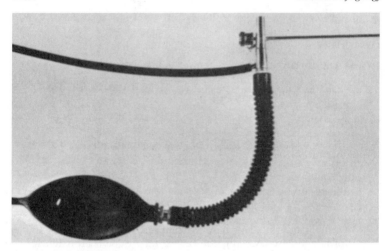

Figure 10–1. Pediatric bronchoscope with attachments for Jackson Rees T-piece, for use during controlled ventilation.

awake or with minimal sedation and topical analgesia. In young children, however, general anesthesia is preferred. In such cases the bronchoscope may be passed through an adapter into the mask and via the mouth or nose of the anesthetized child. Alternatively, an endotracheal tube can be inserted as a conduit for the bronchoscope.

Bronchoscopy for Bronchography

When bronchoscopy is done for bronchography, the child is anesthetized and a bronchoscope is inserted. Under direct vision, a small amount of contrast medium (e.g., a thin solution of barium) is introduced through a catheter into the lobe or lobes to be examined. Radiographs will be of best quality if the contrast medium is introduced during quiet, shallow, spontaneous ventilation. Coughing results in poor-quality films.

Anesthesia Technique

1. Proceed as outlined previously *(see above)*.
2. Before the contrast medium is introduced, give fentanyl (2 μg/kg IV). This produces quiet, shallow ventilation.
3. At the end of the procedure, reverse the narcotic-induced ventilatory depression with naloxone if necessary.

Esophagoscopy

In children, esophagoscopy is usually performed to dilate a stricture or for removal of a foreign body.

Special Anesthesia Problems

1. The child may have undergone esophagoscopy repeatedly and therefore may be very apprehensive.
2. In small infants, passage of an esophagoscope may compress the trachea and obstruct ventilation, even when an endotracheal tube is in place.
3. Coughing, straining, or other movements can result in esophageal perforation during the procedure. Patients must be anesthetized adequately to maintain complete immobility.
4. Lower esophageal strictures or achalasia may have resulted in esophageal dilatation higher up. Food and secretions accumulated in the dilated segment may be aspirated during anesthesia.
5. Rarely, a sharp or potentially damaging foreign body may lodge in the hypopharynx, possibly to be displaced into the airway if the child coughs or strains.

Anesthesia Management

Preoperative

1. Order adequate sedation, especially for children who have undergone esophagoscopy previously (in which case, delay bringing the child to the OR until all preparations have been made).
2. Check whether the radiographs show esophageal dilation and/or retained material.

Perioperative

1. Give 100% O_2 by mask.
2. Induce anesthesia intravenously and secure the airway rapidly. (Use cricoid pressure whenever there is a risk of regurgitation and aspiration—except in the case of a sharp object adjacent to the larynx.)
3. In the case of a sharp foreign body in the hypopharynx, a gentle, smooth inhalation induction of deep anesthesia is indicated.
4. Deepen the anesthesia before permitting the endoscopist to proceed.
5. Monitor the ventilation carefully through a precordial stethoscope.

Postoperative

1. Observe the patient until the patient is fully awake.
2. Be alert for signs of esophageal perforation, especially if difficulty was encountered. These signs include
   a. Tachycardia
   b. Fever
   c. Signs of pneumothorax
   d. Radiographic evidence of pneumothorax or mediastinal air
3. Order nothing by mouth until 2 hours after application of the lidocaine spray.

CROUP

Croup is usually caused by inflammation in the region of the larynx, but other causes must be kept in mind (e.g., a foreign body). The inflammation may be supraglottic (epiglottitis) or subglottic (laryngotracheobronchitis).

Epiglottitis

Since the introduction of a *Haemophilus influenzae* vaccine, epiglottitis has become much less common. It does still occur, however. As the disease becomes rarer, there is a danger that the diagnosis may be missed.

Epiglottitis is most common in children 3–7 years old but may also occur in infants or adults. It is accompanied by severe systemic illness with pyrexia and leukocytosis. In addition to the epiglottitis, all the supraglottic structures are swollen and inflamed, contributing to the obstruction. Blood cultures are almost always positive for the infective agent, which is typically *H. influenzae*, although other organisms have been described. The common symptoms are sore throat, dysphagia, and drooling; severe airway obstruction may develop rapidly. Typically, the patient appears toxic and anxious and sits in a tripod position with chin extended and mouth open. In infants the presentation is less typical, and patients have presented with sudden apnea during investigation of a high fever. Therefore, epiglottitis should be considered in the differential diagnosis of the infant with pyrexia and any respiratory difficulty.

Extraepiglottic infection may occur: pneumonia, cervical adenitis, otitis media, septic arthritis, and meningitis are described in association with epiglottitis.

Anesthesia Management

Preoperative

1. Once the diagnosis is suspected, the child should be disturbed as little as possible. Avoid venipunctures or painful injections, because the child may cry and become acutely obstructed. Do not try to visualize the pharynx, because acute obstruction may result. Gently apply a mask and give O_2.
2. The child must be attended constantly by a physician capable of establishing an emergency airway and equipped to do so.
3. Assemble the team and transfer the patient rapidly to the OR; administer O_2, allowing the child to remain in the chosen posture.
4. Soft-tissue radiographs of the neck may be misleading and are unnecessary in the typical case. If x-ray studies are required to make the diagnosis, the patient must be accompanied to the radiology department by a physician, in case the patient's airway becomes obstructed during the examination. The patient should not be made to lie down for the x-ray examination.

5. The OR should be prepared for emergency bronchoscopy and possible tracheotomy.

If Apnea Occurs (At Any Time)

1. Try to ventilate the patient with O_2 by bag and mask. This is usually successful.
2. If unsuccessful, proceed to an immediate attempt at laryngoscopy and intubation. Also prepare for an emergency tracheotomy if intubation proves impossible.

Perioperative

1. Apply a precordial stethoscope, pulse oximeter, and electrocardiographic electrodes.
2. Do not place the patient in a lying position. Induce anesthesia with O_2 and halothane by placing the mask gently over the child's face while the child is sitting up, either on the OR table or on the anesthetist's or parent's knee.
3. When anesthesia is induced, gently place the patient in the supine position. Assisted ventilation may be necessary at this time.
4. Apply other monitors and establish an intravenous infusion; administer intravenous atropine and obtain a blood culture.
5. Administer lidocaine 1 mg/kg IV to minimize the risk of coughing and laryngospasm; then perform laryngoscopy and orotracheal intubation. In the rare event that the glottis is obscured by swelling and distortion of the supraglottic structures, apply external pressure to the chest. This usually expels a bubble through the larynx, providing a guide to intubation.
6. When the patient is anesthetized and well oxygenated:
   a. Remove the oral tube.
   b. Insert a nasotracheal tube (one size smaller than predicted for age) and tape it securely in position. (The initial passage of a tube will have defined the airway, making replacement by another tube much easier.)
7. Very rarely, pulmonary edema occurs immediately after intubation for epiglottitis. This is thought to be caused by hypoxia, elevated catecholamines, and disturbed alveolar-capillary pressure gradient. Treatment is with controlled ventilation, positive end-expiratory pressure (PEEP), and diuretics.

Postoperative

1. Constant (24 hr/day) nursing care in an intensive care unit is essential. Accidental extubation is a serious early complication and must be prevented by suitable restraints and adequate sedation.
2. Ensure adequate humidification of inspired gases and regular suctioning of the nasotracheal tube. Blockage of the tube may result from tracheal secretions.

3. Commence antibiotic therapy. Cefuroxime, a cephalosporin with a high margin of safety and good penetration of the cerebrospinal fluid, is considered the drug of choice for *H. influenzae* infections.
4. Extubate the patient after the pyrexia has resolved (usually within 12–36 hours). Flexible laryngoscopy may be performed before extubation to examine the state of the supraglottic structures.
5. Observe the patient after extubation for several hours. Very rarely, a patient requires reintubation for recurrent obstruction.

Suggested Additional Reading

Blackstock D, Adderley RJ, and Steward DJ: Epiglottitis in young infants, Anesthesiology 67:97–101, 1987.

Diaz J: Croup and epiglottitis in children: the anesthesiologist as diagnostician. Anesthesiology 64:621–633, 1985.

Hawkins DB, Miller AH, Sachs GB, et al.: Acute epiglottitis in adults. Laryngoscope 83:1211–1220, 1973.

Sendi K and Crysdale WS: Acute epiglottitis: a decade of change—a 10 year experience with 242 children. J Otolaryngol 16:196–202, 1987.

Travis KW, Todres ID, and Shannon DC: Pulmonary edema associated with croup and epiglottitis. Pediatrics 59:695–698, 1977.

Laryngotracheobronchitis

"Acute infectious croup," or laryngotracheobronchitis, is caused by a virus and occurs most commonly in children 2–5 years of age. Inspiratory stridor is the principal symptom.

Therapy varies according to the severity of the disease:

1. In mild cases, conservative measures (e.g., humidification of inspired gases) may be effective.
2. In most other cases, epinephrine inhalations delivered by intermittent positive-pressure breathing (IPPB) results in improvement.
3. Rarely, nasotracheal intubation or tracheotomy is required.

Intermittent Positive-Pressure Breathing with Epinephrine

IPPB with epinephrine is widely reported to be efficacious. It seems that both the positive-pressure ventilation and the inhaled epinephrine contribute to the success.

1. Prepare the nebulizer solution of epinephrine: add 0.5 ml of 2.25% racemic epinephrine to 3.0 ml distilled water.
2. Attach a suitable pediatric-size anesthesia mask to a patient-triggered ventilator. Add the solution to the nebulizer attachment and deliver it at 15–20 cm H_2O pressure and a high inspiratory flow rate.
3. These patients are hypoxic. During IPPB, add at least 40% O_2 to the inspired gases; patients usually then settle well and accept the mask quietly.
4. Monitor ventilation and heart rate via a precordial stethoscope.

Some increase in heart rate may occur, but other arrhythmias are very rare.

5. Give the therapy for 20 minutes, by which time considerable improvement is usually apparent. (If not, the diagnosis of croup should be reconsidered.)
6. After IPPB, observe the patient carefully. Rarely, the stridor increases rapidly, necessitating immediate establishment of an artificial airway.
7. Some patients require more than one therapy. Total failure to respond with any improvement is an indication to review and question the diagnosis. The use of racemic epinephrine is contraindicated in infants with tetralogy of Fallot, because a severe "tet" spell may be precipitated.

Nasotracheal Intubation

If conservative measures and epinephrine inhalations with IPPB fail to relieve symptoms, an artificial airway may be required. Nasotracheal intubation has been used successfully in many centers, with only a small incidence of complications reported. The critical factor seems to be the diameter of the endotracheal tube, which should be very small (e.g., 3.5 mm). The tube is left in place for 7–10 days. Constant (24 hr/day) expert respiratory care is essential; the presence of a small tube and thick secretions renders accidental blockage very likely.

A few patients do not respond as favorably to nasotracheal intubation and cannot be successfully extubated after the standard time. This occurs most commonly in patients younger than 1 year of age, in those with branchial arch deformities or a history of congenital subglottic stenosis, and in those with a history of repeated croup. Tracheotomy may be necessary for these patients.

Tracheotomy

Tracheotomy may become necessary in the therapy of upper airway obstruction or to facilitate respiratory care in other conditions.

Anesthesia Management

Preoperative

1. Give 100% O_2 by mask, and assist ventilation manually as necessary.
2. Do not give sedatives or narcotics.

Perioperative

1. Continue 100% O_2 by mask, induce anesthesia with sevoflurane or halothane and O_2, and assist ventilation as required.
2. Deepen anesthesia, spray lidocaine on the larynx, and allow the surgeon to pass a bronchoscope. (Tracheotomy in children is usually performed after passage of a rigid bronchoscope. This makes it easy for the surgeon to identify the trachea and also enables the anesthesiologist to see immediately that the tracheotomy tube has in fact been passed into the lumen of the trachea.)

3. In case of a "difficult airway" (e.g., Pierre Robin syndrome), anesthesia may be induced with the use of a laryngeal mask airway (LMA), which may then be used as a conduit for subsequent intubation.

Postoperative

1. As soon as possible, obtain a chest radiograph. Check that the tube is positioned correctly and that pneumothorax (a rare complication of tracheotomy) is not present.
2. Be alert to the possibility of accidental extubation before the track into the trachea becomes established. If this happens, it may be very difficult to reinsert the tube. Many surgeons leave long black silk sutures through the edges of the trachea to facilitate emergency reinsertion of the tracheotomy tube.
3. Add an appropriate concentration of oxygen to the inspired gases (to overcome the continuing danger of hypoxemia).
4. Order close, constant observation of the child.
   a. Establishment of the airway does not result in immediate return to normal pulmonary function.
   b. Respiratory arrest may occur during the postoperative period.

Suggested Additional Reading

Adair JC, Ring WH, Jordan WS, and Elwyn RA: Ten-year experience with IPPB in the treatment of acute laryngotracheobronchitis. Anesth Analg 50:649, 1971.

Allen TH and Steven IM: Prolonged nasotracheal intubation in infants and children. Br J Anaesth 44:835, 1972.

Mitchell DP and Thomas RL: Secondary airway support in the management of croup. J Otolaryngol 9:419, 1980.

Newth CJL, Levison H, and Bryan AC: The respiratory status of children with croup. J Pediatr 81:1068, 1972.

SUBGLOTTIC STENOSIS

Subglottic stenosis is one of the most common causes of chronic airway obstruction in infants and children. The stenosis may be congenital or acquired—usually as a complication of prolonged endotracheal intubation. Severe subglottic stenosis requires tracheotomy followed by surgery to reconstruct the subglottic space.

The surgical procedure generally involves division of the cricoid cartilage and insertion of a cartilage graft to increase the diameter. A stent may then be left in place to maintain the lumen.

Associated Conditions (Congenital Type)

1. Congenital heart disease
2. Down syndrome
3. Tracheoesophageal fistula

Anesthesia Management

Preoperative

1. A tracheostomy is in place, and all care and monitoring of the tracheostomy should be continued until the child arrives at the OR.

Perioperative

1. Anesthetize via the tracheotomy tube using sevoflurane or halothane in N_2O/O_2.
2. Remove the tracheotomy tube and insert an armored tube via the stoma; suture it firmly in place. (**Note:** The lumen of the trachea will take a larger tube than is expected!)
3. Check ventilation to both lungs frequently.
4. Maintain anesthesia with N_2O and sevoflurane or halothane, and control ventilation.
5. Blood loss is usually minimal. A stent will be left within the lumen of the larynx.

Postoperative

1. Replace the tracheotomy tube.
2. Administer humidified O_2.
3. Some intravenous fluids may be required for 1–2 days postoperatively until a fluid diet can be taken.
4. A full diet can usually be resumed in a week.
5. The stent is removed and laryngoscopy is performed under general anesthesia 3 months later.
6. The tracheotomy is left in place until the patient is able to tolerate plugging of the lumen of the tube.

Suggested Additional Reading

Crysdale WS: Subglottic stenosis in children: a management protocol plus surgical experience in 13 cases. Int J Pediatr Otorhinol 6:23, 1983.

Friedberg J and Morrison MD: Paediatric tracheotomy. Can J Otolaryngol 3:147, 1974.

Kim IG, Brummit WM, Humphry A, et al.: Foreign body in the airway: a review of 202 cases. Laryngoscope 83:347, 1973.

Maze A and Bloch E: Stridor in pediatric patients. Anesthesiology 50:132, 1979.

Dental Surgery

GENERAL PRINCIPLES

1. Children require general anesthesia more frequently than adults for dental procedures.
2. Many children who present for general anesthesia for dentistry have had previous failed attempts at dental treatment under local analgesia and consequently are very apprehensive.
3. Some children have behavior disorders or mental handicaps and require special consideration.
4. Some children have other medical conditions that require special consideration (e.g., congenital heart disease).
5. Nasotracheal intubation is preferable for children having dental surgery in hospital. (Nasal intubation per se causes bacteremia and is an indication for prophylactic antibiotics if heart disease is present.)
6. The use of air turbine dental drills has been a cause of intraoperative subcutaneous and mediastinal emphysema, leading to airway obstruction and possible pneumothorax. The anesthesiologist must be alert to this danger; if facial swelling occurs, discontinue nitrous oxide (N_2O), check for pneumothorax, and be prepared to support ventilation.
7. Special care must be taken to ensure that no foreign bodies remain in the airway at the end of the procedure (especially throat packs). *All* children should have a gentle, direct laryngoscopy performed before extubation to ensure that the airway is clear.
8. Dental procedures may be prolonged when extensive disease is present. In such instances recovery to a normal appetite is not as brisk as after short operations. Therefore, patients should receive intraoperative intravenous fluids to restore their calculated deficit

and provide maintenance fluids. It is preferred to limit the length of general anesthesia for the outpatient to a maximum of 4 hours and to book surgery for such patients to commence at 8:00 AM.

9. For procedures to be carried out under sedation plus local analgesia, monitoring should be applied as for general anesthesia.

MANAGEMENT FOR GENERAL ANESTHESIA

Preoperative

1. A complete medical history should be obtained and a routine preoperative physical examination performed.
2. Special investigations and treatments, as appropriate, should be ordered for children with other significant disease.
3. Some children do not require premedication. Upset children may benefit from a suitable dose of oral midazolam preoperatively (0.75 mg/kg for children younger than 6 years of age, 0.5 mg/kg for older children). Every effort should be made to reassure and gain the confidence of the upset child.
4. Make sure that all special drugs have been ordered and are administered at the right time (e.g., antibiotics for patients with heart disease).
5. For very upset or uncooperative children who may have behavior disorders or mental handicaps it may be helpful to insert an intravenous line, before admission to surgery, with the parents present.

Perioperative

1. Apply monitors (precordial stethoscope, blood pressure cuff, electrocardiogram, pulse oximeter, and axillary thermistor probe).
2. Induce anesthesia by inhalation or with thiopentone or propofol intravenously.
3. Give a relaxant, oxygenate, and perform nasotracheal intubation. (Soften the distal end of the tube in warm water and lubricate it before insertion.) If succinylcholine is used, children older than 5 years of age should receive d-tubocurarine 0.05 mg/kg IV before the thiopentone to prevent postoperative muscle pain. If such pretreatment is administered, the dose of succinylcholine should be increased to 2 mg/kg to ensure good relaxation for intubation.
4. Maintain anesthesia with N_2O and halothane or sevoflurane in O_2. For short procedures allow spontaneous ventilation. For more prolonged procedures, controlled ventilation may be more appropriate; if so, decrease the inspired anesthetic concentration and monitor blood pressure carefully.
5. Establish an intravenous infusion and give maintenance fluids, including those calculated to replace deficits caused by fasting. After all but very minor dental surgery, a delay in resuming oral intake can be anticipated; therefore, any deficit should be corrected.

6. At the end of the procedure, when all dental instrumentation has been removed, perform a gentle laryngoscopy to ensure that the airway is free of debris or foreign material before extubation.

Postoperative

1. Order analgesics as required. (Dental nerve blocks with local anesthetic reduce the requirement.) Acetaminophen is usually sufficient after dental conservation. After major extractions, a dose of morphine or ketorolac is usually required. Ensure that the patient is provided with analgesic drugs for use after discharge.
2. Continue intravenous fluids until the patient is ready for discharge.

MANAGEMENT FOR SEDATION

1. Barbiturates, benzodiazepines, chloral hydrate, and narcotics have been used. Today, in the hands of an anesthesiologist, propofol is probably the most useful drug, allowing good moment-to-moment control of sedation and ensuring a rapid recovery period.
2. Preoperative care and intraoperative monitoring should be as for general anesthesia *(see above)*.
3. Preoperative medication with midazolam 0.75 mg/kg and prior application of a topical anesthetic cream facilitate insertion of an intravenous catheter.
4. Drugs and equipment for intubation and ventilation with O_2 should be at hand.
5. Sedation should be commenced with a bolus dose of propofol (2.5–3.5 mg/kg) followed by a continuous infusion, beginning with as much as 300 μg/kg/min as required and reducing the rate progressively to 75–100 μg/kg/min as the patient settles. The exact dose requirement for continued sleep varies from patient to patient.
6. Oxygen may be given and end-tidal carbon dioxide sampled by a septate nasal catheter. The airway is usually well maintained, but continuous close monitoring is essential.

Suggested Additional Reading

Berry FA, Blankenbaker WL, and Ball CG: A comparison of bacteremia occurring with nasotracheal or orotracheal intubation. Anesth Analg 52:873, 1973.

Davies JM and Campbell LA: Fatal air embolism during dental implant surgery: a report of three cases. Can J Anaesth 37:112–121, 1990.

Milne B, Katz H, Rosales J, et al.: Subcutaneous facial emphysema complicating dental anaesthesia. Can Anaesth Soc J 29:71, 1982.

Purday JP, Reichert CC, and Merrick PM: Comparative effects of three doses of intravenous ketorolac or morphine on emesis and analgesia for restorative dental surgery in children. Can J Anaesth 43:221–225, 1996.

Puttick N and Rosen M: Propofol induction and maintenance with nitrous oxide in paediatric outpatient dental anaesthesia. Anaesthesia 43:646–649, 1988.

Scott JD and Allan D: Anaesthesia for dentistry in children: a review of 101 surgical procedures. Can Anaesth Soc J 17:391, 1970.

Plastic and Reconstructive Surgery

Many children require plastic surgery to correct congenital deformities, and in most pediatric hospitals this type of surgery constitutes at least 10% of operations. The head and neck are commonly affected, which may introduce special problems for the anesthesiologist. In addition, some children undergo plastic surgery for acquired lesions such as burn scars and contractures or dog bites.

GENERAL PRINCIPLES

1. Many of these children have psychological upsets stemming from both the deformity and multiple surgical procedures. A careful, considerate approach by the anesthesiologist is essential.
2. Smooth general anesthesia with quiet emergence lessens the risk of damage to grafted areas and delicately sutured repairs.
3. Many patients undergoing plastic surgery have potentially serious airway problems that require careful assessment and special management.
4. Congenital structural anomalies commonly affect more than one body system. The child with defects requiring plastic surgery may also have disease affecting other systems. If congenital heart disease is present, ensure that the child is given prophylactic antibiotic therapy preoperatively.

CLEFT LIP AND PALATE

Cleft lip and palate are present in various combinations in as many as 1 of every 1,000 liveborn infants. Their repair constitutes a large part of pediatric plastic surgery. Infants with these lesions may be both anemic and malnourished because of feeding difficulties and may have had repeated respiratory infections.

Associated Conditions

1. Congenital heart disease—not specifically associated with isolated cleft palate, but may be present as part of a syndrome or association
2. Airway anomalies—Pierre Robin syndrome, Treacher Collins syndrome, subglottic stenosis, etc.

Surgical Procedures

1. Cleft lip repair—usually performed at 10–12 weeks
2. Cleft palate repair—usually performed at 12–18 months, but sometimes in younger infants
3. Palatoplasty and pharyngoplasty—usually performed at 5–15 years

Special Anesthesia Problems

1. Airway problems, including difficulty with intubation
2. Blood loss (during cleft palate repair)
3. Problems related to associated conditions (e.g., congenital heart disease)

Anesthesia Management

Preoperative

1. Carry out a very careful assessment.
   a. Direct special attention to the airway, lungs, and other systems that may be affected in congenital syndromes.
   b. Check especially carefully for upper respiratory tract infection; if such an infection is present, surgery should be postponed.
   c. Check for anemia.
2. Check for a history of recent medication with salicylates. If positive, determine the bleeding time; if it is prolonged, surgery should be deferred.
3. For cleft palate surgery transfusion is rarely needed, but check that the patient has been blood-typed and cross-matched for at least 1 unit of blood.

Perioperative

1. If there is any doubt about the ease of endotracheal intubation, perform an inhalation induction.
2. For inhalation induction, administer nitrous oxide (N_2O) and oxygen (O_2) with sevoflurane or halothane until the patient is

anesthetized adequately for laryngoscopy. Then discontinue N_2O and administer halothane in O_2. Give lidocaine 1.5 mg/kg IV before insertion of the laryngoscope to minimize the risk of coughing or laryngospasm.

3. If the cleft is large or bilateral, pack it with moist sterile gauze to prevent trauma during laryngoscopy and intubation.

4. For orotracheal intubation, use an RAE* preformed tracheal tube. Check carefully that bilateral ventilation of the lungs is present after the mouth gag is positioned. Insertion of the gag and flexion of the neck tends to advance the tip of the tube in the trachea, so that it may pass into a bronchus.

5. Monitor air entry continuously during surgery, paying special attention each time the gag is repositioned or the patient is moved.

6. Maintain anesthesia with N_2O and relaxant and controlled ventilation, with a low concentration of halothane (0.75%) or isoflurane (1%) added. This volatile agent should be discontinued before the end of the operation so that the patient awakens promptly on reversal of the relaxant drug.

7. Monitor blood loss carefully and replace if indicated. The infiltration of a local anesthetic with 1:200,000 epinephrine reduces blood loss in cleft palate surgery and also provides some analgesia postoperatively.

8. Inspect the mouth and pharynx gently at the end of surgery; use a laryngoscope and remove all blood and clots. Extubate when the patient is fully awake. After palate repair, acute swelling of the tongue causing obstruction has been reported as a complication of the use of the tongue blade on the mouth gag. Therefore, examine the mouth carefully; if any signs of swelling exist, the patient should be left intubated.

9. A tongue suture is often inserted to facilitate immediate postoperative control of the airway after cleft palate repair.

Postoperative

1. Cleft lip surgery is often performed in the day surgery unit, because the surgery is superficial and postoperative problems are rare.

2. After cleft palate surgery the child is admitted. Ensure constant observation for 24 hours, because airway problems or bleeding may occur. A small percentage of children may have to return to the operating room (OR) for control of bleeding.

3. Order nursing in a croup tent.

4. Order analgesics as necessary but avoid excessive depression.

PHARYNGOPLASTY

Pharyngoplasty is performed to reduce velopharyngeal incompetence and improve speech. The procedure inevitably increases resistance to ventilation. Postoperative airway problems are not uncommon.

---

*Mallinckrodt Inc., St. Louis, MO.

Special Anesthesia Problems

1. Postoperative airway obstruction is a particular danger and may occur in the postanesthesia care unit (PACU).
2. Chronic airway obstruction may persist after the operation and may lead to pulmonary hypertension and/or obstructive sleep apnea.

Anesthesia Management

As for cleft palate *(see above)*.

Postoperative

1. Observe closely in the PACU for airway obstruction and/or bleeding for at least 12 hours.
2. Do not order heavy narcotic sedation—intramuscular codeine is adequate for analgesia.
3. Continuing supervision for signs of obstruction during sleep is suggested, and postoperative sleep studies should be performed.
4. A nasopharyngeal airway may be left in for 24 hours.

Suggested Additional Reading

Bell C, Oh TH, and Loeffler JR: Massive macroglossia and airway obstruction after cleft palate repair. Anesth Analg 67:71–74, 1988.

Doyle E and Hudson I: Anaesthesia for primary repair of cleft lip and palate: a review of 244 procedures. Paediatr Anaesth 2:139–145, 1992.

Halpern L and Roy L: Anesthetic morbidity associated with pharyngoplasty in children: a five year review. Anesthesiology 75:A933, 1991.

Kravath RE, Pollak CP, Borowiecki B, and Weitzman ED: Obstructive sleep apnea and death associated with surgical correction of velopharyngeal incompetence. J Pediatr 96:645, 1980.

Lee JTR and Kingston HGG: Airway obstruction due to massive lingual oedema following cleft palate surgery. Can Anaesth Soc J 32:265–267, 1985.

Levin RM: Anesthesia for cleft lip and cleft palate. Anaesth Rev 6:25–30, 1979.

CYSTIC HYGROMA

Cystic hygroma is in fact a cystic lymphangioma that usually occurs in the neck and less commonly in the axilla. Intraoral extension of this benign tumor may cause airway obstruction. Three percent of cervical tumors extend into the mediastinum.

Special Anesthesia Problems

1. There may be existing airway obstruction.
2. Intubation may be difficult due to distortion of the airway.
3. Complete removal of tumor may involve extensive dissection and be accompanied by major blood loss.

Anesthesia Management

Preoperative

1. Assess the patient carefully, looking especially for evidence of intrathoracic extension of the tumor.
2. Do not give heavy sedation.
3. Ensure availability of blood and blood products for transfusion.
4. Prepare a selection of tubes and laryngoscope blades.

Perioperative

1. Induce anesthesia cautiously by inhalation of N_2O and sevoflurane or halothane. Maintain spontaneous ventilation.
2. When the patient is anesthetized, establish a reliable large-bore intravenous route.
3. Before attempting intubation, discontinue N_2O and give O_2 and halothane for 2 minutes. Coughing and breath-holding and/or laryngospasm during attempts at intubation may be minimized by giving lidocaine 1.5 mg/kg IV.
4. Intubate, preferably using an armored tube, and secure the tube firmly. For some patients, if intraoral dissection is planned, a nasal tube may be preferable. In the case of a difficult intubation, insert an oral tube first, then change to a nasal tube.
5. Maintain anesthesia with N_2O and relaxant and low concentrations of isoflurane (1%) with controlled ventilation.
6. For large tumors requiring extensive dissection, an arterial line should be inserted.
7. Beware of vagal reflexes during dissection in the neck. Give atropine intravenously if these reflexes occur.
8. Replace blood losses carefully with appropriate fluids, guided by the blood pressure and the measured losses.
9. After the operation, extubate the patient smoothly; prevent excessive coughing and bucking, which might cause bleeding at the surgical site.
10. If extensive surgery has been performed adjacent to the airway, extubation should be delayed until the extent of postoperative swelling is determined. If swelling is significant, intubation is required until it resolves. A few patients may require tracheotomy.

Postoperative

1. If extubated:
   a. Order close observation in the PACU overnight (because of the danger of bleeding into the surgical site or compression of the airway).
   b. Avoid large doses of narcotic analgesics.
2. If intubated:
   a. Confirm the position of the endotracheal tube by radiography.
   b. Order appropriate humidified O_2 in air and continuing care.

Suggested Additional Reading

Brooks JC: Cystic hygroma of the neck. Laryngoscope 83:117–128, 1973.

MacDonald DJF: Cystic hygroma: an anaesthetic and surgical problem. Anaesthesia 21:66, 1966.

FRACTURED MANDIBLE

Surgical Procedures

1. Interdental wiring
2. Open reduction and wiring

Special Anesthesia Problems

1. The patient may have a full stomach.
2. Intubation may be difficult because of tissue damage and distortion.
3. Foreign bodies may be present in the airway (e.g., teeth).
4. The mouth is wired closed after the procedure; therefore, postoperative vomiting is virtually lethal.

Anesthesia Management

Preoperative

1. Assess the patient carefully.
2. Determine the more patent nostril for intubation.
3. For patients with a full stomach, delay surgery if possible and give metoclopramide intravenously (to hasten gastric emptying).
4. Do not give heavy sedation.

Perioperative

1. Use a rapid sequence induction with cricoid pressure.
2. Examine the pharynx quickly but carefully during laryngoscopy to search for foreign debris.
3. Use an orotracheal tube initially; then change to a nasotracheal tube. (If you attempt to place the nasotracheal tube initially, you may start a nosebleed—then the patient will have a full stomach plus a nosebleed! Once the oral tube is in place, pass a nasal tube through the nose, repeat the laryngoscopy, and change tubes.)
4. Insert a nasogastric tube and aspirate. Pack the throat with sterile gauze.
5. Maintain anesthesia with N_2O and/or a propofol infusion plus relaxant using controlled ventilation. (This permits rapid reawakening and minimal postoperative nausea.)
6. Before final fixation of the jaws, remove the pack and inspect the pharynx with a laryngoscope; remove blood clots and other debris.
7. Keep the nasotracheal tube in place during transportation to the PACU.
8. Leave the nasogastric tube in place for use during the postoperative period.

Postoperative

1. Order close observation of patient.
2. Do not remove the nasotracheal tube until the patient is fully awake.
3. Ensure that wire cutters are at the bedside at all times.

Removal of Interdental Wiring

General anesthesia is usually required for removal of the wiring and arch bars when the fracture is healed. The wires holding the jaws together can be removed before induction of anesthesia. However, jaw movement remains extremely restricted because of the prolonged immobilization, rendering laryngoscopy and intubation very difficult.

Ensure that the patient has been fasted preoperatively. After removal of the securing wires, induce anesthesia by inhalation of N_2O and halothane until a nasopharyngeal tube can be inserted for maintenance.

Exercise great care to maintain the airway, and have equipment for emergency intubation and/or tracheotomy immediately at hand.

RECONSTRUCTIVE SURGERY FOR BURNS

After the acute phase of injury, children who have extensive burns require repeated anesthesia for plastic and reconstructive surgery.

Special Anesthesia Problems

1. Contractures resulting from burns of the face and neck may make intubation and maintenance of the airway during anesthesia very difficult.
2. Succinylcholine is contraindicated for 2–3 months after severe burns, because it may cause cardiac arrest secondary to hyperkalemia.
3. Severe emotional problems may have resulted from the accident, disfigurement, and repeated surgical procedures.
4. Blood losses may be large during grafting of extensive burns.
5. Temperature homeostasis is impaired, and special measures must be taken to avoid excessive heat loss. Prepare to use a forced-air warming mattress (e.g., Bair hugger*).
6. Infection of burns is a serious hazard at this stage. Observe great care in handling of the patient to prevent cross-infection; use reverse-isolation techniques in the OR and postoperatively.
7. Hepatic dysfunction may occur after burns; recovery takes several weeks.
8. Emergence from anesthesia should be quiet to avoid damage to recently grafted areas.

Anesthesia Management—General Endotracheal Anesthesia

General endotracheal anesthesia may be used, but there are some special considerations:

1. A 40% higher dose of thiopental is required in children with fresh burns and during convalescence. This dose may cause cardiovascular

---

*Augustine Medical, Eden Prairie, MN.

effects if the patient is at all hypovolemic. Ketamine may be preferred for induction of such patients.

2. Succinylcholine is contraindicated in all burn patients.
3. The dose requirements for nondepolarizing muscle relaxants are increased in proportion to the magnitude of the burn. Relaxants should be titrated to achieve the desired effect, and if possible a neuromuscular blockade monitor should be used.
4. If there has been airway involvement in the burn, progressive stenosis may develop, usually in the subglottic area. Carefully select an endotracheal tube, and do not be surprised if a smaller tube is required at a subsequent operation. Severe stenosis may necessitate tracheostomy.
5. Severely ill patients may not tolerate volatile agents; in such cases, narcotic analgesics (e.g., fentanyl) with relaxants and controlled ventilation are preferred.

Preoperative

1. Assess the patient's condition carefully, and review the anesthesia history.
2. Take time to talk with the patient. Encourage questions, answer them honestly, and reassure the patient about the planned procedure.
3. Preoperative fasting must be rigidly observed, even if the use of ketamine is planned. J tube feeds may be given until 3 hours preoperatively.
4. Order adequate sedation (e.g., midazolam) to be given by mouth 30 minutes preoperatively.
5. Make sure that the OR is warmed to 25°C.

Perioperative

1. If no airway problems:
   a. Induce anesthesia intravenously with thiopental or by inhalation of N_2O and halothane or sevoflurane.
   b. Administer relaxant (*not* succinylcholine) and perform intubation after spraying with lidocaine.
   c. Maintain anesthesia with N_2O and halothane or isoflurane with a relaxant and controlled ventilation. Insert a reliable intravenous line.
   d. Monitoring must be adapted to the site and extent of the burn area; that is, a blood pressure cuff is placed on any uninjured limb. An esophageal stethoscope is usually suitable and can incorporate electrocardiogram leads.* Attempt to monitor all the usual parameters. Pulse oximetry can be obtained from the tongue if there is no other site.
   e. Measure blood losses and be prepared to replace them. If massive

---

*For example, Esophagocardioscope, Sims Portex Inc., Keene, NH.

transfusion is required, be alert to the possibility of hypocalcemia, which is more common in burn patients. Monitor coagulation; platelet concentrates and fresh-frozen plasma should be ordered when massive transfusion is required.

2. If there are airway deformities (e.g., cervical contractures):
   a. If the chin cannot be extended or the mouth opened, direct visual intubation may be impossible. Select from the following alternatives:
      i. Perform fiberoptic intubation, either awake and sedated with topical analgesia or after inhalation induction, depending on the patient.
      ii. Perform a blind nasal intubation. Proficiency demands much experience, and this approach may be particularly difficult if scar tissue has distorted the airway.
      iii. After release of scar tissue under local analgesia, induce anesthesia and perform direct-vision intubation.
   b. Once the airway is established, anesthesia can be maintained as described above.

Anesthesia Management—Ketamine

Ketamine is a very valuable agent for use during reconstructive surgery in burned patients, and in some centers it has been used as the sole anesthetic. Provided that emergence reactions are avoided (by appropriate benzodiazepine premedication), ketamine is highly suitable for repeated use in these children; in fact, many request "the same anesthetic as last time" (i.e., ketamine). In addition, this agent causes less disturbance of appetite and feeding than do conventional anesthetics—an important feature for these patients.

Although it is unlikely, airway obstruction may occur during ketamine anesthesia; be prepared to reestablish ventilation.

Other advantages of ketamine in patients with burns are as follows:

1. Profound analgesia is provided without respiratory or cardiovascular system depression. (Cardiac output is increased and is maintained during changes in position.)
2. Analgesics are not usually required postoperatively. Emergence is quiet, with minimal risk to grafted areas.
3. Unlike halothane, ketamine has no immunosuppressive action.
4. Atropine should be given to prevent the copious secretions that may complicate ketamine anesthesia.

Anesthesia Management—Postoperative

1. Emergence from anesthesia should be quiet. Order adequate analgesic drugs if required.
2. If ketamine has been used, be aware of the possibility of psychotic emergence reactions. Order observation until the patient has fully recovered and is fit to return to the ward.

Suggested Additional Reading

Cote GJ and Petkau AJ: Thiopental requirements may be increased in children reanesthetised at least one year after recovery from extensive thermal injury. Anesth Analg 64:1156, 1985.

Martyn JAJ, Liu LMP, Szyfelbein SK, et al.: Pancuronium requirements in burned children. Anesthesiology 59:561–564, 1983.

Martyn JAJ, Matteo RS, and Greenblatt DJ: Comparative pharmacodynamics of d-tubocurarine in burned and non-burned men. Anesth Analg 61:241–246, 1982.

Szyfelbein SK, Drop LG, and Martyn JAJ: Persistent ionized hypocalcemia during resuscitation and recovery phases of body burns. Crit Care Med 9:454–458, 1981.

Tolmie JD, Joyce TH, and Mitchell GD: Succinylcholine danger in the burned patient. Anesthesiology 28:467, 1967.

Wilson RD, Nichols RJ, and McCoy NR: Dissociative anesthesia with CI-581 in burned children. Anesth Analg 46:719, 1967.

Zook EG, Roesch RP, Thompson LW, and Bennett JE: Ketamine anesthesia in pediatric plastic surgery. Plast Reconstr Surg 48:241, 1971.

MAJOR CRANIOFACIAL RECONSTRUCTIVE SURGERY

Extensive reconstruction is now possible for children with severe facial deformities. The improvement in appearance frequently has a major beneficial effect on the child's future life. Much of this surgery is now being performed during infancy or early childhood. The objective is to allow the child to go to school looking as normal as possible.

General Principles

1. A team approach is essential for successful performance of this type of surgery.
2. Operations involving the jaws are usually delayed until dentition is complete (i.e., 13 years or older).
3. Operations not involving dentition (e.g., for craniofacial dysostosis) are usually performed at an earlier age.

Special Anesthesia Problems

1. Intubation of the airway may be difficult if the deformity is severe. Some patients require tracheotomy preoperatively (using local analgesia).
2. Blood loss may be very extensive from the surgical and bone graft donor sites (e.g., pelvic girdle or ribs).
3. Surgery is of long duration, and special precautions must be taken to protect the patient against complications of prolonged anesthesia (e.g., pressure sores).
4. Surgical manipulation involving the orbit and face may initiate the oculocardiac reflex.
5. Surgical manipulations may damage the endotracheal tube intraoperatively (rare).
6. The patient must awaken rapidly after surgery so that the surgeon can check cranial nerve function.

7. Extensive postoperative swelling may dictate the need for prolonged intubation after the operation.

Anesthesia Management

Preoperative

1. Examine the patient very thoroughly, particularly for airway abnormalities and cardiopulmonary disease.
2. Consider the possibility of associated congenital defects or other features of a syndrome that may have implications for anesthesia (*see* Appendix I). Some children (e.g., those with Apert's or Crouzon's syndrome) have sleep apnea, and this possibility should be investigated in a sleep laboratory.
3. Check all laboratory results, especially for indications of coagulopathy.
4. Order any further tests necessary to assess the patient fully before surgery.
5. Ensure that adequate supplies of blood and blood products will be available and that serum has been saved for further cross-matching if necessary.
6. Reassure the patient and explain the planned procedures, including postoperative care.
7. Order preoperative sedation: midazolam 0.5 mg/kg PO (maximum, 20 mg) for children or lorazepam (Ativan) 1–2 mg PO for adolescents.

Perioperative

1. Induce anesthesia:
   a. If there are no intubation problems, induce with intravenous thiopental; then proceed to intubation using a relaxant.
   b. If difficulty is anticipated, use an inhalation induction and proceed to intubation via a laryngeal mask airway (LMA) or other means.
   c. In some cases of extremely difficult airway, a tracheotomy may be performed under local analgesia. This can then be used for anesthesia and as a postoperative airway until swelling subsides.
2. The endotracheal tube should be sutured in position, with due consideration being given to the movements of the facial bones that will accompany the surgery. The tube should either be sutured to a structure that will not be moved or be so positioned in the trachea as to allow for the effects of movement at its point of fixation. An armored tube should be used if possible. The SWAY tube,* which is armored only in the proximal extratracheal segment, may be useful if prolonged intubation is anticipated.
3. Maintain anesthesia with N_2O and narcotic (e.g., fentanyl 2–3 µg/kg/hr) and a suitable relaxant drug.

---

*Phycon SWAY tube, Fuji Systems Corp., Tokyo, Japan.

4. Control ventilation to an arterial carbon dioxide pressure ($PaCO_2$) of 25–30 mmHg.
5. Position the patient with 10°–15° head-up tilt.
6. Pad all pressure areas well, including occiput and areas compressed by the endotracheal tube (e.g., nares, lip).
7. Place ointment in the eyes (the surgeon will usually perform tarsorrhaphy).
8. Monitor:
   a. Ventilation and heart rate via stethoscope
   b. Electrocardiogram, pulse oximeter, and end-tidal carbon dioxide values
   c. Central venous and arterial blood pressure by direct means
   d. Acid-base, blood gas, and hematocrit by serial determinations
   e. Temperatures
   f. Coagulation indices (during transfusion if massive)
   g. Urine output
   h. Precordial Doppler ultrasound—for air embolism during craniectomy
9. Be prepared for massive blood replacement.
10. If reduction in brain mass is required, give furosemide 1 mg/kg IV.
11. When indicated, induce hypotension using either isoflurane or sodium nitroprusside.
11. The patient should be fully awake in the OR at the end of surgery, so that the surgeon can check the patient's vision and ascertain whether cranial nerve injury has occurred during surgery.

Postoperative

1. Order routine postcraniotomy nursing care when applicable.
2. Leave endotracheal tube in place until the patient is fully awake *and* there is no further danger that postoperative tissue swelling might obstruct the airway. (Many patients require intubation for 24–48 hours postoperatively.)
3. Observe caution when using narcotic analgesics.
4. Check hemoglobin and hematocrit to ensure adequacy of blood replacement.

Suggested Additional Reading*

Davies DW and Munro IR: The anesthetic management and intraoperative care of patients undergoing major facial osteotomies. Plast Reconstr Surg 55:50, 1975.

Diaz JH and Henling CE: Pneumoperitoneum and cardiac arrest during craniofacial reconstruction. Anesth Analg 61:146, 1982.

Handler SD: Craniofacial surgery: otolaryngological concerns. Int Anesthesiol Clin 26:61–63, 1988.

---

*For implications for anesthesia in relation to congenital defects, see the relevant entry and references in Appendix I.

Handler SD, Beaugard ME, and Whitaker LA: Airway management in the repair of craniofacial defects. Cleft Palate J 16:16, 1978.

Munro IR: Craniofacial surgery: airway problems and management. Int Anesthesiol Clin 26:73–78, 1988.

Robideaux V: Oculocardiac reflex caused by midface disimpaction. Anesthesiology 49:433, 1978.

Schafer ME: Upper airway obstruction and sleep disorders in children with craniofacial anomalies. Clin Plast Surg 9:555, 1982.

Chapter 13

General and Thoracoabdominal Surgery

GENERAL PRINCIPLES

1. Many of the patients are neonates, some preterm, and therefore demand special considerations.
2. In many cases the pathophysiology of the surgical disease dictates the optimal anesthesia management. The anesthesiologist should understand the effects of the lesion on normal physiology.
3. Surgery is very rarely required immediately; usually some time is available for preoperative resuscitation. The optimum time for surgery must be decided by consultation among anesthesiologist, neonatologist, and surgeon.
4. For emergency abdominal surgery, the problem of the full stomach must be considered. (Even if the patient has not eaten for some time, secretions accumulate in the stomach, and emptying may be delayed by obstruction or ileus.) Children admitted for any emergency surgery may have high volume and acidity of gastric contents. Children with a history of gastroesophageal reflux may be at special risk.
   a. Remember the effects of drugs on the barrier pressure (i.e., lower esophageal pressure [LES] minus gastric pressure). Barrier pressure is reduced by atropine, diazepam, nitrous oxide (N_2O), and volatile anesthetic agents. It is increased by metoclopramide, pancuronium, and vecuronium, and it is little changed by succinylcholine.
   b. Drugs can sometimes be used to reduce the volume and acidity of gastric contents: cimetidine (oral or rectal), ranitidine, metoclopramide, and sodium citrate.
      Possible plans of action:
      i. Whenever possible, pretreat with drugs to reduce the volume and acidity of gastric contents. Pass a gastric tube and aspirate the stomach where appropriate.
      ii. Newborn and small infants at high risk: aspirate stomach contents through a gastric tube, preoxygenate, and perform a rapid-sequence induction or awake intubation.*
      iii. Older children: aspirate stomach contents (if appropriate) and perform a rapid-sequence induction combined with cricoid pressure (Sellick's maneuver). Cricoid pressure must be commenced as soon as any drugs are given that may reduce LES. There is still no relaxant drug that can replace succinylcholine for speed of onset, offset, and intensity of neuromuscular block.
      iv. Make sure that the patient is well anesthetized and well relaxed before intubation is attempted. Struggling during attempts at intubation in an incompletely relaxed child is a common precursor to vomiting and aspiration!

---

*The trend in neonatal anesthesia has been away from awake intubation. The competent neonatal anesthetist now prefers to induce anesthesia and, if indicated, to perform a rapid-sequence induction.

Remember: For rapid-sequence induction, succinylcholine does not increase intra-abdominal pressure in children younger than 10 years of age, and pretreatment with curare is not indicated.

5. During thoracoabdominal surgery, blood loss may be considerable; be prepared to handle major blood transfusion.
6. For major abdominal surgery, always place intravenous lines in the upper limbs or neck. The inferior vena cava (IVC) may rarely have to be clamped or may be otherwise compressed during the operation; in this case, transfusion via the lower limb veins would be useless.
7. N_2O diffuses into the lumen of gas-containing bowel, causing further distention and difficulties for the surgeon. Do not use N_2O when conditions predispose to this condition (e.g., intestinal obstruction).
8. The airways are small and, during lung surgery, bronchial secretions (often sanguineous) may accumulate and interfere with ventilation. Perform tracheobronchial toilet whenever this becomes necessary.
9. During thoracotomy, ventilation-perfusion ($\dot{V}/\dot{Q}$) ratios in the lungs are disturbed; therefore, increase the inspired O_2 concentration to maintain a safe level of oxygen saturation.
10. In infants and small children, retraction of the lungs may obstruct major airways, impairing ventilation, or it may compress the heart and great veins, leading to a precipitous fall in cardiac output and hence in blood pressure (BP). Constant monitoring of breath sounds via stethoscope and observation of the pulse oximeter are essential. In the event of falling saturation, bradycardia, hypotension, or impaired ventilation:
    a. Ask the surgeon to remove all retractors immediately.
    b. Ventilate the patient with 100% O_2.
11. Patients requiring minor surgery (e.g., herniotomy) may be preterm and/or have other conditions (e.g., anemia) that can complicate anesthesia and require special precautions. Remember the special problems of the ex-preterm infant.
12. Many general surgery procedures can now be performed with the use of video-assisted endoscopic techniques. It is anticipated that additional advances in these techniques will further extend the scope of minimally invasive pediatric surgery over the next few years.

Suggested Additional Reading

Cotton BR and Smith G: The lower oesophageal sphincter and anaesthesia. Br J Anaesth 56:37–46, 1984.

Hunt PCW, Cotton BR, and Smith G: Barrier pressure and muscle relaxants. Anaesthesia 39:412–415, 1984.

Kallar SK and Evertt LL: Potential risks and preventive measures for pulmonary aspiration: new concepts in preoperative fasting guidelines. Anesth Analg 77:171–182, 1993.

Phillips S, Daborn AK, and Hatch DJ: Preoperative fasting for paediatric anaesthesia. Br J Anaesth 73:529–536, 1994.

Schurizek BA, Rybro L, Boggild-Madsen NB, et al.: Gastric volume and pH in children for emergency surgery. Acta Anaesthesiol Scand 30:404–408, 1986.

Sehhati GH, Frey R, and Star EG: The action of inhalation anesthetics upon the lower oesophageal sphincter. Acta Anaesth Belg 2:91–98, 1980.

Warner MA, Warner ME, Warner DO, et al.: Perioperative pulmonary aspiration in infants and children. Anesthesiology 90:66–71, 1999.

CONGENITAL DEFECTS THAT MAY NECESSITATE SURGERY DURING THE NEONATAL PERIOD

Congenital Lobar Emphysema

Abnormal distention of a lobe (usually the upper or middle lobe) compresses the remaining normal lung tissue and displaces the mediastinum; respiratory distress and cyanosis result. When severe, this condition manifests as an extreme emergency during the early neonatal period. Less severe forms may pass unnoticed for months or even years.

Obstruction of the bronchus supplying the distended lobe may be extrinsic (e.g., abnormal blood vessels) or intraluminal; or it may be caused by a defect of the bronchial wall (bronchomalacia). More than one lobe may be involved in some patients. The chest radiograph demonstrates a hyperlucent area with sparse lung markings (differentiating it from pneumothorax) and mediastinal shift. The lesion must also be differentiated from congenital diaphragmatic hernia or cystic adenomatoid malformation, which can have a similar radiologic appearance.

Associated Condition

1. Congenital heart disease—an incidence of up to 37% in reported series

Surgical Procedure

1. Lobectomy (if no intraluminal or extrinsic cause can be found and corrected)

Special Anesthesia Problems

1. Severe respiratory failure may occur due to compression of normal lung tissue.
2. There is the possibility of a "ball valve" effect, which further increases the size of the affected lobe during positive-pressure ventilation.
3. N_2O may cause further distention of the lobe and is therefore contraindicated.

Anesthesia Management

1. Observe special precautions for neonates.

Preoperative

1. The patient is nursed while in a semiupright position.
2. Give O_2 by hood. Avoid intermittent positive-pressure ventilation (IPPV) if possible (danger of "ball valve" effect).

3. Insert a gastric tube and apply continuous suction. This prevents gastric distention from further compromising ventilation.
4. Check that blood is available for transfusion.
5. Sudden serious deterioration of the patient's condition may demand immediate emergency thoracotomy to exteriorize the affected lobe and allow the normal lung tissue to ventilate.

Perioperative

1. Bronchoscopy to exclude intraluminal obstruction may be performed before thoracotomy.
2. Give atropine intravenously and induce anesthesia with sevoflurane or halothane in O_2 if the infant's condition permits; otherwise, spray the vocal cords with lidocaine, give O_2 by mask for at least 3 minutes, and then perform laryngoscopy and intubate (or allow the surgeon to pass the bronchoscope).
3. Maintain anesthesia with isoflurane, sevoflurane, or halothane in O_2.
4. After bronchoscopy (if performed) and before thoracotomy, change to an endotracheal tube.
5. Continue with spontaneous or very gently assisted ventilation until the thorax is open. Selective endobronchial intubation of the unaffected lung has been suggested as an alternative to prevent further expansion of the emphysematous lobe or lobes during assisted ventilation. When the chest is open, the affected lobe usually balloons out of the chest and ventilation must be controlled.
6. Once the thorax is open, a nondepolarizing neuromuscular blocking drug can be given to facilitate controlled ventilation and minimize the need for inhaled anesthetic vapors. N_2O can be added to the inspired gases once lobectomy is complete, but the fraction of inspired oxygen (FiO_2) should be maintained at a level that ensures full saturation.
7. After the affected lobe has been excised, the remaining lung tissue will gradually expand to fill the thorax, although a pneumothorax may remain.

Postoperative

1. Discontinue all anesthetic drugs and administer 100% O_2. Reverse relaxant drugs.
2. When the infant is wide awake, suction the endotracheal tube and remove it.
3. Place the infant in a heated incubator and supply O_2 as required to maintain arterial oxygenation.
4. A chest drain (connected to underwater drainage and suction) is required for 48 hours.

Anesthesia Management—Older Children

In approximately 10% of cases, a congenital emphysematous lobe is discovered at an older age. These children should be managed as outlined for younger patients. In some cases a bronchial blocker (e.g.,

Fogarty catheter) may be inserted to isolate the affected side. Do not start controlled ventilation until the chest is open.

Suggested Additional Reading

Cote CJ: Anesthetic management of congenital lobar emphysema. Anesthesiology 49:296, 1978.

Gupta R, Singhal SK, Rattan KN, and Chhabra B: Management of congenital lobar emphysema with endobronchial intubation and controlled ventilation. Anesth Analg 86:71–73, 1998.

Schwartz MZ and Ramachandran P: Congenital malformations of the lung and mediastinum—a quarter century of experience from a single institution. J Pediatr Surg 32:44–47, 1997.

Congenital Diaphragmatic Hernia

The incidence of congenital diaphragmatic hernia is 1 in 4,000 live births. There are several types: anterior through the foramen of Morgagni, posterolateral via the foramen of Bochdalek, and at the esophageal hiatus. The most common lesion is posterolateral, through the foramen of Bochdalek, usually on the left side. Herniation of abdominal contents into the thorax is associated with respiratory distress, mediastinal displacement ("dextrocardia"), and a scaphoid abdomen. Breath sounds are absent over the affected side. Bowel sounds are very rarely heard over the thorax. The radiographic appearance is usually diagnostic but may be indistinguishable from that of congenital lobar emphysema.

In many patients with congenital diaphragmatic hernia, the lungs are severely hypoplastic. It has been thought that compression of the developing lung in the fetus causes this hypoplasia; hence, there have been attempts to correct the defect in utero. However, an alternative theory suggests that this disease results from a primary failure of lung development with associated failure of development of the diaphragm.

The infant is usually in severe respiratory distress at or soon after birth. In recent years the diagnosis has generally been made in utero by fetal ultrasound.

Associated Conditions

1. Malrotation of the gut (40% of cases)
2. Congenital heart disease (15%)
3. Renal abnormalities (less common)
4. Neurologic abnormalities
5. Cantrell's pentalogy

Surgical Procedures

1. Reduction of hernia and repair of the diaphragmatic defect: usually a transabdominal procedure

Special Anesthesia Problems

1. Optimal preoperative preparation of the patient: The trend in recent years is not to rush to surgery. Relief of compression of the lungs by reduction of the herniated abdominal viscera usually does not solve the problem; indeed, there is evidence that respiratory mechanics are worse postoperatively. It is now preferred to treat the respiratory insufficiency by muscle paralysis, controlled ventilation, and therapy to reduce pulmonary vasoconstriction. If these measures fail, extracorporeal membrane oxygenation (ECMO) may be instituted. The operation is performed later, as an elective procedure, when the infant is improving and can be weaned from respiratory support.

Anesthesia Management

Preoperative

Preoperative management requires the facilities and trained staff of a specialist unit. The infant is nursed in a semiupright, semilateral position, facing toward the involved side. A gastric tube is passed and maintained on low suction to prevent further distention of intrathoracic abdominal viscera. All but the exceptionally fit older infant require intubation and ventilation:

1. Muscle paralysis after intubation facilitates controlled ventilation and minimizes struggling, thereby decreasing the O_2 demand. It also reduces airway pressure, minimizes further lung damage, and diminishes the ever-present danger of pneumothorax. (Pneumothorax is a constant danger and must be watched for and immediately treated.)
2. The infant should be hyperventilated, if possible, while avoiding the use of unnecessarily high pressures. In some cases a degree of hypercapnia may be accepted rather than using high pressures that might cause further damage to the hypoplastic lungs.
3. High-frequency ventilation may have a role in facilitating gas exchange while minimizing pressure swings, which might cause further lung damage.
4. Pulmonary vascular resistance may be reduced by general measures such as hyperventilation, fentanyl infusion, and minimal handling of the child. Nitric oxide may be administered by inhalation and may further reduce pulmonary vascular resistance in some patients.
5. The possible role for partial liquid ventilation in managing patients with congenital diaphragmatic hernia is yet to be determined.
6. When all of these measures fail, ECMO is indicated and may permit survival until the pulmonary status improves.
7. In selected cases of extreme pulmonary hypoplasia, lobar lung transplantation may be considered.

Aggressive invasive monitoring using arterial and pulmonary artery lines is required to ensure optimal treatment for the pulmonary status.

The best predictors of the degree of pulmonary hypoplasia, and hence of survival, are the arterial carbon dioxide tension ($PaCO_2$) and the respiratory index (the product of mean airway pressure and respiratory rate). Those patients who are easy to ventilate and not grossly hypercarbic have a better prognosis. Those who are hypercarbic and hypoxic with a high mean airway pressure are less likely to survive. ECMO may increase survival of this latter group. If the child improves on ECMO, surgery is usually performed just before weaning.

Perioperative

1. Induce and maintain anesthesia with appropriate additional doses of fentanyl. Ventilate with O_2/air to maintain oxygen saturation. Low concentrations of isoflurane may be added as required and if tolerated. N_2O is contraindicated. (It could further distend gas-containing herniated viscera.)
2. Monitor airway pressure. This should not exceed 25–30 cmH$_2$O (higher pressures may cause further lung damage).
3. Do not try to expand the lungs after reduction of the hernia (lung damage may result).
4. Monitor blood gas and acid-base status frequently and correct as indicated.

   For patients having surgery on ECMO:

5. Common practice has been to administer additional doses of relaxant and narcotic drugs. However, very often infants on ECMO have developed tolerance to fentanyl and require very large doses to prevent the cardiovascular response to surgery. It is therefore recommended that low concentrations of isoflurane be added to the oxygenator gas supply. Isoflurane can then be carefully titrated to ensure anesthesia and prevent hypertension and tachycardia.
6. Take care that the ECMO cannulas do not become kinked during positioning for surgery.
7. Even though the patient may be heparinized, excessive bleeding usually is not a problem.

Postoperative

1. Return the patient to the intensive care unit (ICU) for continued intensive respiratory care.
2. Some infants who have been salvaged by heroic intensive care measures may remain oxygen-dependent for years.

Suggested Additional Reading

Atkinson J, Hamid R, and Steward DJ: General anesthesia with isoflurane for diaphragmatic hernia repair during ECMO. J ASAIO 40:986–989, 1994.

Bonn D, Tamura M, Perrin D, et al.: Ventilatory predictors of pulmonary hypoplasia in congenital diaphragmatic hernia, confirmed by morphological assessment. J Pediatr 111:423–431, 1987.

Ionoco JA, Cilley RE, Mauger DT, et al.: Postnatal pulmonary hypertension after repair of congenital diaphragmatic hernia: predicting risk and outcome. J Pediatr Surg 34:349–353, 1999.

Iritani I: Experimental study on embryogenesis of congenital diaphragmatic hernia. Anat Embryol (Berl) 169:133–139, 1984.

Langer JC: Congenital diaphragmatic hernia. Chest Surg Clin North Am 8:295–314, 1998.

Redmond C, Heaton J, Calix J, et al.: A correlation of pulmonary hypoplasia, mean airway pressure, and survival in congenital diaphragmatic hernia treated with extracorporeal membrane oxygenation. J Pediatr Surg 22:1143–1149, 1987.

Sakai H, Tamura M, Hosokawa Y, et al.: Effect of surgical repair on respiratory mechanics in congenital diaphragmatic hernia. J Pediatr 111:432–438, 1987.

Somaschini M, Locatelli G, Salvoni L, et al.: Impact of new treatments for respiratory failure on outcome of infants with congenital diaphragmatic hernia. Eur J Pediatr 158:780–784, 1999.

Weinstein S and Stolar CJH: Neonatal surgical emergencies: congenital diaphragmatic hernia and extracorporeal membrane oxygenation. Pediatr Clin North Am 40:1315–1333, 1993.

Tracheoesophageal Fistula and Esophageal Atresia

Tracheoesophageal fistula and esophageal atresia, interrelated conditions, may occur in several combinations. The overall incidence is 1 in 3,000 live births. Maternal polyhydramnios is present, and premature birth is common.

The most common form (approximately 90% of cases) is esophageal atresia with a fistula between the trachea and the distal segment of the esophagus (Fig. 13–1, Type 1). This condition might be detected when the neonate chokes at the first feeding, but ideally it should be diagnosed antenatally by ultrasound or at birth by the inability to pass a soft rubber catheter into the stomach. Plain radiography confirms the diagnosis, showing the catheter curled in the upper esophageal pouch and an air bubble in the stomach, indicating a fistula. Contrast medium should not be used, because it may be aspirated and further damage the lungs.

Esophageal atresia without fistula may occur and is the second most common form of the disease (Fig. 13–1, Type 2); there may be a large gap between the upper and lower segments of the esophagus. In such patients, it is not possible to pass a catheter into the stomach via the esophagus, and there is no gastric air bubble. Aspiration from the upper pouch is an immediate danger. Constant suction of the upper pouch should be instituted pending surgical repair.

The third most common form is the H-type fistula without atresia (Fig. 13–1, Type 3); diagnosis of this type may be more difficult and is often delayed. In such cases, there is usually a history of repeated respiratory infections. The fistula may be difficult to locate even when contrast studies and endoscopy are used. Once the fistula is identified, surgical ligation often can be performed via a neck dissection.

There are other, rarer anatomic variants of this disease, many of which include tracheal stenosis.

Associated Conditions

1. Prematurity (30%–40%)
2. Congenital heart disease (22%)

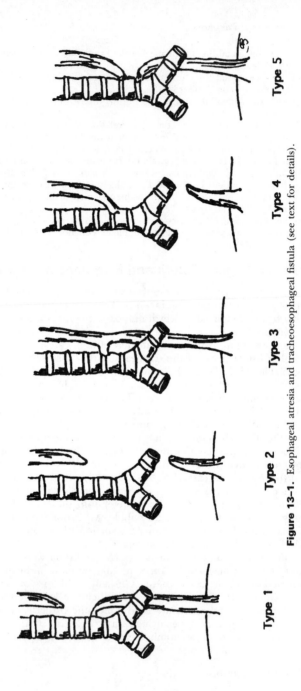

Type 1   **Type 2**   **Type 3**   **Type 4**   **Type 5**

Figure 13-1. Esophageal atresia and tracheoesophageal fistula (see text for details).

3. Additional gastrointestinal abnormalities (e.g., pyloric stenosis)
4. Renal and genitourinary abnormalities
5. The VATER association: vertebral defects, anal atresia, tracheoesophageal fistula, esophageal atresia, radial and renal dysplasia
6. The VACTERL association: with added cardiac and limb defects
7. Tracheomalacia and other abnormalities of the trachea (e.g., stenosis)

Surgical Procedures

The infant's general condition and the anatomy of the defect govern the choice of surgical management:

1. Primary complete repair (ligation of fistula and esophageal anastomosis), which is preferred
2. Staged repair (gastrostomy followed by division of the fistula, followed later by repair of the esophagus)

The current surgical trend is to perform early primary repair. Usually the operation is preceded by a rigid bronchoscopy to define the site of the fistula and exclude other tracheal defects.

Special Anesthesia Problems

1. Prematurity and other associated diseases (congenital heart disease is common) may complicate the case.
2. Pulmonary complications secondary to aspiration may be present.
3. There is a possibility of intubating the fistula.
4. Anesthetic gases may inflate the stomach via the fistula.
5. Surgical retraction during repair may obstruct ventilation.
6. Subglottic or tracheal stenosis may be present.

Anesthesia Management—Primary Repair

1. Observe special precautions for neonates.

Preoperative

1. The baby is nursed in a semiupright position.
2. The proximal esophageal pouch is suctioned continuously to prevent aspiration of secretions.
3. Institute intensive respiratory care to reduce pulmonary complications. (Even so, the lung condition seldom improves until after ligation of the fistula; therefore, surgery should not be delayed in the hope that pulmonary status will markedly improve.)
4. Examination of the infant to detect other associated lesions should be completed (e.g., echocardiography to rule out a congenital heart defect).
5. Establish a reliable intravenous route and ensure that blood is available for transfusion.
6. Give maintenance fluids intravenously, but bear in mind that

dehydration is not a major problem; neonatal fluid requirements are low during the first 24 hours, and fluid and electrolyte depletion does not occur with esophageal obstruction.

7. In the preterm infant with respiratory distress syndrome and poor lung compliance, there is a danger of massive distention of the stomach (or massive leak from a gastrostomy if present) and consequent failure to ventilate. Rupture of the stomach and pneumoperitoneum may occur. Various means to cope with this situation have been suggested:

   a. It has been suggested that the leak through the fistula in such cases may be controlled by a Fogarty catheter passed via a gastrostomy into the lower esophagus.

   b. It has been suggested that a Fogarty catheter may be placed via a gastrostomy and then drawn into the fistula itself with the use of a fiberoptic bronchoscope, thus controlling the leak.

   c. A more common approach is early simple ligation of the fistula in those infants with respiratory distress syndrome who are seen to be developing high airway pressures. The operation is brief and can be followed by esophageal reconstruction after the child's respiratory function has improved.

   d. This problem should be less common since the introduction of surfactant therapy for respiratory distress syndrome.

Perioperative

1. Suction the upper pouch. Apply lidocaine 4% to the gums and palate using a gauze sponge; this lessens the response to intubation.
2. Apply the usual monitors and prepare to monitor ventilation using a precordial stethoscope in the left midaxillary line.
3. Induce anesthesia with sevoflurane or halothane in O_2, maintaining spontaneous ventilation. When anesthesia is established, perform laryngoscopy and spray the larynx with lidocaine (maximum dose, 5 mg/kg). Return to the mask and continue anesthesia for 2 or 3 minutes before allowing the surgeon to pass the bronchoscope. Attach the anesthesia circuit to the side arm of the bronchoscope and continue with spontaneous or gently assisted ventilation. When the bronchoscopy is completed, insert an endotracheal tube with the bevel facing posteriorly (to avoid intubating the fistula). Beware of the possibility of subglottic stenosis; have small tube sizes available. In cases with extreme narrowing of the airway, a large venous cannula has been used as an endotracheal tube.
4. Immediately after intubation, check ventilation throughout the lung fields. *If ventilation is unsatisfactory,* remove the tube, give O_2, and reinsert the tube. It is advantageous to place the tube with its tip just above the carina; this can be done by advancing the tube into the bronchus and then withdrawing it until bilateral ventilation is heard. This should place the tip of the tube below the fistula in most cases, although in some patients the fistula lies at the level of the carina. More complicated methods to position the tube have been described

but are unnecessary in our experience. Always check ventilation again after positioning of the patient is complete.

5. When satisfactory intubation has been achieved, oxygenate and perform tracheobronchial suction to remove any accumulated secretions before the surgery commences.

6. Maintain anesthesia with air, O_2, and sevoflurane or isoflurane with spontaneous or gently assisted ventilation. If the volatile agent is not tolerated, small doses of fentanyl should be substituted (up to 10–12 μg/kg).

7. *If spontaneous ventilation is inadequate:* assist ventilation cautiously, while observing and auscultating over the stomach for inflation.
   a. If inflation occurs, allow the patient to breathe spontaneously (with careful manual assistance) until the chest is open. Then the fistula must be ligated as soon as possible.

8. When the chest is open, give a muscle relaxant and control the ventilation in the usual manner.

9. Monitor ventilation carefully during surgical manipulation: large airways may be kinked by retraction, especially as the fistula is being approached.

Postoperative

1. The patient with a clear chest who is awake and moving vigorously should be extubated in the operating room (OR).

2. If there are pulmonary complications or any doubts about the adequacy of ventilation, continue controlled ventilation.

3. The pharynx is suctioned with a soft catheter that has a suitable maximum length of insertion clearly marked; it must not reach (and damage) the anastomotic site.

4. Prolonged intensive respiratory care may be required. (Swallowing is not normal postoperatively, and aspiration may be frequent.)

5. Prognosis after the repair depends on the maturity of the infant, whether other congenital anomalies are present, and whether pulmonary complications develop. In the absence of these conditions, the mortality rate should be very low.

6. Postoperative analgesia may be provided by a caudal epidural catheter inserted intraoperatively.

Anesthesia Management—Staged Repair

If staged repair is planned, a preliminary gastrostomy is performed under local or general anesthesia. Management of the second stage (ligation of the fistula) should follow the sequence outlined for primary repair. Further surgery (to repair the atresia) may be done later, when the patient's condition is optimal.

Late Complications

1. Diverticulum of the trachea, at the site of the old fistula, is common in patients who had a tracheoesophageal fistula repaired during

infancy. Be aware of this possibility and the danger of intubating the diverticulum during anesthesia in later life.

2. The tracheal cartilage structure is abnormal, and tracheomalacia may cause symptoms during infancy after repair of a tracheoesophageal fistula. Episodes of stridor, dyspnea, and cyanosis ("dying spells") characteristically occur during feeding. This is caused by compression of the soft trachea between the dilated esophagus and the arch of the aorta. Severe symptoms require surgical treatment by aortopexy or tracheoplasty with an external splint.

3. Stricture may develop at the site of the esophageal anastomosis; it may require repeated dilatations and, later, possibly resection with replacement, using the colon or a gastric tube.

Suggested Additional Reading

Bray RJ and Lamb WH: Tracheal stenosis or agenesis in association with tracheo-oesophageal fistula and oesophageal atresia. Anaesthesia 43:654–658, 1988.

Davies MRQ and Cywes S: The flaccid trachea and tracheo-esophageal congenital anomalies. J Pediatr Surg 13:363, 1978.

Filler RM, Rossello PJ, and Lebowitz RL: Life threatening anoxic spells caused by tracheal compression after repair of esophageal atresia: correction after surgery. J Pediatr Surg 11:739, 1976.

Holzki J: Bronchoscopic findings and treatment in congenital tracheo-oesophageal fistula. Pediatr Anaesth 2:297–303, 1992.

Karl HW: Control of life threatening leak after gastrostomy in an infant with respiratory distress syndrome and tracheoesophageal fistula. Anesthesiology 62:670–672, 1985.

Somppi E, Tammela O, Ruuska T, et al.: Outcome of patients operated on for esophageal atresia: 30 years experience. J Pediatr Surg 33:1341–1346, 1998.

Templeton JM, Templeton JJ, Schnauferet L, et al.: Management of esophageal atresia and tracheoesophageal fistula in the neonate with severe respiratory distress syndrome. J Pediatr Surg 20:394–397, 1985.

Tsai JY, Berkery L, Wesson DE, et al.: Esophageal atresia and tracheoesophageal fistula: surgical experience over two decades. Ann Thorac Surg 64:778–783, 1997.

Congenital Laryngotracheoesophageal Cleft

This is a rarer anomaly in which there is a cleft in the posterior wall of the larynx that communicates with the esophagus. Four types are described, depending on the extension of this cleft distally. Type 1 is confined to the larynx, type 2 extends to the trachea, type 3 extends to the carina, and type 4 extends to the bronchi.

Mild type 1 forms of this disease may be missed initially, and the child may later present with a hoarse cry, cyanotic spells during feeding, and repeated episodes of aspiration pneumonia. These minor clefts may be amenable to endoscopic repair.

Severe clefts manifest early with severe respiratory distress, which may be relieved by passage of a gastric tube. Pulmonary damage from aspiration may be severe. Early tracheostomy and gastrostomy may be lifesaving. Definitive repair may involve a combined cervical and thoracic approach; good intraoperative control of the airway is vital and demands close cooperation between anesthesiologist and surgeon in planning the repair. A bifurcated endotracheal tube has been described for use in patients with extensive clefts.

Suggested Additional Reading

Armitage EN: Laryngotracheo-eosophageal cleft: a report of three cases. Anaesthesia 39:706–713, 1984.

Donahoe PK and Gee PE: Complete laryngotracheoesophageal cleft: management and repair. J Pediatr Surg 19:143, 1984.

Kingston HHG, Harrison MW, and Smith JD: Laryngoesophageal cleft—a problem of airway management. Anesth Analg 62:1041–1043, 1983.

Yamashita M, Chinyanga HM, and Steward DJ: Posterior laryngeal cleft—anesthetic experiences. Can Anaesth Soc J 26:502–505, 1979.

Congenital Hypertrophic Pyloric Stenosis

Congenital hypertrophic pyloric stenosis, a common surgical problem of infancy, occurs in up to 1 of every 300 live births in some populations; the incidence has considerable geographic variation. First-born male infants are more commonly affected. Hypertrophy of the muscle of the pyloric sphincter causes obstruction, leading to persistent vomiting. Dehydration, hypochloremia, and alkalosis develop. If the diagnosis is promptly made, severe derangements are avoided.

Diagnosis is made on the basis of the history and by palpation of an olive-sized mass in the region of the pylorus. Confirmation is by abdominal ultrasound examination.

Associated Condition

1. Jaundice (2% of patients), which is caused by glucuronyl transferase deficiency: No special therapy is required, and the jaundice clears after pyloromyotomy.

Surgical Procedure

1. Pyloromyotomy

Special Anesthesia Problems

1. Ensure that dehydration and electrolyte imbalance are fully corrected before surgery (pyloromyotomy is never an emergency surgical procedure).
2. There is a danger of vomiting and aspiration during anesthesia.

Anesthesia Management

1. Observe special precautions for neonates.

Preoperative

1. Insert a gastric tube and apply continuous suction.
2. Rehydrate the patient, correcting the electrolyte imbalance; this may require 24–48 hours.
   a. Give 2:1 dextrose-saline solution and/or normal saline as indicated by serum electrolyte values; patients with greater fluid and sodium deficits require normal saline. Add potassium chloride (KCl supplements, 3 mEq/kg/day) when urine flow is established.
   b. Delay surgery until the infant appears clinically well hydrated and has normal electrolyte levels, acid-base balance, and good urine output.
3. Immediately before surgery, reassess the patient to ensure that the fluid status is now satisfactory:
   a. Check for clinical signs of good hydration (alertness, skin turgor, anterior fontanel, normal vital signs, moist tongue, urine output).
   b. Check biochemistry. Values before surgery should be pH, 7.3–7.5; sodium (Na), greater than 132 mmol/L; chloride (Cl), greater than 88 mmol/L; potassium (K), greater than 3.2 mmol/L; and bicarbonate, less than 30 mmol/L.

Perioperative

1. Give atropine intravenously.
2. Place the patient in the left lateral position, oxygenate, and then aspirate the stomach with a soft catheter—even if the patient has been on continuous gastric suction.
3. Give 100% O_2 by mask.
4. Use a rapid-sequence induction with cricoid pressure.
5. Maintain anesthesia with N_2O and a potent inhaled agent.
6. Give a muscle relaxant and control the ventilation. (This permits the use of minimal amounts of anesthetic agents.) The choice of relaxant is dictated by the probable duration of surgery (i.e., the speed of the surgeon). Rocuronium (0.5–1.0 mg/kg) is useful for short procedures.
7. Ensure that the infant is well relaxed and immobile while the pyloric tumor is being split. (Coughing or movement could result in surgical perforation of the mucosa.)
8. At the end of the operation, the patient must be wide awake and in a lateral position for extubation.
9. Infiltration of the abdominal incision with bupivacaine with epinephrine provides good postoperative analgesia and reduces the requirement for other analgesic therapy.

Postoperative

1. Acetaminophen (20–40 mg/kg P.R. in a single loading dose) should be administered in the postanesthesia care unit (PACU). If analgesia is insufficient, administer small doses of intravenous morphine

(0.02–0.03 mg/kg). Oral feeding is started with clear fluids 6–12 hours postoperatively.

2. Maintain intravenous infusion of fluids until oral intake is adequate (usually 24 hours). Hypoglycemia has been reported when intravenous fluids containing glucose were discontinued before oral intake was adequate.

3. Postoperative respiratory depression may occur as a result of the effect of preoperative alkalosis on the pH of the cerebrospinal fluid. Apnea has been reported to occur in full-term infants after pyloromyotomy. The incidence of this problem and its causes are unclear, but it is suggested that infants should be carefully observed, if possible with apnea monitoring, for 24 hours postoperatively.

Suggested Additional Reading

Andropoulos DB, Heard MB, Johnson KL, et al.: Postanesthetic apnea in full term infants after pyloromyotomy. Anesthesiology 80:216–219, 1994.

Bissonnette B and Sullivan PJ: Pyloric stenosis. Can J Anaesth 38:668–672, 1991.

Cook-Sather SD, Tulloch TV, Liacouras CA, et al.: Gastric fluid volume in infants for pyloromyotomy. Can J Anaesth 44:278–283, 1997.

Fujimoto T, Lane GJ, Segawa O, et al.: Laparoscopic extramucosal pyloromyotomy versus open pyloromyotomy for infantile hypertrophic pyloric stenosis: which is better? J Pediatr Surg 34:370–372, 1999.

Habre W, Schwab C, Gollow I, et al.: An audit of postoperative analgesia after pyloromyotomy. Paediatr Anaesth 9:253–256, 1999.

Hulka F, Harrison HW, Campbell TJ, et al.: Complications of pyloromyotomy for infantile hypertrophic pyloric stenosis. Am J Surg 173:450–452, 1997.

Omphalocele and Gastroschisis

In omphalocele and gastroschisis, there is herniation of abdominal contents through the anterior abdominal wall. In gastroschisis, the defect is lateral to the umbilicus (usually on the right side), the umbilical cord is situated normally, and other congenital defects are rare. In omphalocele, the umbilical cord is continuous with the apex of the sac, and associated congenital defects are common (75%). The incidence of these conditions is 1 in 30,000 live births for gastroschisis and 1 in 5,000–10,000 live births for omphalocele.

Gastroschisis is often an isolated defect, whereas omphalocele is usually accompanied by other conditions. The physiologic consequences of the abdominal wall defect are, however, similar in both lesions.

Associated Conditions

1. Prematurity: 30%
2. Other gastrointestinal malformations (malrotation, diaphragmatic hernia, etc.): 25%
3. Genitourinary anomalies: 25%
4. Congenital heart disease: 10%
5. Beckwith-Wiedemann syndrome (omphalocele, macroglossia, and

severe hypoglycemia). These infants are usually large and have visceromegaly of the liver, kidney, and pancreas.

Surgical Procedures

The size of the abdomen in relation to the lesion determines the surgical procedure.

1. Primary closure is preferred if possible, because there is less risk of infection and other gastrointestinal complications. However, primary closure usually increases intra-abdominal pressure, which, if excessive, may lead to impaired ventilation, reduced cardiac output, hypotension, and splanchnic ischemia, with impaired hepatic, renal, and bowel function. It has been recommended that the intragastric pressure be measured and used as a guide to the safety of primary closure: pressures higher than 20 mmHg are poorly tolerated.
2. Skin closure only.
3. Staged procedure: This approach involves initial closure using a prosthetic pouch, followed by progressive daily reduction of the pouch to the level of the abdominal wall and subsequent full-thickness closure.

Special Anesthesia Problems

1. Heat and fluid loss from exposed viscera
2. Severe fluid and electrolyte disturbance and hypovolemic shock from transudation of fluid into the bowel (hypoproteinemia may occur)
3. High intra-abdominal pressure after closure, which may lead to compromised ventilation, decreased cardiac output, renal failure, and hepatic impairment (including delayed clearance of narcotic drugs)
4. The possibility of hypoglycemia in those infants with visceromegaly

Anesthesia Management

1. Observe special precautions for neonates.

Preoperative

1. The patient is nursed in a semiupright position with exposed viscera wrapped in sterile plastic film and covered by towels; this is done to prevent infection and minimize heat and fluid losses.
2. A gastric tube should be inserted to decompress the bowel.
3. Monitor the blood glucose frequently; if the patient is hypoglycemic (less than 40 mg/dl), infuse glucose continuously (6–8 mg/kg/min).

   N.B. Patients with Beckwith-Wiedemann syndrome have an increased insulin response; severe rebound hypoglycemia may occur if bolus doses of glucose are given.

4. Rehydrate the patient and correct the hypovolemia as well as electrolyte and oncotic status. Initial fluid requirements are high (up

to 140 ml/kg/24 hr); normal saline plus colloid (plasma or albumin) is required to correct the hypovolemia.
5. Order blood for transfusion (250 ml).

Perioperative

1. Ensure that the OR is warmed to at least 24°C and that heating lamps and forced-air warming devices are available.
2. Aspirate the gastric tube.
3. Give 100% O_2 by mask.
4. Perform a rapid-sequence induction with cricoid pressure.
5. Induce and maintain anesthesia with halothane (0.5%–1.0%) or sevoflurane (1%–2%) in O_2 and air.
   a. N_2O is contraindicated because it distends the bowel.
   b. Narcotic analgesics (e.g., fentanyl) may not be metabolized as rapidly as expected due to the effect of high intragastric pressure on hepatic blood flow.
6. Muscle relaxants may or may not be required to control ventilation.
7. Intragastric pressure should be transduced during abdominal closure to determine whether a primary closure will be tolerated. If the intragastric pressure exceeds 20 mmHg, hemodynamic instability and renal insufficiency may follow.

Postoperative

1. Assess spontaneous ventilation; if in doubt, change to a nasotracheal tube and continue controlled ventilation.
2. Continue nasogastric suction.
3. Continue intravenous fluids and glucose. Some infants require a prolonged period of intravenous hyperalimentation, because bowel function may be impaired for a long period (even weeks or months).

Suggested Additional Reading

Dillon PW and Cilley RE: Newborn surgical emergencies: gastrointestinal anomalies, abdominal wall defects. Pediatr Clin North Am 40:1289–1314, 1993.

Dunn JC and Fonkalsrud EW: Improved survival of infants with omphalocele. Am J Surg 173:284–287, 1997.

Gurkowski MA and Rasch DK: Anesthetic considerations for Beckwith-Wiedemann syndrome. Anesthesiology 70:711–712, 1989.

Langer JC: Gastroschisis and omphalocele. Semin Pediatr Surg 5:124–128, 1996.

Mollitt DL, Ballantine TVN, Grosfeld JL, and Quinter P: A critical assessment of fluid requirements in gastroschisis. J Pediatr Surg 13:217, 1978.

Snyder CL: Outcome analysis for gastroschisis. J Pediatr Surg 34:1253–1256, 1999.

Yaster M, Buck JR, Dudgeon DL, et al.: Hemodynamic effects of primary closure of omphalocele/gastroschisis in human newborns. Anesthesiology 69:84–88, 1988.

Biliary Atresia

Biliary obstruction in the newborn most commonly results from neonatal hepatitis or biliary atresia. Atresia of the intrahepatic and extrahepatic bile ducts may be congenital, or it may be caused by postnatal inflammation. As these bile ducts progressively obstruct, the infant becomes increasingly jaundiced. The incidence of biliary atresia is 1 in 25,000 live births. The problem in the persistently jaundiced newborn with direct (mixed) hyperbilirubinemia is to rule out other causes and confirm the diagnosis of atresia of the bile ducts. This is usually achieved by radioisotope studies and percutaneous liver biopsy.

Associated Anomalies

1. Malrotation
2. Situs inversus

Surgical Procedure

1. Hepatic portoenterostomy (Kasai's procedure). The extrahepatic bile ducts are resected, and the porta hepatis is dissected to a depth of 2–3 mm; then a Roux-en-Y jejunal anastomosis is performed. The major preoperative survival determinant seems to be the age at which the operation is performed. If the infant is older than 12 weeks of age, success is less likely. These older infants are often listed for liver transplantation.

Anesthesia Problems

1. Hepatic function is impaired, especially in the older child.
2. Hypoprothrombinemia develops and leads to impaired coagulation, especially in older infants.
3. Blood loss may be extensive, but this is unusual.
4. Intraoperative radiographs may be needed in some patients.

Anesthesia Management

Preoperative

1. Observe all considerations for the neonate.
2. Check the coagulogram, and verify that the patient has received a vitamin K_1 injection.
3. Check that adequate blood and fresh-frozen plasma are available for transfusion.

Perioperative

1. Administer 100% O_2 by mask and place monitors.
2. Induce anesthesia intravenously or by inhalation of sevoflurane.
3. Administer a muscle relaxant and intubate. *Cis*-atracurium is preferred in patients with uncertain hepatic function.

4. Induce and maintain anesthesia with low concentrations of sevoflurane or isoflurane in an O_2/air mixture.
5. Supplement relaxant drugs as necessary and continue to control the ventilation.
6. Insert large-bore intravenous lines into upper limbs or neck.
7. Monitor the BP carefully; be alert to the possibility of sudden hypotension due to IVC obstruction during surgical manipulation of the liver. Placing the infant in a slight head-down position may minimize falls in BP during manipulations of the liver.
8. Monitor the temperature; if necessary, use an overhead heater or a hot air mattress (or both) in addition to all other measures, to maintain normothermia.

Postoperative

1. Prolonged intravenous hyperalimentation may be required.
2. Ascending cholangitis is common, and portal hypertension may develop.
3. Many children develop esophageal varices and have repeated episodes of bleeding.
4. The use of salicylates is very dangerous and is contraindicated in these children.

Suggested Additional Reading

Barkin RM and Lilly JR: Biliary atresia and the Kasai operation: continuing care. J Pediatr 96:1015, 1980.

Bates MD, Bucuvalas JC, Alonso MH, et al.: Biliary atresia: pathogenesis and treatment. Semin Liver Dis 18:281–293, 1998.

Hicks BA and Altman RP: The jaundiced newborn. Pediatr Clin North Am 40:1161–1175, 1993.

Kasai M, Kimura S, Asakura Y, et al.: Surgical treatment of biliary atresia. J Pediatr Surg 3:665, 1968.

Intestinal Obstruction in the Newborn

Intestinal obstruction in the newborn may result from various lesions (e.g., duodenal atresia, duplication, midgut volvulus, malrotation) or from accumulation of viscid meconium ("meconium ileus").

Associated Conditions

1. Prematurity
2. Down syndrome—and hence congenital heart disease (18%)
3. Cystic fibrosis (invariably accompanies meconium ileus)
4. Subglottic stenosis with duodenal atresia

Special Anesthesia Problems

1. Hypovolemia; acid-base and electrolyte imbalance
2. Gross abdominal distention in some cases
3. Risk of regurgitation and aspiration

Anesthesia Management

1. Observe special precautions for neonates.

Preoperative

1. Check that the patient has had adequate fluid volume replacement.
2. Check acid-base and electrolyte status and correct any imbalance as far as possible.
3. Ensure that the gastrointestinal tract has been decompressed as much as possible (via an indwelling gastric tube).

Perioperative

1. Give atropine intravenously.
2. Aspirate the stomach contents via the gastric tube.
3. Give 100% O_2 by mask.
4. Intubate the trachea with the patient awake or after a rapid-sequence induction. Beware of the possibility of subglottic stenosis.
5. Induce and maintain anesthesia with isoflurane (0.5%–1%) or sevoflurane (1%–3%) in an air/O_2 mixture. Do not give N_2O, because it may cause further bowel distention.
6. Give small doses of relaxant drugs and control the ventilation.
7. Despite apparently adequate preoperative fluid resuscitation, some patients become hypotensive once the abdomen is open, especially those with small bowel atresia or midgut volvulus. They may need surprisingly large volumes of intravenous fluid (even blood or plasma) to restore the BP. Be prepared!

Postoperative

1. Do not extubate the trachea until the infant is fully awake and vigorous. Then extubate with the patient in the lateral position.
2. Prolonged intravenous or gastrostomy feeding may be required.
3. After meconium ileus, problems including prolonged bowel dysfunction, sepsis, and pneumonia must be anticipated.

Suggested Additional Reading

Lynn HB: Duodenal obstruction: atresia, stenosis, and annular pancreas. In Ravitch MM, Welch KJ, Benson CD, et al. (eds.): Pediatric Surgery, 3rd ed. Year Book, Chicago, 1979.

Sears BE, Carlin J, and Tunnell WP: Severe congenital subglottic stenosis in association with congenital duodenal obstruction. Anesthesiology 49:214, 1978.

Stevenson RJ: Neonatal intestinal obstruction in children. Surg Clin North Am 65:1217–1234, 1985.

OTHER MAJOR THORACOABDOMINAL LESIONS AND PROCEDURES

Neuroblastoma and Ganglioneuroma

Neuroblastoma is the most common solid malignant tumor of infancy. More than 50% of such tumors appear in the retroperitoneal space, but they may occur anywhere along the sympathetic chain. Four stages of the disease are described: stage 1, limited to the primary site; stage 2, extension from primary but not across the midline; stage 3, beyond the midline; and stage 4, with metastases. Metastases are present at diagnosis in more than 50% of cases.

The diagnosis is sometimes made on fetal ultrasound. In neonates and young infants, the diagnosis may be made by palpation of an abdominal mass. The older child frequently has evidence of chronic disease, including fever, weight loss, and anemia. The tumor secretes catecholamines, which may cause hypertension, and a vasoactive intestinal peptide (VIP), which may cause watery diarrhea, dehydration, and electrolyte disturbance. The tumor may also cause symptoms as a result of its extension to involve other tissues; for example, the extradural space may be involved and neurologic signs may appear. Most patients have increased levels of catecholamines and metabolites in the urine. Computed tomography (CT) and magnetic resonance imaging (MRI) permit localization of the tumor and identification of metastases.

Treatment of stage 1 or 2 disease is by surgical excision. Stage 3 or 4 disease is treated by initial chemotherapy or radiotherapy, or both. Patients with widespread disease may be treated by total body radiation, chemotherapy, and bone marrow transplantation.

Special Anesthesia Problems

1. Massive blood loss may occur during surgery, especially in those patients who have had preoperative radiotherapy. Major vessels (e.g., IVC) may be invaded by tumor and may be a source of rapid blood loss or tumor emboli.
2. Catecholamine levels are usually increased and hypertension may be present, but cardiac arrhythmias are very unusual. Those very rare patients with severe hypertension should be assumed to have a contracted blood volume and may benefit from preoperative preparation as outlined for pheochromocytoma.
3. Thoracic tumors may compress the lungs and produce respiratory failure. Cervical tumors may displace the trachea and compress the airway.
4. Patients with extension to the extradural space (dumbbell tumor) may need a combined abdominal and neurosurgical approach with laminectomy.

Anesthesia Management

Preoperative

1. Carefully assess the systemic effects of the disease on the child. Check the hemoglobin level and serum electrolytes. Check the results of CT or MRI for evidence of major blood vessel involvement.
2. Assess the extent of hypertension and its control by preoperative therapy.
3. Order appropriate sedation (e.g., midazolam 0.5 mg/kg PO).
4. **Important:** Adequate supplies of blood for transfusion must be

available, together with facilities to measure (and replace) large
blood losses.

Perioperative

1. Observe all special considerations for infants.
2. Place monitors and induce anesthesia.
3. Maintain anesthesia with N_2O and isoflurane; the latter can be
   titrated to control BP easily.
4. Vecuronium is preferred for relaxation; it provides cardiovascular
   stability and minimal histamine release.
5. Establish reliable large-bore intravenous routes in the upper limbs or
   neck.
6. Routine monitors should be supplemented with an arterial line and
   a urinary catheter. A double-lumen line via the jugular vein provides
   for infusions and monitoring of central venous pressure (CVP).
7. During surgical manipulations of the tumor, fluctuations in BP may
   occur. These can usually be treated by increasing the inspired
   concentration of isoflurane. Rarely, it may be necessary to use small
   doses (0.2 mg/kg) of phentolamine or an infusion of sodium
   nitroprusside.
8. Be prepared to provide rapid infusions of warmed blood. There is
   usually a decline in BP as the tumor is removed, which may have to
   be corrected by fluid infusion. Be alert to the fact that hypotension
   might also be caused by surgical retraction compromising IVC flow.
9. If major blood transfusion becomes necessary, check coagulation
   indices and prepare to correct deficiencies.

Postoperative

1. Most patients can be extubated at the end of the procedure;
   however, if the patient is unstable, plan to continue artificial
   ventilation.
2. Plan for optimal postoperative pain management; epidural analgesia
   is ideal for many patients.
3. Continue to monitor volume status and urine output carefully to
   ensure adequate continuing replacement.

N.B. Ganglioneuromas are benign tumors arising from sympathetic
ganglia. They do not invade other tissues but gradually enlarge and
may produce symptoms because of their size or pressure on adjacent
structures. They do not generally secrete significant amounts of
catecholamines or other active peptides. Surgical excision is usually
simpler than for neuroblastomas, but it may be complicated by the
tumor's location and size.

Suggested Additional Reading

Grosfeld JL: Neuroblastoma: A 1990 review. Pediatr Surg Int 6:9–13, 1991.
Haberkern CM, Coles PG, Morray JP, et al.: Intraoperative hypertension during

surgical excision of neuroblastoma: case report and review of 20 years experience. Anesth Analg 75:854–858, 1992.

Kain ZN, Shamberger RS, and Holzman RS: Anesthetic management of children with neuroblastoma. J Clin Anesth 5:486–491, 1993.

Lung Surgery

Lung surgery may be indicated for the following conditions:

1. Lung abscess
2. Bronchiectasis
3. Lung cysts
4. Bronchogenic cysts
5. Diagnostic biopsy (in children, usually to confirm or exclude infection by a virus or other pathogen)
6. Pulmonary arteriovenous malformation
7. Sequestrated pulmonary lobe
8. Pulmonary neoplasm
9. Chronic pulmonary infection

Special Anesthesia Problems

1. Once the thorax is open, major inequalities of ventilation and perfusion should be anticipated; increase the FIO_2 and monitor saturation. Blood and secretions within the bronchial tree may compound this problem; if so, suction the endotracheal tube frequently.
2. Major hemorrhage may occur suddenly if large vessels are inadvertently cut or torn. Therefore, reliable large-bore infusion routes must be established and blood for transfusion must be immediately available in the OR while the patient's chest is open.
3. Postoperative pain limits coughing and deep breathing, especially in older children, predisposing to atelectasis. Plan for optimal analgesia (e.g., thoracic epidural catheter).
4. Pulmonary function may be seriously impaired, resulting in respiratory failure in some patients (e.g., those admitted for lung biopsy). In such patients, even minor fluid overload can precipitate serious deterioration in lung function postoperatively; be extremely cautious with fluid therapy.
5. Pus from purulent lesions (e.g., lung abscess, bronchiectasis) may become dispersed during surgery unless a lobe or lung can be isolated. Preoperative bronchoscopy to remove accumulated secretions is useful for some patients.
6. Pulmonary arteriovenous malformation results in a very large right-to-left shunt, with consequent arterial desaturation that cannot be corrected by increasing the FIO_2.

Methods for Single Lung Ventilation

Double-lumen tubes are not available for infants and small children. However, there are patients in whom it is highly desirable to ventilate

Table 13–1. Approximate Size of Endobronchial Tube versus Age

Age (yr)	Tube Internal Diameter* (mm)
0.5–1	3
1–2	3.5
2–4	4
4–6	4.5–5.0
6–8	5.0–5.5

*For right main bronchus; use one size smaller tube for left main bronchus intubation.

only one lung (e.g., for thoracoscopic surgery) or to isolate a lung (e.g., lung abscess, bronchopulmonary fistula). In such cases some alternatives are available:

1. Selective intubation of the right or left main bronchus may be appropriate in some small patients (e.g., those with bronchopleural fistula, those in whom it is necessary to collapse one lung to facilitate the surgery). A tube of suitable size to fit into the bronchus should be chosen (Table 13–1). The direction that the endotracheal tube will take can usually be predetermined by selecting the direction of the bevel. If the bevel faces to the left and the patient's head is turned toward the left, the tip will usually advance down the right bronchus, and vice versa. Alternatively and preferably, a small fiberoptic bronchoscope may be used to direct the tip of the tube into the desired bronchus. The bevel of the endobronchial tube should be rotated in a direction away from the midline to ensure that the upper lobe bronchus is ventilated.

   If it is necessary to isolate a lung segment in a small child, a Fogarty catheter (positioned during bronchoscopy) can be used as a blocker. However, the Fogarty catheter does not have a central lumen, so it cannot be used to suction or collapse the blocked segment. A new bronchial blocker for small infants has recently been introduced. The Arndt bronchial blocker set* has a central lumen and can be accurately introduced down the endotracheal tube with the use of a fiberoptic bronchoscope.

2. Double-lumen tubes are available for older children (Table 13–2). The smallest easily available size is 26F; it may be suitable for children 8–10 years old. The tube should be positioned using the same principles as in adults. The position should always be checked using a small fiberoptic bronchoscope passed down each lumen. Always recheck the location of the tube after repositioning the patient.

3. The Univent tube,† which incorporates a bronchial blocker, may be applicable to some older patients (Table 13–3). Currently the smallest size available has a 3.5-mm diameter blocker; this fits most 6- to 8-year-old children.

*Cook Critical Care, Bloomington, IN.
†Univent Tube, Vitaid Ltd., Lewiston, NY.

Table 13–2. Double-lumen Tube Size versus Age

Age (yr)	Size of Tube* (French)
8–11	26
11–13	28
14–16	32
16–18	35

*These are approximate sizes; the actual tube that will fit must be judged on examination of the patient.

Note: A final alternative in the case of unilateral purulent disease, thoracotomy may be performed with the patient in the prone (Parry-Brown) position. In this position, purulent secretions tend to drain out via the endotracheal tube and do not contaminate the dependent lung.

Anesthesia Management

Preoperative

1. Assess the patient very carefully, considering the history, physical examination, laboratory results, and other studies.
   a. Evaluate pulmonary function as fully as possible (only limited data may be obtainable for children too young or otherwise unable to cooperate in the full range of tests).
   b. Check the results of blood gas and other available studies. In summary, ascertain whether the patient is in the best possible condition for the planned surgery.
2. Ensure that adequate supplies for transfusion have been ordered and serum has been saved for further cross-matching.
3. Ensure that appropriate respiratory care is ordered. For older patients, explain the value of preoperative breathing exercises and the need for postoperative respiratory care.
4. Order appropriate preoperative sedation, taking care to avoid causing respiratory depression in patients with impaired pulmonary function. Oral midazolam, 0.5 mg/kg, is often ideal.

Perioperative

1. Apply monitors.
2. Give 100% O_2 by mask.

Table 13–3. Size of Univent Tube versus Age

Age (yr)	Tube Internal Diameter (mm)
6–10	3.5
10–14	4.5
14–16	6.0
16–18	7.0

3. Induce anesthesia, usually with intravenous thiopental followed by vecuronium.
4. Ventilate with 100% O_2 until the patient is fully relaxed, then perform intubation, using the appropriate endotracheal tube. This may be preceded by bronchoscopy when indicated. In such cases, intermittent ventilation via the bronchoscope while monitoring saturation is usually quite satisfactory.
5. Insert an esophageal stethoscope and thermistor probe.
6. Establish a reliable wide-bore (18-gauge or larger) intravenous route.
7. Insert an arterial line (except for "minor" procedures in healthy children).
8. Maintain anesthesia with N_2O and sevoflurane or isoflurane, or N_2O with narcotic, adding sufficient O_2 to maintain the saturation at 95%–100%.
9. Give nondepolarizing muscle relaxant and control the ventilation (aim to maintain the $PaCO_2$ at 35–40 mmHg).
10. After the patient has been positioned for thoracotomy, recheck the ventilation of all areas of the lungs.
11. Suction the endotracheal tube as necessary to remove secretions during surgery.
12. If one-lung anesthesia is used, monitor arterial saturation and increase the inspired oxygen concentration as necessary to maintain pulse oximetry value greater than 95%.
13. Periodically inflate the lungs fully during thoracotomy and as the chest is being closed.
14. When the chest is closed, ensure that chest drains are connected to a Heimlich valve or underwater drain.
15. At the end of surgery, before extubation, ensure that the patient is awake and responding and has adequate spontaneous ventilation. If in doubt, leave the endotracheal tube in place and continue artificial ventilation until it is safe to withdraw this support.

Postoperative

1. Provide analgesia: A thoracic epidural block using bupivacaine with fentanyl is ideal and may be left in place for up to 72 hours postoperatively. Otherwise, intercostal nerve blocks plus a narcotic infusion or patient-controlled analgesia may be used.
2. Ensure that chest drains are patent and are connected to an underwater seal and suction.
3. Order arterial blood gas determinations as necessary to assess the adequacy of ventilation.
4. Ensure that chest radiography is performed, and check the films for pneumothorax or atelectasis.
5. Order hemoglobin (Hb) and hematocrit (Hct) determinations to assess the adequacy of blood replacement.

Suggested Additional Reading

Baraka A, Dajani A, and Maktabi M: Selective contralateral bronchial intubation in children with pneumothorax or bronchopleural fistula. Br J Anaesth 55:901, 1983.

Borchardt RA, LaQuaglia MP, McDowall RH, et al.: Bronchial injury during lung isolation in a pediatric patient. Anesth Analg 87:324–325, 1998.

Hammer GB, Fitzmaurice BG, and Brodsky JB: Methods for single-lung ventilation in pediatric patients. Anesth Analg 89:1426–1429, 1999.

Hammer GB, Brodsky JB, Redpath JH, et al.: The Univent tube for single-lung ventilation in paediatric patients. Paediatr Anaesth 8:55–57, 1998.

Haynes SR and Bonner S: Anesthesia for thoracic surgery in children. Paediatr Anaesth 10:237–251, 2000.

Tan PPC, Chu J-J, Ho ACY, et al.: A modified endotracheal tube for infants and small children undergoing video-assisted thoracoscopic surgery. Anesth Analg 86:1212–1213, 1998.

Mediastinal Tumors

Relatively common tumors of the mediastinum in children include

1. Lymphoma, Hodgkin's disease, etc.
2. Dermoid cysts
3. Neuroblastoma and ganglioneuroma
4. Thymoma (less common)

These children may need general anesthesia for excision of the mediastinal tumor or for cervical node or other biopsies to establish a diagnosis.

Special Anesthesia Problems

1. Acute airway obstruction may occur during anesthesia, even in patients with no history of dyspnea. Endotracheal intubation may fail to relieve the obstruction, and endobronchial intubation may be required to maintain ventilation. This is especially likely in patients with massive enlargement of hilar glands secondary to lymphoma or other tumor. Even during the simple procedure of cervical node biopsy, general anesthesia may be extremely dangerous.
2. The hilar mass may compress the heart, compromise ventricular filling, and cause acute hypotension.
3. Major blood loss may occur during mediastinal surgery.
4. Myasthenic patients require special consideration.

Anesthesia Management

Preoperative

1. Assess the patient carefully, and anticipate potential airway and cardiovascular problems. Inquire about any postural dyspnea—orthopnea is a sign of potential impending disaster! Look for signs of superior vena cava obstruction.

2. Examine radiologic studies and pulmonary function tests:
   a. CT scans to define the extent of airway compromise; if the area of the airway is decreased by more than 50%, extreme caution is recommended (i.e., consider preoperative steroids or operation under local anesthesia). Examine the potential for heart and great vessel compression by the tumor mass.
   b. Flow-volume curves; if expiratory flow rates are deceased by 50% or more, extreme caution is recommended (*see above*).
3. If the child has a massive mediastinal mass, dyspnea and/or orthopnea, or findings of concern on radiologic studies or pulmonary function tests (as just described), administer steroid hormones for 24–48 hours preoperatively to shrink the mass (the histology should not be compromised, and tissue necrosis should not occur). These agents usually induce rapid regression of hilar node enlargement and lessen the danger of airway obstruction or cardiac compression.
4. For mediastinal surgery, ensure that blood is available for transfusion and that serum is saved for cross-matching any necessary additional units.
5. If there is any danger of airway obstruction, do not order sedative premedication.
6. If airway problems are anticipated, prepare a full range of endotracheal tubes and laryngoscope blades and have a bronchoscope available.

Perioperative

N.B. Cervical lymph node biopsy in the older child with a symptomatic large mass at the hilum may be most safely performed using a local anesthetic with the patient in the sitting position.
   For general anesthesia:

1. Check that the awake patient can tolerate the position chosen for surgery. Anesthesia should be induced by inhalation while maintaining spontaneous ventilation. Breath sounds and oxygen saturation should be monitored continuously.
2. Establish reliable intravenous routes for infusion.
3. Monitor ventilation continuously (using breath sounds and capnography), and check carefully after any changes in the patient's position. If obstruction develops:
   a. Turn the child to the left decubitus position to relieve pressure on the tracheobronchial tree and heart. If that fails to restore cardiac output, turn the child prone.
   b. Intubate and advance the tube until it is past the obstruction—endobronchial if necessary!
   c. If this fails, perform rigid bronchoscopy.
   d. In extreme cases, emergency thoracotomy may be required.
4. Maintain anesthesia with N_2O and sevoflurane or isoflurane; spontaneous ventilation is preferable.
5. Monitor the cardiac rhythm closely during surgical dissection.

6. At the completion of surgery, check adequacy of ventilation before extubation.

Postoperative

1. If applicable, ensure that the nurses in the PACU are aware that airway obstruction or cardiac compromise might occur in certain positions.
2. Order maintenance fluids and appropriate analgesia.
3. If blood replacement was required, check the Hct.
4. Obtain a chest radiograph in the PACU; check for pneumothorax.

Suggested Additional Reading

Azizkhan RG, Dudgeon DL, Buck JR, et al.: Life threatening airway obstruction as a complication to the management of mediastinal masses in children. J Pediatr Surg 20:816–822, 1985.

Cheung S and Lerman J: Mediastinal masses. Anesthesiol Clin North Am 16:893–909, 1998.

Keon TP: Death on induction of anesthesia for cervical node biopsy. Anesthesiology 55:471–472, 1981.

Shamberger RC: Preanesthetic evaluation of children with anterior mediastinal masses. Semin Pediatr Surg 8:61–68, 1999.

Vas L, Naregal F, and Naik V: Anaesthetic management of an infant with anterior mediastinal mass. Paediatr Anaesth 9:439–443, 1999.

Myasthenia Gravis

Myasthenia presents in three forms in infants and children:

1. *Transient neonatal myasthenia* occurs in babies of myasthenic mothers. The child presents within a few hours of birth, usually with hypotonia and difficulty in feeding. Improvement occurs within a few weeks, but therapy with anticholinesterases is needed meanwhile.
2. *Juvenile myasthenia gravis* (autoimmune myasthenia) usually manifests in childhood or adolescence. The disease may be generalized or limited to the ocular muscles. Abnormal fatigability, limb weakness, and ptosis are the usual features. The diagnosis is confirmed by the demonstration of a decreased compound muscle action potential on repetitive nerve stimulation, or by improved muscle power after injection of an anticholinesterase drug (edrophonium).
3. *Congenital myasthenic syndromes* due to various defects of neuromuscular transmission may cause symptoms during infancy or childhood and are difficult to distinguish from autoimmune myasthenia without complex testing.

Associated Condition

1. Hyperthyroidism may be present.

Treatment

1. Anticholinesterase therapy produces symptomatic improvement, but secretions may become a problem; pyridostigmine is the drug of choice.

2. Plasmapheresis or intravenous immunoglobulin results in temporary improvement in many patients and may reduce the requirement for surgery.
3. Prednisone and azathioprine have been demonstrated to improve some patients.
4. Thymectomy may increase the probability of remission, especially if it is performed early after the symptoms appear.

Surgical Procedure

Thymectomy is performed in some patients with severe generalized myasthenia gravis who fail to respond to other treatment, even if there is no thymoma. The best remission of symptoms is seen in young patients who have thymic hyperplasia.

Special Anesthesia Problems

1. Muscle weakness may lead to ventilatory failure.
2. Treatment with anticholinesterases increases the respiratory tract secretions, which may accumulate.
3. Potential sudden deterioration in muscle power may be caused by either of the following:
   a. A myasthenic crisis
   b. A cholinergic crisis induced by excessive dosage with anticholinesterase
4. Postoperative pain may limit ventilation and coughing, compounding the problem. Regional analgesia for postoperative pain is ideal (e.g., epidural analgesia).
5. Chest physiotherapy postoperatively rapidly fatigues the patient if it is too vigorous.
6. There are abnormal responses to neuromuscular blocking drugs. Anesthesia solely with inhaled agents has proved very successful for pediatric patients.

Anesthesia Management

Preoperative

1. The patient should be admitted to the hospital for a period of rest, and anticholinesterase drugs should be reduced or withdrawn.
2. Ensure that blood is available for transfusion.
3. Do not give heavy premedication—*no narcotic analgesics.*

Perioperative

1. Induce anesthesia by inhalation of sevoflurane or with a small dose of thiopental (3–4 mg/kg IV) or propofol (3–5 mg/kg).
2. Deepen anesthesia with N_2O and sevoflurane or halothane.
3. Do not give any muscle relaxants; intubate when the patient is adequately anesthetized with halothane or sevoflurane and after applying topical analgesic to the larynx.
4. Control ventilation.

5. Ensure reliable intravenous infusion routes.
6. At the completion of surgery, allow the patient to waken and resume spontaneous ventilation with the endotracheal tube in place. Check the vital capacity; if this is adequate (more than 20 ml/kg), proceed with extubation.

Postoperative

1. Close observation and respiratory care in the ICU is essential. Optimal pain management must be provided (e.g., epidural catheter).
2. Reduce or discontinue anticholinesterase therapy (to lessen the likelihood of a cholinergic crisis).
3. Edrophonium testing may be performed periodically as a guide to anticholinesterase therapy (i.e., administer a small dose of edrophonium to confirm that this produces an improvement in muscle power). If there is no improvement, an impending cholinergic crisis is indicated.
4. Use caution with narcotic analgesics—regional nerve block is preferable.
5. Plan physiotherapy very carefully to avoid overtiring the patient. (Time the therapy sessions to take advantage of the increased muscle power after each edrophonium test.)
6. If fatigue and/or serious retention of secretions occurs, perform nasotracheal intubation and institute IPPV.

Suggested Additional Reading

Andrews PI: A treatment algorithm for autoimmune myasthenia gravis in childhood. Ann N Y Acad Sci 841:789–802, 1998.

Davies DW and Steward DJ: Myasthenia gravis in children and anaesthetic management for thymectomy. Can Anaesth Soc J 29:253, 1973.

Drachman DB: Present and future treatment of myasthenia gravis. N Engl J Med 316:743, 1987.

Kiran U, Choudhury M, Saxena N, and Kapoor P: Sevoflurane as a sole anaesthetic for thymectomy for myasthenia gravis. Acta Anaesthesiol Scand 44:351–353, 2000.

Seybold ME: Thymectomy in childhood myasthenia gravis. Ann N Y Acad Sci 841:731–741, 1998.

Splenectomy

See Idiopathic Thrombocytopenic Purpura (page 467) and Trauma (page 413).

Pheochromocytoma

Pheochromocytoma is rare in children (fewer than 5% of all cases); when it appears, it is usually in the adrenal medulla and is bilateral in 20% of patients or more. The principal symptoms are headache, nausea, and vomiting, with sustained or, less commonly, episodic hypertension.

Abdominal pain may occur. If undiagnosed, this might prompt an unnecessary and dangerous exploratory operation in an unprepared patient. The diagnosis is confirmed by the finding of increased catecholamines (or their metabolites) in the urine. Sustained hypertension with vasoconstriction contracts the intravascular volume and elevates the Hct.

Associated Conditions

1. Neurofibromatosis
2. Thyroid tumor
3. Multiple endocrine adenomatoses (e.g., Sipple's syndrome)

Special Anesthesia Problems

Note: Anesthesia is very dangerous in the unprepared patient—violent swings in BP may occur.

1. Management of the BP and volume status of the patient can be difficult.
2. Major blood loss may occur from extensive surgery performed to locate and remove multiple tumors.
3. It is necessary to avoid anesthetic drugs that might increase the release of catecholamines (e.g., succinylcholine) or sensitize the heart to these substances (e.g., halothane). Pancuronium or droperidol may cause a hypertensive crisis. Drugs that release histamine (e.g., *d*-tubocurarine, atracurium, rapacuronium) should be avoided.
4. Good preoperative sedation and a smooth induction are essential to prevent release of catecholamines.

N.B. The potential for dangerous cardiac arrhythmias is extremely rare in children.

Anesthesia Management

General anesthesia may be required for special investigations to locate the tumor, as well as for its extirpation, and must be conducted with the same considerations.

Preoperative

1. The patient should be treated with α-blocking drugs (e.g., phenoxybenzamine HCl, 0.25–1.0 mg/kg/day) for several days, until
   a. BP is consistently normal or there are signs or symptoms of postural hypotension.
   b. Hct has fallen (indicating expansion of intravascular volume). It is not necessary to administer a β-blocker to children, and this is contraindicated in the almost inevitable presence of incomplete α-blockade. (β-blockade without α-blockade may lead to cardiac failure.)
2. Ensure that adequate supplies of blood for transfusion are available.

3. Check that drugs are at hand to treat any disturbance of BP or cardiac rhythm, including
   a. Phentolamine—to lower BP (usually necessary)
   b. Propranolol—to treat arrhythmias
   c. Isoproterenol—to increase heart rate
   d. Norepinephrine—to increase BP
4. Give premedication on the ward (e.g., midazolam, 0.75 mg/kg PO).

Perioperative

1. If the patient appears apprehensive on arrival in the OR anteroom, give small doses of midazolam intravenously and wait 5 minutes before taking the patient into the OR.
2. Attach monitors.
3. Induce anesthesia intravenously with thiopental 5 mg/kg, adding atropine 0.02 mg/kg.
4. Give rocuronium 0.5–1.0 mg/kg IV.
5. Ventilate with N_2O, O_2, and 1% isoflurane.
6. Give lidocaine 1.5 mg/kg IV; when the patient is fully relaxed, intubate the trachea.
7. Maintain anesthesia with N_2O, O_2, and 0.75% isoflurane with controlled ventilation.
8. Insert arterial and CVP lines. An epidural catheter may be inserted for postoperative pain control and to supplement intraoperative analgesia and improve hemodynamic stability. If so, be prepared to infuse intravenous fluids as necessary as the block becomes established.
9. Infuse fentanyl 5 μg/kg when surgery commences and continue with an infusion of 2 μg/kg/hr.
10. Monitor arterial and venous pressures closely throughout.
11. When the tumor has been excised:
    a. Transfuse fluids rapidly to maintain arterial pressure. Large volumes may be required.
    b. Maintain CVP at 9–11 cmH_2O, and check the Hct periodically.
    c. If hypertension persists, suspect additional tumors.
12. When the tumor or tumors have been removed:
    a. Discontinue isoflurane.
    b. Continue anesthesia with N_2O, O_2, fentanyl, and rocuronium until the end of surgery.

Postoperative

1. Check blood glucose levels frequently. (Hypoglycemia may occur as a result of the fall in catecholamine level and a secondary rebound hyperinsulinism.)
2. Anticipate a rise in Hct as the effect of phenoxybenzamine wears off.
3. Maintain epidural analgesia or order analgesics as required.
4. Order maintenance intravenous fluids; these should contain added dextrose.

Suggested Additional Reading

Bittar DA: Innovar induced hypertensive crises in patients with phaeochromocytoma. Anesthesiology 50:366, 1979.

Channa AB, Mofti AB, Taylor GM, et al.: Hypoglycaemic encephalopathy following surgery on phaeochromocytoma. Anaesthesia 42:1298–1301, 1987.

Jones RB and Hill AB: Severe hypertension associated with pancuronium in a patient with pheochromocytoma. Can Anaesth Soc J 28:394, 1981.

O'Riordan JA: Pheochromocytomas and anesthesia. Int Anesthesiol Clin 35:99–127, 1997.

Pullerits J and Balfe JW: Anaesthesia for phaeochromocytoma. Can J Anaesth 35:526–533, 1988.

Stringel G, Ein SH, Creighton RE, et al.: Pheochromocytoma in children—an update. J Pediatr Surg 15:496, 1980.

Wilms Tumor (Nephroblastoma)

Wilms tumors constitute 50% of the retroperitoneal masses in children and cause 6%–8% of deaths from cancer in persons younger than 12 years of age. These tumors vary histologically but may grow large and usually manifest as an abdominal mass. Some 5% are bilateral. Abdominal pain and fever are common symptoms. Hypertension may develop, possibly as a result of ischemia of renal tissue adjacent to the tumor, but the BP may remain elevated after removal of the entire affected kidney.

Associated Conditions

1. Hemihypertrophy
2. Congenital absence of the iris (aniridia)

Special Anesthesia Problems

1. Massive blood loss may occur during surgery. Full hemodynamic monitoring should be instituted (arterial and CVP lines).
2. Surgical manipulations may kink the IVC and cause abrupt falls in cardiac output.
3. A thoracoabdominal approach may be required for large tumors.
4. The size of the tumor and previous whole-body radiation may impair pulmonary function.
5. Hypertension may be present (60% of cases) secondary to renin secretion. It may be severe in some patients and may require preoperative and intraoperative therapy. Angiotensin-converting enzyme (ACE)–inhibiting drugs (e.g., captopril) have been suggested as most appropriate preoperatively. Vasodilating drugs such as sodium nitroprusside may be required during surgery.
6. Rarely, tumor may invade the IVC; in such cases intraoperative pulmonary tumor embolism may occur.
7. A coagulopathy, acquired von Willebrand's disease, may occur in association with Wilms tumor. This improves after resection of the tumor. Factor VIII concentrates may be required to reduce the bleeding time.
8. Anemia is commonly associated with nephroblastoma.

9. Large intra-abdominal tumors may predispose to delayed gastric emptying and regurgitation on induction of anesthesia.

Anesthesia Management

Preoperative

1. Check that blood is available for transfusion (at least 2,000 ml for large tumors) and that serum is saved for further cross-matching.
2. Be prepared for probable massive transfusion; check coagulation.
3. Do not palpate the patient's abdomen.
4. Consider the use of antacids and metoclopramide to reduce the danger of acid aspiration on induction.

Perioperative

1. Apply monitors and induce anesthesia. A rapid-sequence induction is preferred.
2. Start intravenous infusions into an upper limb or neck vein using a large-bore cannula (at least 18-gauge).
3. Maintain anesthesia with isoflurane and a relaxant (rocuronium is preferred).
4. Beware of abrupt declines in BP (due to surgical compression of the IVC). Notify the surgeon to desist immediately if this occurs.
5. If hypertension is a problem (unusual), control it by increasing the concentration of inspired isoflurane.

N.B. Significant blood losses may occur during wound closure: continue transfusion to match losses. (Do not relax as soon as the tumor is out!)

Postoperative

1. Hypertension may continue and may require therapy (e.g., hydralazine).
2. Blood loss into the wound may continue, requiring continued transfusion.

Suggested Additional Reading

Charlton GA, Sedgwick J, and Sutton DN: Anesthetic management of renin secreting nephroblastoma. Br J Anaesth 69:206–209, 1992.

Cobb ML and Vaughan RW: Severe hypertension in a child with Wilms' tumor: a case report. Anesth Analg 55:519, 1976.

Jenking RDT: The treatment of Wilms' tumor. Pediatr Clin North Am 23:147, 1976.

Noronha PA, Hruby MA, and Maurer HS: Acquired von Willebrand disease in a patient with Wilms tumor. J Pediatr 95:997–999, 1979.

"Acute Abdomen"

In children, an "acute abdomen" most commonly represents acute appendicitis, intussusception, or perforated Meckel's diverticulum.

Appendicitis

Appendicitis is the most common cause of acute abdomen in childhood. The concerns for the anesthesiologist are possible fluid and electrolyte disturbance (secondary to nausea and vomiting) and the presence of sepsis and high fever. Adequate fluid resuscitation should be ensured before proceeding to general anesthesia.

Intussusception

Intussusception is the most common cause of obstruction between infancy and 5 years of age. A segment of bowel passes into more distal bowel and may become ischemic and gangrenous. Enlarged Peyer's patches, caused by viral infection, may precipitate this lesion by providing the lead point. The diagnosis is confirmed by contrast enema, which may also serve to reduce the intussusception. If this fails, a second attempt at hydrostatic reduction under general anesthesia may be successful; inhalation anesthetics may facilitate the process by relaxing abdominal muscles, decreasing smooth muscle activity, and reducing splanchnic blood flow. Pneumatic pressure of air or oxygen has also been used to reduce intussusception. In this case there is a risk of gas embolism, so N_2O should be omitted from the anesthesia technique. Laparotomy is indicated for peritonitis, failed reduction, and repeated episodes.

Suggested Additional Reading

Collins DL, Pinckney LE, Miller KE, et al.: Hydrostatic reduction of ileo-colic intussusception: a second attempt in the operating room with general anesthesia. J Pediatr 115:204, 1989.

Guo J, Ma X, and Zhou Q: Results of air pressure enema reduction of intussusception: 6396 cases in 13 years. J Pediatr Surg 21:1201, 1986.

Hadidi AT and El Shal N: Childhood intussusception: a comparative study of nonsurgical management. J Pediatr Surg 34:304–307, 1999.

Meckel's Diverticulum

Meckel's diverticulum is partial persistence of the omphalomesenteric duct, which is present in 2% of the population; it may provide a site for bleeding, perforation, or intestinal obstruction. Severe bleeding may occur from ectopic gastric mucosa within the diverticulum and may result in hypovolemic shock.

Special Anesthesia Problems

1. Full stomach: even if the child has not eaten or drunk anything for several hours (and even if the child has vomited), do not assume that the stomach is empty. Gastric secretions accumulate rapidly when intestinal ileus is present.
2. Fluid and electrolyte disturbances may occur secondary to vomiting.
3. The patient may have a high temperature; this increases the metabolic rate for oxygen and compounds the risk should any

interruption of ventilation occur. It also increases the maintenance fluid requirements by 10%–12% per 1°C increase in body temperature.

Anesthesia Management

Preoperative

1. Assess the patient's general condition carefully. Check the volume status, fluid intake, serum electrolytes, and urine output. Ensure that fluid replacement is sufficient to correct deficits and produce good urine output.
2. If the patient's temperature is elevated, the patient should not be given atropine or hyoscine intramuscularly, because doing so may lead to serious hyperthermia.
3. Prepare and check all equipment for a rapid-sequence induction and have suitable assistance available.

Perioperative

1. Check that a reliable intravenous route is available.
2. Attach monitors.
3. Give 100% O_2 for 4 minutes.
4. Inject induction drugs directly into a free-running intravenous line; give thiopental with atropine, followed immediately by succinylcholine.
5. Have an assistant apply cricoid pressure.
6. Do not ventilate via mask.
7. Insert an endotracheal tube as soon as the patient has fasciculated and relaxed.
8. Maintain anesthesia with N_2O and isoflurane with a nondepolarizing muscle relaxant.
9. Patients with high fever may benefit from intraoperative cooling, facilitated by the use of volatile agents and muscle relaxants.
10. At the end of surgery, withdraw all anesthetic agents, reverse the relaxants, and ensure that the patient is fully awake.
11. Place the patient in a lateral position for extubation.

Postoperative

1. Order analgesics as required.
2. Order maintenance fluids to be given intravenously.

Testicular Torsion

Testicular torsion requires immediate surgery. Therefore, in most cases, it is not possible to prepare the patient. The volume and contents of the stomach in these patients are similar to those of the child with an acute abdomen. Therefore, beware of the risk of regurgitation and aspiration at induction.

Anesthesia Management

Preoperative

1. Prepare and check all equipment for a rapid-sequence induction and have suitable assistance available.

Perioperative and Postoperative

1. As for "Acute Abdomen."

Neonatal Necrotizing Enterocolitis

Neonatal necrotizing enterocolitis (NEC), a disease of low-birth-weight infants (usually those with less than 34 weeks' gestation), is characterized by intestinal mucosal injury secondary to ischemia of the bowel. It may lead to perforation and peritonitis. Severe fluid and electrolyte disturbance, endotoxic shock, and coagulopathy due to thrombocytopenia may develop. As the disease progresses, multiple system organ failure may occur. The etiology of NEC is uncertain, but the disease usually affects infants with a history of birth asphyxia, respiratory distress syndrome, and shock. Other possible etiologic factors include enteral feeding, infection, and umbilical artery catheterization.

The clinical picture is one of abdominal distention, bloody diarrhea, temperature instability, and lethargy; apnea may occur. Abdominal radiography may show intramural bowel or portal venous gas.

The medical management of NEC includes cessation of feeding and institution of continuous gastric suction, use of intravenous fluids and alimentation, administration of antibiotics, and correction of anemia and/or coagulopathy. Steroids and inotropes may be used to treat shock. Bowel perforation is the usual indication for surgery.

Special Anesthesia Problems

1. Prematurity and respiratory distress
2. Shock, hypovolemia, electrolyte disturbance, and coagulopathy
3. Sepsis, acidosis, and congestive cardiac failure
4. Interstitial gas in the bowel wall
5. Interaction of antibiotics with relaxant drugs

Anesthesia Management

Preoperative

1. Restore blood and fluid volumes: blood, plasma, and crystalloid solutions may be required; third space losses are considerable. If volume replacement does not improve the BP, inotropes are indicated. Check Hct, blood gases, electrolytes, and the blood glucose level.
2. Check coagulation: thrombocytopenia must be corrected by platelet infusions.

3. Exchange transfusion may be required for severe sepsis. Correct the acid-base status.
4. Monitor carefully for apnea.

Perioperative

1. Observe all special precautions for the premature infant. Reliable intravenous routes and an arterial line are essential. Ensure that all monitors are functioning well before surgery commences.
2. Use of fentanyl (10–12 μg/kg) and ventilation with appropriate concentrations of O_2 is the preferred method. (Do not use N_2O, because doing so may expand intramural bowel gas.)
3. Administer doses of vecuronium as required for relaxation.
4. Continue fluid resuscitation throughout surgery as dictated by clinical status and laboratory studies. Warm all intravenous fluids.
5. Anticipate that major fluid infusions may be required to maintain cardiovascular homeostasis when the abdomen is opened. Carefully monitor the BP and infuse adequate volumes of appropriate crystalloid and colloid to correct hypotension.

Postoperative

1. Return the patient to the neonatal ICU for continued respiratory care.

Suggested Additional Reading

Brown EG and Sweet AY: Neonatal necrotizing enterocolitis. Pediatr Clin North Am 29:1149, 1982.

Haselby KA, Dierdorf SF, Krishna G, et al.: Anaesthetic implications of neonatal necrotizing enterocolitis. Can Anaesth Soc J 29:255, 1982.

Organ Transplantation

Transplantation of solid organs is now becoming commonplace in pediatric practice. Though transplantation (apart from kidneys) is limited to a few specialist centers, organ procurement may be performed in many hospitals. The anesthesiologist has a major role to play in the care of the donor, to ensure that donated organs remain in optimal condition until harvesting.

Determination of Brain Death

Determination of brain death has been based on the following: the presence of deep coma, lack of brain-stem function, unresponsiveness to stimuli, together with

1. Exclusion of potentially reversible causes of coma (e.g., metabolic causes, drug ingestion)
2. Isoelectric electroencephalogram
3. Absence of cerebral blood flow on angiography or scan
4. Lack of heart rate response to intravenous atropine

These criteria should be reviewed by independent practitioners who are not members of the transplantation team before a "brain dead" designation is assigned. Infants and children have demanded special consideration: it has been suggested that at least two electroencephalograms and cerebral blood flow studies, 24 hours apart, should be performed, with continuous intervening observation to ensure the irreversibility of the state. This is still an area of some controversy.

Care of the Donor

When cerebral death occurs, a sequence of physiologic changes follow throughout the body that may compromise the survival of organs destined for transplantation. Hence, intensive measures to support these organs are indicated. The anesthesiologist will be involved in caring for the donor during organ retrieval.

After cerebral death the following occur:

1. Hypotension: Widespread vasodilation occurs, and the patient tends to become pink and hypotensive. This hypotension may be compounded by hypovolemia secondary to the use of diuretics for previous attempts at cerebral resuscitation. Myocardial function may also be depressed.
2. Central diabetes insipidus leads to polyuria, dehydration, hyperosmolarity, and hypernatremia.
3. Arrhythmias, atrial or ventricular, are frequent owing to intracranial pressure changes, electrolyte disturbances, and myocardial injury.
4. Hypothermia is present owing to loss of central thermoregulation.
5. Coagulopathy occurs secondary to disseminated intravascular coagulation as a result of released substrates from necrotic brain.

To counter these changes the following management regimen is suggested:

1. The circulating volume should be restored rapidly. Large volumes of fluid may be required (20–40 ml/kg), but overhydration should be avoided.
   a. Lactated Ringer's solution and 5% dextrose in normal saline. Use 5% dextrose in water if the Na concentration is greater than 150 mEq/L.
   b. Albumin 5% for refractory hypotension.
   c. Packed red blood cells for an Hct less than 30. Adequate volume expansion is indicated by a CVP value greater than 8 cmH$_2$O and a continuing satisfactory urine output. Warm all fluids to prevent hypothermia.
2. If hypotension persists despite adequate volume expansion, vasopressor therapy should be commenced:
   a. Dopamine is the drug of first choice, in a dose of 5–15 µg/kg/min.
   b. Epinephrine up to 0.1 µg/kg/min.
      Vasopressors should, if possible, be discontinued before organs are harvested to minimize the chance of ischemic injury. The use

of dopamine in cardiac donors is controversial, because it is claimed that dopamine may deplete and damage the myocardium.

3. Renal function should be maintained by fluid loading:
   a. If urine output drops to less than 2 ml/kg/hr, give furosemide 1 mg/kg as necessary.
   b. For diabetes insipidus, give *either* 1-deamino-8-D-arginine vasopressin (DDAVP), 1–4 µg IV, *or* pitressin infusion, 0.01–0.02 units/kg/hr titrated to maintain the desired output.
   c. Suitable electrolyte solutions should be administered to correct hypernatremia and hypokalemia.
4. Hepatic function should be preserved by maintaining oxygenation and perfusion.
5. Other measures:
   a. Measure esophageal and rectal temperature and maintain normothermia.
   b. Determine and correct acid-base and electrolyte status.
   c. Continue optimal ventilation (beware of pulmonary changes).
   d. Use careful aseptic technique. Prophylactic antibiotics may be used. Blood cultures are taken immediately before organs are harvested.

All the these measures should be continued throughout the surgical procedure of organ procurement.

Suggested Additional Reading

Ali MJ: Essentials of organ donor problems and their management. Anesthesiol Clin North Am 12:655–671, 1994.

Jordan CA and Snyder JV: Intensive care and intraoperative management of the brain dead organ donor. Transplant Proc 19(Suppl 3):21–25, 1987.

Liver Transplantation

Major advances in the control of rejection and in surgical and anesthesia techniques have made liver transplantation an option for infants and children. A limitation is imposed by the lack of suitably sized donor organs, but transplantation of a portion of a living related donor organ has become a useful alternative. Common indications for pediatric liver transplantation include the following:

1. Biliary atresia
2. Metabolic disease (e.g., α_1-antitrypsin deficiency)
3. Liver tumors—The results are significantly better in infants and children older than 1 year of age who weigh more than 10 kg.

Special Anesthesia Problems

1. Major blood losses may occur, requiring massive blood transfusion.
2. Intraoperative cardiovascular instability may result from preexisting myocardial disease, plus mechanical factors (surgical manipulation),

electrolyte disturbances (K^+, Ca^{++}), acidosis, and release of vasoactive and cardiotoxic factors on reperfusion.

3. Coagulation defects may preexist secondary to impaired preoperative hepatic function and are compounded by massive blood losses and transfusion.

4. Metabolic derangements may occur, including hypothermia, hypoglycemia (rare), hyperglycemia (more common), hypernatremia secondary to bicarbonate therapy, ionized hypocalcemia secondary to citrate, and hyperkalemia on reperfusion.

5. Pulmonary function may be impaired secondary to liver disease (hepatopulmonary syndrome), and severe hypoxemia may be present. However, this condition improves after successful transplantation. Restrictive disease may be present secondary to ascites.

6. Renal dysfunction may be present, as may hepatorenal syndrome, due to previous renal tubular damage.

Anesthesia Management

Preoperative

1. Preoperative angiography to assess the vascular connections of the liver may require general anesthesia. Urgent admission at the time a donor organ becomes available is then the normal process.

2. Examine the patient carefully to exclude the presence of acute disease that might influence anesthesia. Assess coagulation status and correct as possible.

3. Bowel preparation is performed.

4. Immunosuppressive therapy is initiated: high-dose steroid therapy and cyclosporin A administration.

5. Anticipate increased blood losses in patients younger than 2½ years of age and in those with elevated prothrombin times, acute liver disease, bleeding varices, or encephalopathy.

6. Avoid intramuscular injections in patients with coagulopathy. Oral midazolam premedication is preferred.

7. Many patients are at risk for aspiration; possible recent feeding, delayed gastric emptying, and abdominal distention may be present.

8. Appropriate psychological support must be provided for the child and the family.

Perioperative

First Stage

The first stage includes mobilization of the diseased liver before its removal.

1. Apply basic monitors and induce anesthesia using a rapid-sequence induction. If a small intravenous infusion must be started for induction, insert the catheter in a lower extremity.

2. Continue anesthesia using heated humidified air/O_2/isoflurane as tolerated, with fentanyl supplementation. N_2O is contraindicated

because it may cause bowel distention and increase the risk should intraoperative air embolization occur. Apply controlled ventilation to produce normocapnia with positive end-expiratory pressure (PEEP) to prevent atelectasis.

3. Maintain neuromuscular block with pancuronium. All drugs, including fentanyl, pancuronium, dopamine (renal concentrations), and magnesium sulfate, should preferably be administered as continuous infusions via a central vein.

4. Insert at least three large-bore intravenous routes into the upper limbs and neck, and prepare rapid blood transfusion and warming devices. Insert an arterial line, preferably in the radial artery (the abdominal aorta may have to be clamped); a CVP line; and a urinary catheter. Place esophageal and rectal temperature probes.

5. The patient should be carefully positioned and padded on an eggshell crate mattress. A forced air warmer should cover the legs and head. Inspired gases should be heated and humidified.

6. Prepare to monitor blood gases, electrolytes, glucose, ionized calcium, Hct, platelet count, prothrombin time, and partial thromboplastin time at frequent intervals, performing as many tests as possible on equipment in the OR suite. Other studies of coagulation (e.g., thromboelastogram) may be helpful to guide replacement therapy.

7. During mobilization of the liver, major bleeding may occur (especially in the postoperative Kasai patient), depending on the extent of intra-abdominal adhesions from previous surgery. The intravascular volume should be replaced as necessary to maintain the CVP, BP, urine flow, and the Hct.

8. Hypotension may occur as a result of manipulation of the liver on its pedicle and compromise of IVC flow, but it may also be a result of low ionized calcium levels. Mannitol (0.5 g/kg) may be administered before clamping to establish a brisk diuresis.

Second (Anhepatic) Stage

1. When the IVC is clamped, venous return from the lower body becomes dependent on collateral anastomotic channels unless a venovenous bypass system is used. In this case, venous return is maintained but hazards of hypothermia, thromboembolism, and air embolism may be introduced. Venovenous bypass may, however, reduce blood loss and improve intraoperative splanchnic and renal blood flow, with associated reduced morbidity. Venovenous bypass is not usually used in infants weighing less than 10–15 kg, because it is difficult to maintain flow in small cannulas and small infants seem to tolerate IVC clamping.

2. Hypoglycemia had been postulated as a problem of the anhepatic stage, but it is unusual because the dextrose content of infused blood and fluids maintains high blood levels. Monitor blood glucose levels.

Third Stage

1. When the donor liver is reperfused, the most worrisome physiologic changes may occur. Severe hypotension, arrhythmias, heart block, and cardiac arrest may result. These changes are thought to stem from combined acute changes in acid-base and electrolyte levels and the effects of vasoactive and cardiotoxic factors released from reperfused, previously ischemic tissues.
2. In order to minimize these changes, the following steps should be taken:
   a. Before reperfusion, the ionized calcium and bicarbonate (pH) levels should be increased.
   b. Volume expansion with crystalloid or colloid solutions to maintain a CVP greater than 10 mmHg should be established. Further volumes should be immediately available for infusion.
   c. Rapid evaluation and correction of adverse electrolyte changes must be performed.
   d. Vasopressors should be prepared for instant infusion as required.
3. During the third stage, large blood losses may continue. Platelet transfusions are usually withheld until this stage to minimize the risk of vascular thrombosis in the transplanted liver.
4. The need to treat coagulopathy is based not only on coagulation studies but also on observation of the surgical field; if oozing occurs, replacement therapy must be instituted.
5. Hypertension is common late in the operation and is often unresponsive to additional narcotics and antihypertensive medication. It is thought to be caused by multiple factors: volume overload, impaired renal function, cyclosporine, and steroid therapy. Treatment with salt restriction, diuretics, and ACE inhibitors is advised.
6. There may be difficulty in closing the abdomen because of the size of the implanted liver and distention of the bowel. Ventilation may be compromised, and in extreme cases the use of a Silastic pouch to close the abdomen temporarily (as in patients with omphalocele) may be required.

Postoperative

1. The patient is returned to the ICU, intubated, and maintained on IPPV for at least 12 hours. Pulmonary problems are common and require aggressive therapy.
2. In many cases, return to the OR is necessary to reexplore for continued bleeding, impaired liver perfusion, or biliary obstruction.
3. Renal function is often impaired, and hypertension may be a continuing problem. Acid-base and electrolyte disturbances must be anticipated and treated.
4. There is a high risk of infection, and careful aseptic precautions are essential.
5. Neurologic complications, manifesting as seizures, are not uncommon.

6. Acute rejection—evidenced by headache, fever, malaise, nausea, and abdominal pain—may occur in 7–14 days. Liver enzyme levels may rise and synthetic functions diminish. Modification of the immunosuppressive drug regimen is required. The use of living related donors may decrease the immunologic problems associated with liver transplantation.

Suggested Additional Reading

Carton EG, Plevak DJ, Kranner PW, et al.: Perioperative care of the liver transplant patient: part 2. Anesth Analg 78:382–399, 1994.

Davis PJ and Cook DR: Anesthetic problems in pediatric liver transplantation. Transplant Proc 21:3493, 1989.

Frankville DD: Special considerations for pediatric transplantation. Anesthesiol Clin North Am 12:767–787, 1994.

Goss JA, Shackleton CR, McDiarmid SV, et al.: Long-term results of pediatric liver transplantation: an analysis of 569 transplants. Ann Surg 228:411–420, 1998.

Lichtor JL, Edmond J, Chung MR, et al.: Pediatric orthotopic liver transplantation: multifactorial predictions of blood loss. Anesthesiology 68:607, 1988.

Reding R, de Goyet J de V, Delbeke I, et al.: Pediatric liver transplantation with cadaveric or living related donors: comparative results in 90 elective recipients of primary graft. J Pediatr 134:280–286, 1999.

COMMON MINOR SURGICAL PROCEDURES

N.B. Some children who require minor elective surgery have conditions that may complicate anesthesia and require special attention:

1. Anemia or an upper respiratory infection.
2. A history of prematurity and respiratory distress syndrome. These infants must not be considered absolutely normal even if they are now apparently healthy. Their pulmonary function is impaired during at least the first year of life. Apnea may occur postoperatively, especially in infants who are still at less than 45 weeks of postconceptional age. To be safe, it is usually advised that the infant born prematurely who is still at less than 50 weeks' postconceptional age be admitted to hospital after any minor surgical procedure.

Division of "Tongue-Tie"

If the frenulum is so short that the patient has difficulty passing the tongue around the buccal sulcus, surgical division of the "tongue-tie" probably is advised. This is usually done as an outpatient procedure.

Special Anesthesia Problems

1. This is a very short, minor procedure, but the surgeon must have good access to the oral cavity and a good airway must be ensured.

Anesthesia Management

Preoperative

1. Premedication: sedative premedication (oral midazolam) if required

Perioperative

1. Induce anesthesia by inhaled sevoflurane or intravenous propofol. Intubate using succinylcholine (preceded by atropine!) or mivacurium.
2. Maintain anesthesia with a propofol infusion or sevoflurane and N_2O.
3. Suction the pharynx to remove blood. Apply lidocaine gel to the sublingual wound.
4. The patient should be fully awake before extubation and transfer to the PACU.

Postoperative

1. Further analgesics are not usually required.

Inguinal Herniotomy

Inguinal hernia is common during childhood, usually a result of patent processus vaginalis; its repair is the most common elective general surgical procedure in children. Because these hernias readily become incarcerated during the first year of life, their repair should not be unduly delayed in this age group. Once incarceration has occurred, conservative treatment is usually instituted. Virtually all of these hernias can be reduced, and then, after 24–48 hours, herniotomy can be performed.

If emergency surgery is to be performed as an outpatient procedure, select suitable anesthesia techniques.

The small preterm infant may benefit from spinal analgesia for herniotomy, especially if there is a history of residual pulmonary disease.

Anesthesia Management

Preoperative

1. Assess the patient's general condition carefully.
2. Infants at risk, with a history of prematurity, should be admitted for postoperative apnea monitoring (*see above*).

Perioperative

The choice of anesthesia technique for hernia repair depends on the surgeon. There are pediatric surgeons who can perform a unilateral inguinal herniotomy in 10 minutes—there are also those who can stretch this procedure out to last well over an hour! For the faster surgeon, general inhalational anesthesia delivered by mask is ideal; for longer procedures it is probably wise to intubate the patient.

1. For general anesthesia, induce anesthesia by inhalation or with intravenous thiopental or propofol. Maintain anesthesia by mask with spontaneous ventilation and halothane or sevoflurane in N_2O/O_2.
2. Alternatively, for longer procedures, intubate after administration of a muscle relaxant, and maintain anesthesia with N_2O and halothane or sevoflurane and controlled ventilation.
3. Perform an ilioinguinal and iliohypogastric nerve block on the operative side (or sides) or a caudal block. Acetaminophen, 30–40 mg/kg PR, may be given to augment postoperative analgesia. Narcotic analgesics should generally be avoided, because they increase the incidence of PONV.
4. Ensure that analgesia is adequate before allowing surgery to commence and during traction on the peritoneum.

Postoperative

1. Order additional analgesics as required.

Suggested Additional Reading

Langer JC, Shandling B, and Rosenberg M: Intraoperative bupivacaine during outpatient hernia repair in children: a randomised double blind trial. J Pediatr Surg 22:267–270, 1987.

Orchidopexy

Anesthesia management for orchidopexy is the same as for inguinal herniotomy.

A caudal block should be performed after induction of anesthesia, before the surgery commences, to provide for postoperative analgesia.

Circumcision

Indications for circumcision vary in different communities and from time to time. It remains a common (often outpatient) procedure in pediatric surgery.

Special Anesthesia Problems

1. Management of postoperative pain

Anesthesia Management

Preoperative

1. Assess the patient's general condition carefully.

Perioperative

1. Induction and maintenance of anesthesia as for herniotomy. Mask anesthesia is usually adequate.

2. Provide for analgesia postoperatively. Perform either or both of the following:
   a. Block the dorsal nerve of the penis using 0.25% bupivacaine without epinephrine; maximal dose, 2 mg/kg.
   b. Apply lidocaine jelly to the wound.

Postoperative

1. If regional anesthesia is unsatisfactory, order opioid analgesia (e.g., morphine 0.05–0.10 mg/kg), which can be repeated in the PACU as required until the patient is comfortable.

Suggested Additional Reading

Bacon AK: An alternative block for post-circumcision analgesia. Anaesth Intensive Care 5:63, 1977.

Tree-Trakarn T and Pirayavaraporn S: Postoperative pain relief after circumcision: comparison among morphine, nerve block, and topical analgesia. Anesthesiology 62:519–522, 1985.

Endoscopic and Minimally Invasive Pediatric Surgery

Advances in optical systems, video equipment, and surgical instrumentation over the past decade have allowed the extensive development of endoscopic surgery techniques, many of which are now applied to infants and children. Surgery is performed using very short, well-placed incisions that permit the insertion of an endoscope and each of the necessary surgical instruments. Endoscopic surgery is followed by less pain, reduced requirements for analgesic drugs, and less pulmonary compromise, thereby permitting earlier hospital discharge and a rapid return to normal activity.

Many abdominal procedures, including appendectomy, splenectomy, bowel resection, and fundoplication, may be performed endoscopically. Thoracic procedures include biopsy of mediastinal or pulmonary lesions, closure of ductus arteriosus, cervical sympathectomy, and anterior spinal fusion.

Special Considerations

1. All procedures planned as endoscopic may require urgent open operation should unexpected complications arise; always be prepared for emergency laparotomy or thoracotomy.
2. Bleeding may occur and may be difficult to rapidly control until open operation is performed; ensure that reliable large-bore intravenous routes are established.
3. For laparoscopic surgery, general endotracheal anesthesia with controlled ventilation is required. During the instillation of carbon dioxide into the peritoneal cavity, the following changes can be anticipated:
   a. Intra-abdominal pressure will increase by 8–15 mmHg and will

progressively tend to limit the excursion of the diaphragm, requiring higher pulmonary inflation pressures.

b. Limitation of diaphragmatic excursion may be expected to reduce the functional residual capacity and increase the tendency to airway closure and hypoxemia. During controlled ventilation the peak inspiratory pressure (PIP) can be expected to increase by 30%. If the patient is placed in the Trendelenburg position, a further 25% increase in PIP may occur.

c. Movement of the diaphragm in a cephalad direction may elevate the carina and result in endobronchial migration of a low-placed endotracheal tube.

d. Arterial carbon dioxide tensions will increase due to absorption of insufflated gas, requiring an increased minute ventilation to maintain normocarbia. Positioning, pneumoperitoneum, and the requirement for increased ventilation may cause the PIP to double. Absorption of carbon dioxide may be greater in children than in adults owing to the physiologic properties of the peritoneum.

e. End-tidal carbon dioxide monitoring may not be reliable during laparoscopy because of increased ventilatory dead space.

f. As the pneumoperitoneum is established, heart rate and BP may increase. If the intra-abdominal pressure exceeds 20 mmHg, a fall in BP may occur. Maintenance of adequate hydration and normovolemia minimizes the risk of hypotension, which should be treated by intravenous infusions and release of the pneumoperitoneum.

g. Reflex bradycardia due to vagal stimulation may occur and require treatment with atropine.

h. N_2O should not be used, because it may lead to distention of the bowel and increase the danger should air embolism occur.

i. Beware of the possibility of pneumothorax as a complication of laparoscopy.

j. Carbon dioxide embolism is very rare, but it has occurred during laparoscopy, causing cardiovascular collapse. Monitor carefully throughout the procedure and notify the surgeon immediately if there are any sudden unexplained physiologic changes.

4. For thoracoscopic surgery, general endotracheal (or endobronchial) anesthesia is required.

a. Single-lung ventilation is required so that the lung in the hemithorax to be operated may collapse and permit good surgical vision and access. See page 303 for methods to achieve single-lung ventilation.

b. During instillation of carbon dioxide to the hemithorax, cardiorespiratory functions should be carefully monitored, and the surgeon should be informed of any significant changes.

c. Adequate hydration and normovolemia should be ensured by appropriate intravenous fluid therapy. Hypovolemia may lead to severe hypotension as a pneumothorax is established.

d. Ventilation and inspired oxygen concentrations must be adjusted to maintain safe parameters throughout the procedure.

   e. Anesthetic agents that interfere with normal hypoxic pulmonary vasoconstriction (e.g., halothane) should be avoided in order to ensure that pulmonary blood flow is optimally distributed away from the collapsed lung. Low concentrations of isoflurane or intravenous agents (e.g., propofol, fentanyl) are preferred.

Suggested Additional Reading

Ivani G, Vaira M, and Mattioli G: Paediatric laparoscopic surgery; anaesthetic management. Paediatr Anaesth 4:323–325, 1994.

Manner T, Aantaa R, and Alanen M: Lung compliance during laparoscopic surgery in paediatric patients. Paediatr Anaesth 8:25–29, 1998.

Sfez M, Guerard A, and Desruelle P: Cardiorespiratory changes during laparoscopic fundoplication in children. Paediatr Anaesth 5:89–95, 1995.

Tobias JD: Anaesthetic implications of thoracoscopic surgery in children. Paediatr Anaesth 9:103–110, 1999.

Chapter 14

Cardiovascular Surgery and Cardiologic Procedures

Heart surgery in children is performed almost exclusively for congenital heart disease (CHD). The incidence of CHD is approximately 6 per 1,000 live births. The lesions listed in Table 14–1 account for more than 90% of all congenital heart defects. There are various classifications of CHD, but that given in the table is most useful for the anesthesiologist.

THE CHILD WITH CONGENITAL HEART DISEASE

Infants with CHD usually present early with respiratory distress and/or cyanosis and difficulty with feeding, or later with failure to thrive. Some malformations cause severe congestive cardiac failure during the neonatal period, evidenced by marked hepatomegaly. Cardiac failure results from the high pressures needed to compensate for obstruction to blood flow (valve stenosis or coarctation) or from high-volume flow through intracardiac or extracardiac shunts (e.g., ventricular septal defect [VSD], patent ductus arteriosus [PDA]). Dyspnea may result from cardiac failure and/or changes in pulmonary blood flow.

The diagnosis of CHD in infants may be difficult; innocent murmurs are common, but serious lesions may be present without a loud murmur. The physiology of the neonatal cardiovascular system may obscure significant lesions; for example, the high pulmonary vascular resistance (PVR) may limit left-to-right shunts, and a PDA may mask coarctation of the aorta. An echocardiogram is essential to make a definitive diagnosis in many cases and should be requested whenever CHD is suspected.

Older infants and children with CHD may present with reduced exercise tolerance, chest pain, or syncope. Alternatively, a murmur may

Table 14–1. Incidence of Congenital Heart Disease

Type of Lesion	Frequency (%)*
Lesions with Increased Pulmonary Blood Flow	
Ventricular septal defect (VSD)	16.6
Patent ductus arteriosus (PDA)	6.5
Endocardial cushion defect (AV canal)	5.3
Atrial septal defect (ASD)	3.1
Truncus arteriosus	1.5
Cyanotic Lesions	
Hypoplastic left ventricle	7.9
Tetralogy of Fallot	3.5
Transposition of great arteries	2.5
Tricuspid atresia	1.5
Obstructive Lesions	
Coarctation of the aorta	8.0
Pulmonary stenosis	3.5
Aortic stenosis	2.0

*Frequency of lesions symptomatic in the first year of life.
(From Fyler DC, Buckley LP, Hellenbrand WE, et al.: Report of the New England Regional Infant Cardiac Program. Pediatrics 65(Suppl):388, 1980, with permission.)

be discovered on routine medical examination. Children with CHD often experience repeated respiratory infections.

General Systemic Effects of Congenital Heart Disease

Usually the child is small; height and weight are often below average. Children with CHD, and especially those with cyanotic CHD, may also demonstrate some developmental delay. The underweight child with CHD, however, has a metabolic rate that is considerably higher than predicted from size or weight. Infants with cyanotic CHD are not able to increase their metabolic rate to meet the demands of physiologic stress (e.g., cooling) and hence tolerate such stress poorly.

Effects on the Respiratory System

CHD can have major effects on pulmonary function. Enlarged vessels or chambers of the heart may compress major airways. Increased pulmonary blood flow results in small airway obstruction, decreased compliance, increased resistance, and ventilation-perfusion ratio ($\dot{V}/\dot{Q}$) imbalance. Excess pulmonary blood flow eventually results in irreversible pulmonary hypertension owing to structural changes in the vessels; these include medial hypertrophy and peripheral extension of the muscle layer into normally nonmuscular arterioles. These vascular changes may be prevented by pulmonary artery (PA) banding or total repair during early life.

Patients with decreased pulmonary blood flow have less efficient ventilation, requiring increased minute ventilation to eliminate carbon dioxide. The gradient between end-tidal and arterial carbon dioxide levels is increased. The uptake of inhaled anesthetic agents into the blood (but not into the alveoli) is delayed. Cyanosis is associated with a reduced ventilatory response to hypoxemia.

Effects on the Heart

In addition to the special characteristics of the child's heart, CHD may impose other changes:

1. Obstructive lesions impose a pressure load on the affected ventricle. This ventricle then hypertrophies—becomes less compliant and less able to accept any increase in stroke volume—and is subject to myocardial ischemia and consequent arrhythmias.
2. Large shunts or valvular incompetence impose a volume load on the ventricle. This ventricle initially responds with an increased stroke volume but later dilates and fails. The dilated ventricle requires a high wall tension to effect pressure change within the chamber (Laplace's law); it therefore is vulnerable to myocardial depressants and cannot cope with additional loads.
3. Myocardial ischemia may result from low aortic diastolic pressures and rapid heart rates in some patients (e.g., those with a PDA).

Effects on the Blood

Cyanosis induces compensatory changes in the blood: polycythemia occurs, and the blood volume increases. The high hematocrit (Hct) may lead to thrombosis (especially cerebral) and abscess formation. Cyanotic CHD is also commonly accompanied by coagulopathy secondary to thrombocytopenia, impaired platelet function, and decreased vitamin K–dependent factors.

Effects on Hepatic and Renal Function

These functions are impaired in cyanotic CHD and especially in those patients with congestive heart failure (CHF). Splanchnic blood flow is reduced. Clearance of drugs via the liver or kidneys is delayed (e.g., morphine clearance is reduced in patients with CHD).

GENERAL PRINCIPLES OF ANESTHESIA MANAGEMENT

1. Children with CHD and their parents are often very apprehensive and deserve careful and considerate attention. Older children and their families may have had to endure repeated surgery.

2. The techniques used must minimize demands on the cardiovascular system.
   a. Give adequate premedication to reduce anxiety, activity, and O_2 requirements.
   b. A rapid, smooth induction of anesthesia, with no crying or struggling, is very desirable.
   c. Give adequate doses of analgesics or general anesthetic agents perioperatively. Prevent tachycardia and/or hypertension. High-dose narcotic anesthesia together with good postoperative analgesia may favorably influence the neuroendocrine and metabolic responses to surgery and improve survival.
   d. Apply controlled ventilation but maintain normocarbia unless there is a specific indication to adjust the CO_2 tension. Avoid producing inadvertent hypocarbia, which may
      i. Reduce cardiac output.
      ii. Cause vasoconstriction and increase systemic resistance.
      iii. Decrease PVR and increase left-to-right shunts.
      iv. Shift the hemoglobin/oxygen (Hb/O_2) dissociation curve to the left and limit O_2 transfer.
      v. Decrease myocardial blood flow.
      vi. Decrease the serum K level, resulting in arrhythmias.
      vii. Decrease cerebral blood flow.

   Decide on an optimal level of ventilation for each patient and maintain this level.

   e. Give adequate doses of muscle relaxants to prevent any risk of movement or ventilatory efforts, especially when the heart is open (danger of air emboli).
   f. Maintain the patient's body temperature and avoid cold stress except when induced hypothermia is indicated.
   g. When appropriate, consider left ventricular (LV) afterload reduction and/or measures to reduce PVR (*see below*).
3. Optimal myocardial function and cardiac output must be maintained during surgery:
   a. Do not give agents that cause excessive myocardial depression.
   b. Adjust the fluid balance to maintain optimal cardiac filling pressures.
4. Detrimental changes in cardiac shunts must be prevented.
   a. Use anesthetic drugs that have minimal effect on SVR.
   b. Be aware of the possible effects of intermittent positive-pressure ventilation (IPPV) on shunts; avoid high intrathoracic pressures, but maintain the lung volume as necessary by the use of optimal positive end-expiratory pressure (PEEP). PVR is minimal at an optimal lung volume and increases at greater or lesser volumes.
   c. Drugs that produce a controllable degree of myocardial depression (e.g., halothane) may be useful when ventricular muscle is causing dynamic obstruction to blood flow (e.g., tetralogy of Fallot).
   d. Patients who are dependent on systemic-to-pulmonary shunts will desaturate if the systemic arterial pressure is allowed to fall.

e. Anemia may increase left-to-right shunts. Conversely left-to-right shunting may be reduced by increasing the Hct, because the increased blood viscosity has a greater effect on PVR than on systemic vascular resistance (SVR).

f. Be prepared to use drugs or other methods to manipulate PVR or SVR as may become necessary.

5. Conditions that favor optimal myocardial perfusion must be maintained throughout surgery to avoid ischemic damage to the heart and subsequent impairment of cardiac function postoperatively.

   a. The duration of diastole and the diastolic pressure are important factors in maintaining perfusion of the myocardium, which is especially vulnerable if left-to-right shunting and ventricular hypertrophy are present. Inadequate anesthesia and analgesia produces tachycardia, which shortens diastole and therefore may impair myocardial perfusion. Replace blood and give adequate fluids to maintain the diastolic pressure.

   b. Maintain an optimal Hct to preserve oxygen transport to the myocardium. Anemia may compromise subendocardial blood flow.

   c. During cardiopulmonary bypass (CPB), it is preferable to maintain a regular rhythm until the aorta is cross-clamped and cardioplegia is induced; this preserves myocardial perfusion. If ventricular fibrillation occurs, higher perfusion pressures and an LV vent are needed to ensure adequate myocardial perfusion.

6. The cardiac work load must be minimized:

   a. Prevent hypertension and tachycardia during anesthesia by ensuring adequate levels of analgesia and by using vasodilators and/or β-adrenergic blocking drugs when appropriate.

   b. Do not give excessive doses of drugs that may produce hypertension (e.g., Neo-Synephrine).

   c. Pulmonary hypertension must be controlled.

7. Heparin has a larger volume of distribution and a more rapid plasma clearance in infants than in adults. Therefore, larger doses may be required initially, an activated clotting time (ACT) of 400 seconds or more is required before CPB, and the level of heparinization should be checked frequently (every 30 minutes).

8. During CPB, the myocardium may be protected by

   a. Cardioplegic solutions that are infused at a pressure of 100–150 mmHg into the coronary circulation after aortic clamping. Controversy still exists concerning the most advantageous type of solution, and this may differ in infants and adults. Most solutions contain high levels of potassium with added dextrose and buffers. The addition of free radical scavenger agents and calcium ion channel blockers has been suggested. The ideal cardioplegic solution

      i. Produces immediate arrest and avoids energy depletion.

      ii. Provides substrate for anaerobic metabolism.

      iii. Buffers metabolic acidosis in the tissue.

      iv. Minimizes tissue edema by osmolar effects.

      v. Stabilizes cell membranes.
      vi. Minimizes reperfusion injury.

Blood cardioplegia is preferred by many institutions. Repeated doses of cardioplegic solution are normally given at 15- to 20-minute intervals.

    b. Hypothermia. But remember that the heart has a great tendency to rewarm because of surgical manipulation and heat from operating room (OR) lights. Therefore, during prolonged surgery, cold cardioplegic solutions should be repeatedly applied, and a pericardial cooling bath should be used.

    c. Pre-CPB systemic corticosteroids may help preserve myocardial tissue during periods of ischemic arrest, but this is controversial.

    d. An optimal reperfusate solution may be used after a period of ischemic arrest. This may flush out metabolites and prevent reperfusion injury. This solution should be warmed and alkaline and should contain a low concentration of ionized calcium and a slightly elevated potassium concentration. In practice, a repeat dose of warmed cardioplegic solution is often given just before reperfusion.

9. After CPB, small infants and children may bleed excessively owing to dilutional thrombocytopenia and low levels of coagulation factors. This is primarily a result of the large pump-priming volume in relation to the child's blood volume. Be prepared to administer platelets and other factors as required. Fresh whole blood, if available, may be particularly advantageous in small infants. Make sure that infants do not cool after weaning from CPB; coagulopathy may result.

SPECIAL PROBLEMS

1. *Large shunts* may be present. Right-to-left shunts result in
    a. Low arterial oxygen tension (PaO_2). This is often only minimally improved by increasing the fraction of inspired oxygen (FiO_2).
    b. Delayed uptake of inhaled anesthetic agents.
    c. Extreme danger of systemic emboli from venous air embolism.
    d. Short arm-brain circulation time, with no pulmonary transit; therefore, there is a danger of overdose with intravenous drugs.
    e. Less efficient ventilation and gas exchange; increased ventilation is necessary to maintain a normal arterial carbon dioxide tension ($PaCO_2$), whether the patient is awake or anesthetized.
    f. An increased arterial to end-tidal CO_2 tension gradient; end-tidal CO_2 levels underestimate arterial levels.

2. Left-to-right shunts result in
    a. Pulmonary vascular overperfusion but good ventilatory efficiency and gas exchange initially.
    b. Later, pulmonary hypertension develops and progresses to irreversible increased vascular resistance, which may limit the operability of associated cardiac lesions.
    c. Eventual CHF.

3. *Obstructive lesions* may result in
   a. Fixed cardiac output, and therefore very limited ability to compensate for changes in metabolic demand or a decline in peripheral vascular resistance.
   b. Myocardial hypertrophy, with possible inadequacy of myocardial perfusion, especially to the subendocardium. Reduced ventricular compliance results in dependence on a high cardiac filling pressure.
   c. CHF.
   d. Sudden serious arrhythmias.
4. *Heart failure* is common in infants with CHD and is worsened by drugs that depress the myocardium (e.g., halothane).
5. *Electrolyte disturbance*
   a. Serum electrolyte (especially K^+) levels may be low, particularly in patients who have had prolonged diuretic therapy. (Hypokalemia predisposes to cardiac arrhythmias, particularly with digitalis therapy and during hypothermia.)
   b. Neonates with CHD may have low Ca^{++} and glucose levels.
   c. Low serum magnesium levels may occur and predispose to arrhythmias.
6. *Drugs* essential for CHD therapy can cause problems:
   a. Digitalis: the therapeutic index is low, and toxicity is an ever-present hazard, especially in young children. Check a recent serum digitalis level (therapeutic range, 0.8–2 ng/ml). Hypothermia increases the risk of digitalis toxicity because the K^+ concentration falls.
   b. Diuretics: may deplete K^+, further increasing the risk of digitalis toxicity.
   c. β-Adrenergic blocking agents: they may impair cardiac contractility; however, this is not usually a problem with therapeutic doses. If being used in the treatment of cyanotic spells, these drugs should be continued until the day of surgery.
   d. Calcium channel–blocking agents: these are not commonly used in pediatric patients. If used in infants, they may cause severe, persistent myocardial depression. The combination of β-blocking agents with calcium channel blockers is very dangerous and should be avoided.
7. *Polycythemia.* A high Hct (greater than 55% in cyanotic lesions) results in
   a. Increased viscosity of the blood—and therefore increased cardiac work
   b. Increased tendency to thrombosis
   c. Further increased risk of thrombosis if dehydration or venous stasis develops
   d. Coagulopathy
   e. Predisposition to cerebral abscess

Despite the dangers of polycythemia, these children are very dependent on a high Hct to ensure adequate O_2 transport. Hemodilution to normal Hct levels may be followed by severe cardiovascular collapse.

Hemodilution before surgery, if thought to be indicated, must be very carefully controlled and the Hct not taken lower than 40%–45%.

8. Some infants with large left-to-right shunts are at extreme risk of pulmonary hypertensive crises during and after surgery (e.g., truncus arteriosus, arteriovenous [AV] canal). It is important to prevent such crises, because they are difficult to reverse. The measures taken may include
   a. Adequate anesthesia/analgesia during surgery, and minimal handling of the child postoperatively.
   b. Controlled hyperventilation ($PaCO_2 = 25$–30).
   c. Fentanyl infusion (e.g., 25 μg/kg loading dose plus 2 μg/kg/hr).
   d. Sodium nitroprusside (SNP) infusion 0.5–5 μg/kg/min.
   e. Inhalation of nitric oxide (NO). NO has specific pulmonary vasodilating properties and is a very useful drug to control PVR. It does require special equipment for its administration. It must be mixed in the gases delivered to the patient in a concentration of 20–80 ppm; this requires equipment to monitor its final concentration in the mixture. It cannot be premixed in oxygen containing mixtures of gases, because nitrogen dioxide (NO_2) will be formed, which is damaging to the lungs. It should be mixed with the lowest FiO_2 that ensures adequate Hb saturation, in order to minimize NO_2 formation. NO must not be suddenly withdrawn, because severe rebound pulmonary hypertension may result.

9. Some infants are dependent on the patency of the ductus arteriosus as a route for shunting of blood until surgery can be performed (e.g., transposition of the great arteries with intact septum, interrupted aortic arch). Prostaglandin E_1 (PGE_1) is used to keep the ductus open in such infants. An infusion of 0.05–0.1 μg/kg/min should be continued until the appropriate surgical procedure is completed.

10. *Associated malformations.* Many children with CHD have additional defects (e.g., cleft palate, Down syndrome, subglottic stenosis) that may complicate anesthesia and require special considerations.

11. *Induction of anesthesia.* Different methods do not have markedly different effects on oxygen saturation, even in cyanotic patients; therefore, the anesthesiologist may choose whatever seems best and most appropriate for a given patient. In our practice, an intravenous induction using a narcotic analgesic, a very small dose of barbiturate, and an intubating dose of a nondepolarizing relaxant is usually preferred; this allows for good ventilation, rapid airway control, and very stable conditions. Use of EMLA or amethocaine cream and suitable sedation facilitate the ease of venous cannulation. Beware of using halothane or other myocardial depressant vapors in other than very low concentrations. Ketamine has been commonly used, but an intramuscular injection always upsets the child and leads to stress and crying.

12. *Muscle relaxants.* Nondepolarizing agents take longer to have their

full effect in patients with CHD; a longer period of mask ventilation should be applied before intubation is attempted.

13. *Temperature control.* Temperature control may be especially poor in neonates with cyanotic CHD, because these children cannot respond to heat losses as well as normal infants do. Body temperature falls rapidly if they are exposed to a cool environment. Vasoconstriction in the cold child impairs efforts at insertion of intravenous lines and may result in metabolic acidosis. Keep the child warm until all the lines are in place.

14. *Sepsis.* This is a major threat to the success of cardiac surgery; great care must be taken to observe strict asepsis when invasive monitoring or infusion lines are being inserted. In patients undergoing transplantation, all lines should be inserted with the use of very careful technique and each site covered with povidone-iodine (Betadine) ointment and a Tegaderm dressing.

15. *Repeated surgery.* Some children need repeated surgery, which imposes a severe psychological stress on them and their parents. A very considerate, careful approach by the anesthesiologist is essential.

ROUTINE PREOPERATIVE, PERIOPERATIVE, AND POSTOPERATIVE CARE

Preoperative Assessment and Preparation

Review all the medical records, obtain a history from the parents, and perform an independent physical examination, especially of the cardio-vascular and respiratory systems, ears, nose, throat, teeth, and veins.

If the child has had a significant recent lower respiratory infection, elective surgery should be postponed, if possible, for 2–3 weeks, because an increased susceptibility to pulmonary complications is possible during this period.

Look for evidence of associated disease or dysmorphic features that might complicate anesthesia management. Look carefully for signs of cardiac failure: tachypnea, sweating, and hepatomegaly in infants. Carefully determine the respiratory status to exclude acute disease that might compromise the patient perioperatively.

Review the cardiology notes, echocardiogram, cardiac catheterization, and angiographic data. Aim to fully understand the current pathophysiology. Note salient abnormalities and findings on the anesthesia chart. Review previous anesthesia experience.

Many patients with CHD take several medications regularly. Propranolol and other β-blockers should be continued up to the day of surgery. With rare exceptions, digitalis and diuretics should be withheld on the day of operation. Calcium channel–blocking drugs are very infrequently used in children but, if they are used, they should be discontinued the day before surgery.

If the patient requires O_2 therapy and/or maintenance of the sitting position during transit to the OR, order these specifically.

Plan in advance for postoperative pain management. In those patients who may be extubated early, spinal or epidural opioids may be most useful. In most other cases, pain can be managed by an intravenous infusion of a narcotic analgesic and/or patient-controlled analgesia.

Blood Supplies

During any type of cardiac surgery, blood must be immediately available in the OR. In many centers, ordering blood is the responsibility of the surgical service. However, the day before surgery, the anesthesiologist should ensure that adequate supplies of blood and blood products will be available by operation time.

Some patients have special requirements. For example:

1. For cyanotic patients with an Hb greater than 16 g/dl, plasma should be available.
2. For all infants, check that the blood to be supplied is less than 3 days old and has been tested for cytomegalovirus. Washed cells should be ordered for small infants to avoid the danger of hyperkalemia.
3. For infants undergoing CPB, ensure that appropriate quantities of packed cells, fresh-frozen plasma, and platelets (1 unit/5 kg) and cryoprecipitate have been ordered. Alternatively, fresh whole blood is considered especially advantageous, and is reported to reduce bleeding after CPB, but may be difficult to obtain.
4. For all patients likely to require prolonged CPB (longer than 1.5 hours), ensure that fresh-frozen plasma and platelets have been ordered.
5. Where "relatively minor" surgery is planned for older children and those with an initially high Hct, the use of hemodilution with a clear fluid prime in the pump oxygenator may avert the need for blood transfusion. At the end of CPB, modified ultrafiltration may be used to remove the fluid prime and restore the Hct. Alternatively, the contents of the pump circuit may be collected to be reinfused into the patient postoperatively. (Blood should be ordered to be available on a standby basis.)

Premedication

1. Children with CHD require adequate preoperative sedation to reduce excitement, anxiety, and crying (and thus reduce O_2 consumption). Order a hypnotic to be given the evening before surgery for anxious older children and preoperative sedation for all children older than 6 months to 1 year of age.
2. In recent years, an oral regimen has come to be preferred:
   a. Midazolam 0.5–0.75 mg/kg PO (maximum 20 mg), taken in cherry syrup to mask the taste, is very effective; allow 10–30 minutes for the peak effect to be achieved.
   b. The child who will not take liquid midazolam may be persuaded to accept a fentanyl Oralet. A dose of up to 15 µg/kg produces

good sedation without respiratory depression. The pulse oximeter should be monitored during the onset of sedation.
c. Lorazepam 1–2 mg PO is effective for the adolescent patient. These regimens of premedication do not usually cause significant declines in O_2 saturation levels preoperatively, even in cyanotic patients. However, the child should be supervised as sedation occurs, and a pulse oximeter may be used as the patient becomes settled.

EMLA cream or amethocaine gel should be applied to a predetermined site for intravenous cannulation, covered with an occlusive dressing, and allowed to remain in place for as long as possible before induction.

3. For cyanotic children with a high Hct, ensure that oral fluids are regularly offered up to 2 hours before the operation to prevent dehydration. Alternatively, if oral fluids cannot be taken, order maintenance intravenous fluids before surgery.

ANESTHESIA MANAGEMENT

Routine Anesthesia Management

Preoperative

1. Check all anesthesia and monitoring equipment before having the patient brought into the OR.
2. Make available for use, in case of emergency, syringes containing the following drugs:
   a. Sodium bicarbonate, 8.4% solution: 20 ml
   b. Atropine solution, diluted to 0.1 mg/ml: 4 ml
   c. Calcium chloride, 10% solution: 10 ml
   d. Epinephrine, 1:10,000 preparation: 10 ml
   e. Neo-Synephrine, 0.1 mg/ml

Solutions of inotropic drugs should be prepared. These should be made in a concentration that will permit their infusion at a therapeutic rate without adding an excessive fluid load. In practice, for small infants and children, it is useful to use a dilution that will deliver the required dose when infused at 1–2 ml/hr (*see* Appendix III, p 526).

3. Check that preoperative medication has been given as ordered and is effective.
4. On arrival in the OR, gently apply basic monitors: pulse oximeters (one probe to a finger, thumb, or ear and one probe to a toe), precordial stethoscope, blood pressure (BP) cuff, and electrocardiogram (ECG) electrodes. Record heart rate and rhythm as well as BP. Do not prolong this process, especially if the child is apprehensive, but proceed carefully and rapidly.

Perioperative

1. Administer O_2 by mask. Often the child will be happier if the mask is held slightly away from the face. Use a high flow.
2. Induce anesthesia, preferably intravenously, particularly in patients with a right-to-left shunt, which slows inhalation induction. For most patients, fentanyl 2–5 μg/kg followed by thiopental given slowly intravenously (2–4 mg/kg) produces a smooth induction with minimal cardiovascular effects. In small infants, precede the fentanyl by a small dose of atropine (0.01 mg/kg) or an appropriate dose of pancuronium to avoid bradycardia. For the very unstable patient, omit thiopental but give fentanyl slowly up to 30 μg/kg IV with midazolam up to 0.2 mg IV for induction.
3. Drugs given intravenously should be administered in small doses, *slowly*. (If a right-to-left shunt is present, they act very rapidly; but if the circulation time is slow, their effect may be less rapid.) Be patient and wait for the desired effect. Beware of overdose.
4. For intubation: give an initial dose of nondepolarizing relaxant and ventilate the patient until relaxation is adequate; pancuronium 0.1 mg/kg, vecuronium 0.1 mg/kg, or rocuronium 1 mg/kg produces good conditions for intubation within 3 minutes (*see also* item 9 in this list).
5. Use a cuffed endotracheal tube to ensure ability to ventilate well. Carefully position the tube and check ventilation to all areas.
6. Maintain anesthesia with a suitable mixture of N_2O/O_2 or air/O_2. (It is rarely necessary to use more than 50% O_2. If a large right-to-left shunt is present, an increase in the FiO_2 has very little effect on the PaO_2.) It is probably advisable to avoid N_2O in the patient with pulmonary hypertension, although the effect on PVR is not large.
7. If myocardial function is good, for simple lesions, low concentrations of a volatile agent (e.g., isoflurane 0.5%–0.75%) may be used. Otherwise, for all complex lesions add narcotics in adequate doses (e.g., fentanyl, sufentanil).
8. Control ventilation to produce desired carbon dioxide tension. Note that end-tidal carbon dioxide is a satisfactory means to monitor $PaCO_2$ in acyanotic patients but may underestimate the $PaCO_2$ in children with cyanotic CHD. Always check the end-tidal carbon dioxide against the $PaCO_2$; the end-tidal level can then be used to follow trends.
9. The choice of muscle relaxant for use during maintenance of anesthesia should be influenced by the following points:
   a. Vecuronium has very little effect on cardiovascular parameters, has an intermediate duration of action, and, if properly dosed, can readily be reversed for early extubation. It is probably the agent of choice for many infants and children.
   b. Pancuronium with fentanyl is a useful combination to use in the very unstable small infant with a complex lesion.
10. Insert a nasopharyngeal and rectal or bladder thermometer. An esophageal stethoscope cannot be inserted if a transesophageal echocardiogram (TEE) probe will be used.

11. Insert adequate-bore intravenous routes, an arterial line, a double-lumen central venous line (*see* Chapter 4), and a urinary catheter. In older children who may be extubated early, it is preferred if possible to place the arterial line and the intravenous line into the same upper limb (usually the left). The other hand can then be used to operate the patient-controlled analgesia machine!
12. Give maintenance fluids as outlined on page 114. If the child was polycythemic preoperatively, plasma may be preferable to blood as replacement fluid, especially if a systemic-pulmonary shunt is being performed. An Hct of at least 35%–40% by the end of surgery is usually desirable. Use a blood warmer for all infusions.
13. For those patients who may be extubated early after surgery, consider the use of epidural or spinal narcotics.

Open Heart Surgery

1. Follow routine management (*see above*). A cerebral function monitor may be useful during CPB.
2. If a TEE probe is to be inserted, monitor ventilation, saturation, the end-tidal carbon dioxide curve, and the BP very carefully. Passage of the probe may compromise ventilation and/or the major vessels, especially in small infants; it may also trigger autonomic reflexes.

The TEE has proved most useful intraoperatively for pediatric patients. The exact anatomy and pathophysiology can be defined and the adequacy of repair assessed immediately. Residual shunts can be detected intraoperatively and valve function, ventricular filling, and contractility assessed. The flow in conduits or shunts can be examined. TEE probes are available that can be inserted into infants weighing 3 kg or less.

3. Maintain anesthesia with the following:
   a. N_2O/O_2 in suitable proportions to ensure oxygen saturation at an acceptable level. Use air/O_2 for patients for whom N_2O may be contraindicated. Very occasionally, it may be necessary to deliver an FiO_2 below 0.21 to maintain pulmonary vasoconstriction and avoid overperfusion of the lungs. In this instance, it is desirable to be able to mix nitrogen with the inspired gases.
   b. If tolerated, isoflurane 0.5%–0.75% or halothane 0.5%, depending on the lesion, may be given and supplemented with generous doses of fentanyl.
   c. Patients with a history of failure who may benefit from afterload reduction will probably do well with minimal isoflurane (e.g., VSD with left-to-right shunt). Patients with dynamic ventricular outflow obstruction who may benefit from a degree of controlled myocardial depression usually do well with minimal (0.5%) halothane (e.g., tetralogy of Fallot, subaortic stenosis).
4. Give incremental doses of relaxant drugs as needed. Administer an

additional generous bolus just before bypass to ensure complete immobility.

5. Give maintenance fluids, such as lactated Ringer's solution according to body weight to replace the calculated deficit during fasting (if any) and maintain urine output at greater than 1 ml/kg/min. Additional "fluid loading" before CPB has not been shown to be advantageous. Avoid dextrose-containing fluids; hyperglycemia might result in increased neurologic damage in case of cerebral hypoxia/ischemia, but monitor blood glucose levels in small infants to prevent hypoglycemia.

6. Blood loss from sponges, suction, drapes, *and specimens* must be assessed carefully, and the volume replaced. It is seldom necessary to transfuse blood before CPB unless major blood loss occurs during opening of the chest or dissection around the heart (e.g., during repeat operations). In such repeat cases, an infusion of lactated Ringer's solution through a blood warmer should be prepared and connected to the patient, ready to run, before sternotomy.

   a. Aim to maintain the Hct near the preoperative level and the intravascular volume high enough to maintain the central venous pressure (CVP).

   b. If the Hct was very high preoperatively, replace initial losses with plasma, but beware of too much hemodilution before CPB.

   c. During venous cannulation in small infants, a significant volume of blood may be lost into the cannulas. Ensure that this volume is replaced, usually by transfusion from the pump oxygenator circuit via the aortic cannula.

7. Patients with cyanotic CHD may benefit from the administration of ϵ-aminocaproic acid (Amicar), an antifibrinolytic agent, to reduce bleeding. A loading dose of 200 mg/kg should be infused, preferably before sternotomy. Alternatively, tranexamic acid, 50–100 mg/kg, may be administered before skin incision.

8. In patients having repeat procedures, blood losses may be reduced by the administration of aprotinin. A test dose of 1 ml should be administered after all monitoring is established. After 10 minutes, if no reaction (e.g., hypotension, bronchospasm) occurs, a loading infusion of 120 mg per square meter of body surface area (BSA) may be infused over 30 minutes via a central line. This is followed by a maintenance infusion of 28 mg/m^2 BSA.

9. During dissection around the heart, watch the BP closely; arrhythmias are common, although most are innocuous. If hypotension or arrhythmia persists, ask the surgeon to desist until the condition corrects itself. Continuing hypotension suggests hypovolemia; in this case, a fluid infusion is required so that the patient can tolerate essential manipulations around the heart.

10. If N_2O is given, discontinue it before cannulation in case any air embolism should occur.

11. Before the heart is cannulated, give the initial dose of heparin.

Preferably, determine the dose by plotting a dose-response curve (Fig. 14–1).

a. Take a blood sample and determine the control ACT.
b. Give heparin 1 mg/kg (100 units/kg).
c. Repeat the ACT and plot a graph (Fig. 14–1).
d. Give a further dose of heparin 1 mg/kg (100 units/kg).
e. Again determine and plot the ACT.
f. Draw the dose-response curve and determine the additional dose of heparin required to prolong the ACT to 600 seconds.
g. Give this dose and recheck the ACT after 2–3 minutes.

Alternatively, a single dose of 3 mg/kg (300 units/kg) may be given and the ACT checked; this should be at least 400 seconds before initiation of CPB. Small infants may require more heparin and demonstrate more variation in dose requirements than older patients.

12. Once CPB is established, the pump flow should be increased to establish a satisfactory perfusion. Indicators of adequate perfusion are the cerebral function monitor, urine output, and repeated acid-base studies. In patients with cyanotic CHD, perfusion pressures may be low during early bypass, because of the patient's increased vascular bed and the use of a low-viscosity perfusate. Patients with tetralogy of Fallot may also have extensive collateral flow into the lungs. High flows may be required initially, but the systemic pressure will increase progressively, especially as cooling progresses. The use of vasoconstrictors is not usually necessary but should be considered if hypotension persists. When the perfusion pressure is low, it is of vital importance that the superior vena cava (SVC) pressure should be at or near zero. Any increase in jugular venous pressure in these circumstances may have a serious effect on

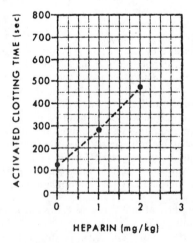

Figure 14–1. Heparin dose-response curve.

    cerebral blood flow. Monitor CVP carefully to detect any
compromise of SVC venous return due to obstruction of the
cannulas.

13. During partial bypass, ventilate the lungs with O_2. Never give any
N_2O because of the possibility of exacerbating air embolism.

14. During total bypass:
    a. Keep the lungs inflated at a low pressure.
    b. Add 0.5% isoflurane to the oxygenator to continue anesthesia
    and improve perfusion during normothermic bypass, or give
    additional doses of fentanyl. Remember that fentanyl is bound
    to the plastic components of the CPB circuit, so blood levels fall
    precipitously on bypass. Do not add volatile agents to the
    oxygenator during hypothermic bypass; the increased tissue
    solubility of the agent at low body temperatures may result in
    residual cardiac depressant effects after rewarming and during
    weaning from CPB. Discontinue any volatile agents 15 minutes
    before the end of bypass.

15. Hypertension in the adequately anesthetized patient may be treated
by injection of phentolamine (0.2 mg/kg). During hypothermic
CPB, it has been demonstrated that children secrete
catecholamines; phentolamine, by its α-adrenergic blocking action,
improves perfusion and delays the development of metabolic
acidosis.

16. During bypass (partial and total), repeat the ACT every 30 minutes
and give additional doses of heparin as necessary to prolong the
ACT to more than 600 seconds.

17. Take blood samples for acid-base, electrolyte, and Hct
determinations every 30 minutes and just before CPB is
discontinued. Monitor glucose levels in small infants.

18. Before discontinuing CPB:
    a. Inflate the lungs, suction the endotracheal tube, and check
    ventilation by observing the movement of both lungs.
    b. Commence pacing if the heart rate is slow or if sinus rhythm is
    absent; infants and children need an atrial contraction to
    maintain a good cardiac output at this stage. Atrial pacing can
    be used for slow heart rates with normal conduction. AV
    sequential pacing is required if conduction is abnormal. If AV
    block is present, it is possible to sense the atrial contraction and
    use it to pace the ventricle.
    c. If the cardiac action is impaired, inotropic agents should be
    commenced at a time well before weaning. A combination of
    dopamine 5 μg/kg/min with dobutamine 5 μg/kg/min is a
    common initial routine.
    d. If the cardiac action is severely depressed, prepare an infusion
    of epinephrine 0.1 μg/kg/min.
    e. All neonates should have a calcium chloride infusion established
    at 5 mg/kg/hr.

19. For patients with pulmonary hypertension, the following should be
established before weaning:
    a. A PA line to monitor pressure

    b. Hyperventilation with oxygen

    c. Correction of any preexisting metabolic acidosis

    d. NO available to be added to inspired gases if necessary

In some patients with mild elevation of pulmonary artery pressure, it may be useful to commence an infusion of SNP at 0.5–2 μg/kg/min before weaning from bypass.

20. As CPB is discontinued:

    a. Administer calcium chloride (10 mg/kg) to improve cardiac action if necessary. (Calcium should never be given until the heart has resumed a good regular rhythm.)

    b. Request infusion of blood from the pump, and infuse cells until the left atrial pressure is adequate (8–12 mmHg, depending on the cardiac lesion). The Hct on bypass is usually lower, and it is advisable to infuse a mixture of cells to increase the Hct to 30%–35% as CPB is discontinued. In small infants, fresh whole blood is preferred; otherwise, an appropriate mixture of packed red blood cells and recently thawed fresh-frozen plasma may be infused to restore the Hct and administer coagulation factors. Older children, especially those having more minor procedures, may be weaned at a lower Hct, given a diuretic (furosemide), and have the pump contents reinfused over the ensuing period. In this way it may be possible to avoid the need for blood transfusion.

21. If the patient remains hypotensive despite a good rate and rhythm:

    a. Adjust the dopamine infusion (5–10 μg/kg/min). Higher doses of dopamine are often required in infants compared with older children and adults.

    b. Dobutamine 5–10 μg/kg/min may be added. This drug also increases inotropy, but it may also increase heart rate and decrease SVR in pediatric patients.

    c. Calcium infusion may improve performance in some patients, especially small infants. It is required in patients with DiGeorge syndrome.

    d. If all else fails, an infusion of epinephrine 0.1–0.5 μg/kg/min may be indicated.

22. Modified ultrafiltration may be employed after CPB has been discontinued. The bypass circuit is modified to withdraw blood from the aortic cannula, pass it through an ultrafiltration unit, and return it to the right atrium. Ultrafiltration removes fluid and filters substances from the blood. This increases the patient's Hct. In addition, it may remove inflammatory substances released during CPB. It has been suggested that modified ultrafiltration may reduce bleeding and enhance postoperative cardiopulmonary function.

23. When the patient's condition is stable and the cannulas have been removed, give protamine slowly, preferably via a peripheral intravenous route. To determine the dose, repeat the ACT and plot it on the line of the heparin dose-response curve; drop a line to

determine the heparin equivalent and modify this value by the protamine neutralization factor (PNF) for the vial of heparin used. (For example, if the ACT at the end of CPB represents 3 mg of heparin per kilogram, give protamine, 3 mg/kg, adjusted by the appropriate PNF [Fig. 14–1].) If hypotension occurs with protamine, it usually can be reversed by administration of calcium.

24. At 20 minutes after CPB, take blood samples for coagulation studies, electrolytes, and blood gases. Repeat ACT and give more protamine if indicated.

25. If bleeding persists, give platelets (1 unit/5 kg), fresh-frozen plasma (20 ml/kg), and/or cryoprecipitate, according to coagulation indices.

N.B. Anticipate continued bleeding due to platelet and other factor deficiencies:

a. After a long pump run
b. In children with cyanotic CHD
c. In small babies, in whom the pump-priming volume is very large in relation to blood volume

All bleeding must be well controlled before the chest is closed.

26. In some patients after complex intracardiac repairs, a decision may be made to delay sternal closure and to cover the heart with a plastic membrane. When myocardial edema is present, this avoids the constricting effects of sternal closure on cardiopulmonary function and has been shown to increase BP and urine output while decreasing CVP. The sternum is closed when the patient develops a negative fluid balance several days postoperatively.

27. At the end of surgery, the decision must be made whether to extubate the patient immediately or to continue with ventilatory support. The choice depends on the disease that was present and the intraoperative course.

28. The trend toward "fast-tracking" of some pediatric cardiac patients is now well established; it may be combined with minimally invasive surgical approaches. After simple procedures (e.g., closure of atrial septal defect [ASD], resection of subaortic membrane), the patient may be extubated in the OR and may be expected to have a very short stay in the intensive care unit (ICU). In such cases:

a. Employ an anesthesia technique that ensures early brisk recovery; avoid heroic doses of narcotics or ultra-long-acting relaxants.
b. Plan for good postoperative analgesia*; a single-shot caudal morphine injection is safe, effective, and easy.
c. Ensure that excess pump priming fluid is removed by means of modified ultrafiltration after CPB is discontinued.

---

*The place of epidural catheters for patients undergoing CPB is highly controversial. The benefits may have been documented, but the risks remain undetermined.

It may be more appropriate for some patients to be transferred to the ICU for extubation on arrival or soon thereafter, depending on local circumstances.

29. Many pediatric patients require postoperative ventilatory support.
    a. These include patients with
        i. Hypoxemia despite a high FIO_2
        ii. Low cardiac output
        iv. Pulmonary hypertension
        v. Diminished lung compliance
        vi. Persistent arrhythmias
        vii. Hypothermia (lower than 34°C)
        viii. Continuing hemorrhage
    b. In such patients:
        i. Plan for continuing IPPV and/or continuous positive airway pressure (CPAP) or pressure support ventilation. Controlled ventilation and CPAP are particularly beneficial during the immediate postoperative period; at this stage, the patient predictably has a tendency toward reduced lung volume and increased lung water (especially the infant). IPPV also permits excellent pain control by narcotic infusion.
        ii. *Do not reverse the muscle relaxants.*
        iii. The choice of a nasal versus an oral endotracheal tube for postoperative ventilation has varied from unit to unit. Children tolerate nasal tubes extremely well; they are less likely to kink within the patient and cannot be occluded by the teeth. They are also easier to secure in place accurately. It has been suggested that nasal tubes might predispose to middle ear or sinus disease; this has not proved to be a major problem. The continued use of the oral tube removes the need to change the tube and proves quite satisfactory in some units.

N.B. It is preferable to change tubes at the end of the procedure rather than pass a nasotracheal tube initially: this could cause a nosebleed perioperatively, especially when the patient is heparinized. During some types of surgery, blood-stained secretions may accumulate in the tube. The change is then considered advisable to provide the child with a clean tube before transfer to the ICU. Ensure that the nasotracheal tube does not exert pressure on the margins of the nares or the nasal septum; necrosis, ulceration, and scarring can occur. The change to a nasotracheal tube should be made only if the patient's condition is judged to be stable; otherwise, ventilation via the orotracheal tube is advised.

30. During transportation to the ICU (all patients):
    a. Attach a full bag of blood to the IV line to ensure immediate availability in case of sudden hemorrhage.
    b. Cover the patient with warm blankets.
    c. Give O_2 by mask or, if the patient is still intubated, continue

controlled ventilation with O_2. Make sure that an adequate supply of O_2 is available for the journey to the ICU.

d. Use a battery-powered monitor to provide for the following:
   i. Pulse oximeter
   ii. ECG
   iii. All intravascular pressures
e. Continue the infusions of inotropic drugs and/or vasodilators using a battery-powered syringe pump. Beware of interruptions to the flow of these drugs during and after transport to the ICU.

Postoperative Management in the Intensive Care Unit

1. Ensure that the patient's ventilation is adequate when placed on the ventilator, by auscultating the chest. Order a suitable FIO_2 concentration, and confirm ventilation and oxygenation by blood gas determination as soon as the patient is settled.
2. Ensure good analgesia; if regional analgesia has not been provided, order suitable narcotic analgesic and sedative drugs:
   a. Morphine may be given intravenously every 2 hours or, preferably, as a continuous infusion (10–30 µg/kg/hr for children, 5–15 µg/kg/hr for infants).
   b. Midazolam 0.1 mg/kg IV every 2 hours as needed or midazolam infusion 1–2 µg/kg/min.
3. Order maintenance fluids: 5% dextrose with 0.3 N saline initially (with added KCl 2 mEq/kg/24 hr, provided that urine output is 1 ml/kg/hr or more; otherwise, withhold the KCl).
4. Check blood loss via drainage tubes; instruct the nurses to replace this and further losses with "reconstituted whole blood."
5. A chest radiograph should be obtained. Examine it carefully, looking for pneumothorax, hemothorax, and atelectasis, and ensure that the tip of the endotracheal tube is well above the carina. Check placement of all other indwelling lines; ensure that the tip of the CVP line is positioned at the level of the junction of the SVC and right atrium. (Cardiac perforation may complicate lines placed too low in the atrium.)
6. If bleeding persists, order coagulation studies. Based on the results, administer fresh-frozen plasma or platelet concentrates as indicated.

Profound Hypothermia with Circulatory Arrest

Profound hypothermia with circulatory arrest is used for some neonates and infants undergoing cardiac surgery. It is particularly advantageous when surgery involves the aortic root.

Hypothermia is now usually achieved by means of bloodstream cooling on CPB. The debate concerning the safety of profoundly hypothermic circulatory arrest versus continued perfusion is ongoing. It is evident, however, that many infants have been managed by this method and have shown no evidence whatsoever of cerebral impairment as they grow to adulthood.

Anesthesia Management

Anesthesia management is as described previously, with the following modifications:

1. No dextrose-containing solutions should routinely be given, because hyperglycemia may increase the risk of cerebral damage during total circulatory arrest. However, the blood glucose level should be monitored to detect and treat hypoglycemia should it occur. Large doses of fentanyl (more than 50 µg/kg) should be given and may limit the increase in blood glucose concentration that occurs as a metabolic response during hypothermic CPB.

2. Give methylprednisolone (Solu-Medrol) 15–25 mg/kg IV slowly, before cooling on CPB. Ensure that the patient is given adequate doses of relaxant drugs. (Once circulatory arrest has occurred, no further drugs can be given.)

3. Add phenytoin (Dilantin) 5 mg/kg to the CPB prime solution.

4. After CPB is begun, ensure that the difference between the esophageal temperature and the temperature of the pump's output does not exceed 10°C. Set cooling mattresses to 10°C. Turn the temperature of the room down. Place ice bags around the head.

5. The optimal management of blood gas tensions and acid-base balance during profound hypothermia has been the subject of much debate.
   a. The "alpha stat" approach (i.e., pH alkalotic when corrected for the actual body temperature) has been favored in many centers. Blood gas analysis should show a normal or low carbon dioxide tension during cooling. The advantages are that this approach may maintain cerebral autoregulation during cooling and may also result in improved postoperative cardiac function.
   b. The "pH stat" (hypercarbic) approach requires that carbon dioxide be added to the oxygenator gases during cooling. This has the theoretical advantages of increased cerebral blood flow and improved oxygen delivery and has been demonstrated to improve neurologic outcome in infants. It is the recommended strategy in many pediatric centers.

6. Administer phentolamine 0.2 mg/kg to improve tissue perfusion, ensure rapid even cooling, and minimize acidosis on rewarming.

7. When the esophageal temperature is 16°C and the rectal temperature is lower than 20°C, CPB is discontinued, blood is drained to the oxygenator, and the venous cannulas are removed.

8. Record the duration of circulatory arrest. The duration of safe circulatory arrest at a given temperature is unknown, but it is generally preferred to limit it to 60 minutes at 15°–18°C core temperature.

9. Keep the lungs slightly inflated at 5 cmH$_2$O with an air/O$_2$ mixture.

10. When the repair is complete, the venous cannulas are replaced and the patient is rewarmed until the esophageal temperature reaches 37°C. The temperature of the blood from the pump should never

exceed 39°C, and the patient's temperature should not be raised to more than 37°C.

11. Do not correct the metabolic acidosis often seen during rewarming. It will spontaneously correct as the patient's metabolism resumes. Administration of sodium bicarbonate usually results in postoperative metabolic alkalosis.

12. It is suggested that the use of Hct levels of 30% during CPB cooling and rewarming may preserve neurologic functions better than occurs with more hemodilution.

PRINCIPLES OF POSTOPERATIVE CARDIAC CARE

Respiratory System

The status of the respiratory system after cardiac surgery in infants and children may be determined by the following factors:

1. Preexisting status
   a. Immaturity of respiratory system in young patients (especially infants)
   b. Effects of the cardiac disease on the lungs
2. Effects of anesthesia, operation, and CPB on the respiratory system
   a. Decreased lung volume
   b. Increased lung water

Most children benefit from a period of controlled ventilation and/or PEEP or CPAP. This assists in restoring the lung volume to normal and improves gas exchange. Levels of added O_2 and PEEP or CPAP can be reduced as the pulmonary status improves. Diuretic therapy may be indicated to reduce lung water. Special measures to control PVR may be required in patients with pulmonary hypertension.

Cardiovascular System

After cardiac surgery, the cardiovascular status is determined by

1. Preexisting status
   a. Immaturity of the heart and circulatory system in infants
   b. Effects of the cardiac disease on the cardiovascular system
2. Effects of anesthesia, surgery, and CPB, which are dictated by
   a. The duration of anesthesia and surgery
   b. The duration of CPB
   c. The duration of induced cardiac arrest
   d. The success of myocardial protection techniques

After all but the most minor cardiac operations, a deterioration in cardiac function is to be expected. This deterioration progresses for the first few hours after the operation, probably associated with edema of the myocardium and other changes. The result is a decrease in compliance of the ventricles and a decrease in contractility. Treatment at this time must be directed to

1. Ensuring optimal filling pressures. Because the compliance of the ventricles is low in infancy and reduced in all patients after cardiac surgery, high filling pressures (e.g., 8–12 mmHg) will probably be required.
2. Producing an optimal cardiac rate and rhythm. This is most effectively achieved by the use of sequential pacing when necessary. Sinus rhythm (i.e., atrial contraction) significantly augments cardiac output.
3. Reducing the afterload. The use of vasodilators in patients with ventricular dysfunction increases cardiac output with little change in cardiac work or arterial BP. When vasodilators are used, the preload must be maintained by infusion of appropriate fluids; SNP infusion is commonly used to produce vasodilation (infusion rates start at 0.5–2 µg/kg/min and increase up to 5 µg/kg/min). Alternatively, phenoxybenzamine may be administered to produce a long-lasting adrenergic blockade. Some patients do not tolerate LV afterload reduction well—for example, those with impaired RV function (e.g., after tetralogy repair).
4. Inotropic agents: If a low cardiac output persists despite these measures, resort to an inotropic agent becomes necessary:
   a. Dopamine is infused at 5–10 µg/kg/min by infusion pump. In infants and children, dopamine has been shown effective in increasing cardiac output, *but*
      i. Higher doses are required than in adults.
      ii. The vasodilating effect is less than in adults. Hence, the concurrent infusion of a vasodilator (SNP) is usually warranted. The combined administration of dopamine and SNP may also be effective in reducing PVR in patients with pulmonary hypertension, but it must often be given as soon as the patient is weaned from bypass.
   b. Calcium is infused to maintain the serum Ca^{++} at a high-normal level (1–1.2 mmol/dl).
   c. If serious low output persists despite these measures, an epinephrine infusion 0.05–1 µg/kg/min may be needed.

Fluid and Electrolyte Therapy

1. Blood should be administered to maintain the hemoglobin level at near-normal levels (14–15 g/dl), especially when cardiac dysfunction is present.
2. Acid-base status should be monitored and acidosis corrected by sodium bicarbonate infusions.
3. Dextrose-containing electrolyte solutions should be infused at low maintenance rates:
   a. 5% dextrose plus 0.3 N saline for older children.

   b. 10% dextrose plus 0.3 N saline for infants, to provide dextrose 4–6 mg/kg/min.
4. KCl 2 mEq/kg/day should be added, *provided* that the urine output is greater than 1 ml/kg/hr.
5. Hypomagnesemia may occur perioperatively, especially with aggressive diuretic therapy. Magnesium sulfate 1 mEq/kg/day may be added to the intravenous fluid regimen if necessary.
6. If urine output falls (to less than 1 ml/kg/hr) in the absence of hypotension, fluid orders should be reviewed to ensure an adequate intake, and a "fluid challenge" may be administered. If there is no result, a diuretic may be ordered (furosemide, 1–2 mg/kg IV).

SPECIAL CONSIDERATIONS FOR ANESTHESIA IN NEONATES

Cardiac surgery in neonates should be performed only where the most expert, comprehensive medical and nursing care and all requisite facilities are available.

The general principles of anesthesia in neonates are as follows:

1. Assess the patient's condition carefully and ensure that the status is the best that can be achieved before surgery.
2. Ventilation may be indicated preoperatively, especially if heart failure or metabolic acidosis is severe. (Respiratory care is as important preoperatively as postoperatively.)
3. Metabolic acidosis must be corrected as far as possible by infusion of sodium bicarbonate together with efforts to improve the effective cardiac output.
4. CHF must be controlled as far as possible. The following therapy should be instituted:
   a. Optimal digitalization (check serum level)
   b. Diuretic therapy: furosemide infusion
   c. Place in a neutral thermal environment.
   d. Maintain slight head-up position.
   e. O_2 therapy to maintain PaO_2 at 70–90 mmHg
   f. Correction of any acidosis
   g. In addition, if these measures fail:
      i. Intubation and controlled ventilation
      ii. Use of other inotropic agents (e.g., dopamine)
5. If the infant is severely hypoxic or in shock, correct the acid-base status, oxygenate, and administer methylprednisolone sodium succinate (25 mg/kg) with induction of anesthesia.
6. Control of body temperature is very important; avoid unintentional hypothermia.
7. If bradycardia occurs, assume it is caused by hypoxia until proved otherwise. Respond immediately:
   a. Discontinue anesthetics.
   b. Request removal of packs and retractors from the chest.
   c. Expand the lungs with 100% O_2.

8. If cardiac function deteriorates, suspect metabolic acidosis. Determine acid-base status and correct as necessary.
9. Ensure optimal postoperative care; all neonates require meticulous attention to respiratory care and constant, highest-quality nursing care, including
   a. Maintenance of body temperature at about 37°C
   b. Avoidance of cold stress
10. Neonates should be nursed with a slight head-up tilt and moved frequently from side to side. Dressings and chest drains should be so located as to cause minimal restriction.
11. Controlled ventilation may be required for long periods. The infant with a soft chest wall is particularly vulnerable to declines in lung volume and ventilatory muscle fatigue. PEEP or CPAP usually improves arterial oxygenation.
12. Atelectasis, particularly of the upper lobes, is a common complication. It is treated by aspiration of lung secretions and application of chest physiotherapy.
13. If the period of intensive care is prolonged, special attention must be paid to ensuring adequate nutrition.
14. Unexpected difficulty in weaning from ventilator support must raise the possibility of phrenic nerve damage during surgery.
15. The appearance of a pleural effusion in the early postoperative period suggests the possibility of thoracic duct injury.

SPECIAL CONSIDERATIONS FOR SPECIFIC OPERATIONS

Ligation of Patent Ductus Arteriosus

Older Infants and Children

1. PDA as the sole lesion in older infants and children usually presents few problems. The child is asymptomatic but ligation is necessary to prevent potential later complications (i.e., pulmonary hypertension and cardiac failure, subacute bacterial endocarditis, or aneurysm).
2. Routine anesthetic management as for thoracotomy is appropriate. Prophylactic antibiotics should be administered. An arterial line is not considered essential. The BP must be monitored in the right arm; in the unlikely event of bleeding from the ductus, it may be necessary to clamp the left subclavian artery. Monitor saturation from the right hand and from a foot.
3. A single-shot dose of caudal morphine after induction provides for good postoperative analgesia when combined with intercostal nerve blocks by the surgeon.
4. During the procedure, monitor carefully
   a. For bradycardia during dissection near the vagus nerve.
   b. For vital signs after ligation; normally the continuous murmur ceases and a soft systolic murmur remains. The BP (especially diastolic) may rise slightly at this time, but large changes are unusual.

Major changes in BP might suggest that the wrong vessel has been ligated! If the aorta has accidentally been ligated, hypertension and loss of the oximeter signal from the foot will occur. If a PA has accidentally been ligated, the continuous murmur of the ductus will remain. If a bronchus has been ligated, airway pressures will increase and the murmur will persist unchanged.

5. Blood loss is usually minimal, seldom necessitating transfusion, but it may be sudden and massive if a major vessel is torn. Therefore, establish a reliable large-bore intravenous infusion line (18-gauge cannula if possible) and check that blood is immediately available in the OR during the operation.

Postoperative Care

1. Routine post-thoracotomy care should be applied. Good analgesia facilitates deep breathing exercises.
2. Rarely, the thoracic duct may be injured during PDA ligation. The resulting chylothorax may require drainage, and continued losses of chyle may impose a severe nutritional challenge.
3. Damage to the left recurrent laryngeal nerve in the region of the ductus is also a rare complication.

N.B. PDA closure is now sometimes performed via a thoracoscope. In such cases, the patient should be managed as for open operation; this may become necessary should bleeding occur. Intraoperative TEE may be used to monitor the closure. PDA closure may also be performed in the cardiac catheter laboratory by placing a transcatheter occlusive device. General anesthesia is usually required for such procedures to ensure absolute patient immobility.

Premature Infants

Persistence of the ductus arteriosus may occur in preterm infants, especially those weighing less than 1,500 g. In addition to prematurity, respiratory distress syndrome, excessive fluid therapy, neonatal asphyxia, hypoxia, and acidosis predispose to this condition. PDA results in a large left-to-right shunt, with pulmonary vascular engorgement and CHF. Clinical signs include tachypnea, hepatomegaly, and "bounding pulses."

Diagnosis is confirmed by auscultation of the typical murmur, radiographic evidence of increased vascularity, and echocardiogram findings of a large left atrium:aorta ratio. PDA may prevent weaning from ventilatory support of infants with respiratory distress syndrome.

Treatment for Patent Ductus Arteriosus

1. *Medical treatment.* Administration of indomethacin, a prostaglandin inhibitor, 0.1–0.4 mg/kg IV daily for several days may induce closure of the PDA. Indomethacin may also cause renal damage and suppress bone marrow. Therefore, it is contraindicated in patients with renal failure or coagulopathy. Very small infants (those weighing less than 1,000 g) do not respond as well with closure of the PDA as do larger, less immature infants.

2. *Surgical treatment (ligation).* This is necessary if indomethacin therapy fails or is contraindicated.

Special Anesthesia Problems

1. Observe all special precautions for the preterm infant.
2. Be prepared for sudden blood loss; the ductus is very thin and tears easily!
3. In some circumstances it may be preferable to operate on very small preterm infants in the neonatal ICU. This avoids all the problems of transportation but requires that the anesthesiologist adapt routines to safely administer adequate anesthesia and analgesia in the ICU setting.

Preoperative

1. Assess the patient carefully. Anemia, if present, may predispose to CHF. In such circumstances, transfusion of erythrocytes may result in considerable improvement. The increased Hct improves myocardial oxygenation and may also reduce the extent of left-to-right shunting.
2. For those patients to be transferred to the OR, ensure that all arrangements are made to transfer the patient in a heated transport incubator with a ventilator.
3. No premedication is required.

Perioperative

1. Ensure that the OR is heated and all warming devices are in position before transferring the patient to the OR table.
2. Attach monitors. Monitor saturation in a preductal site (right hand) and in the foot; measure the BP in the right arm (*see above*).
3. Intubation
   a. If the patient is intubated, ensure that the tube is firmly fixed, absolutely patent, and optimally positioned; otherwise, reintubate.
   b. If the patient is not intubated, give atropine 0.02 mg/kg, fentanyl 10 μg/kg, vecuronium 0.1 mg/kg, or rocuronium 1 mg/kg. Ventilate with O_2 for 3 minutes and intubate.
4. Induce and maintain anesthesia with N_2O (in a concentration appropriate to ensure saturation) and isoflurane 0.5%–1.0% or fentanyl 10–12 μg/kg.
5. Vecuronium (0.1 mg/kg) may be used to facilitate ventilation and prevent movement.
6. Establish a reliable intravenous line. Blood loss is usually minimal but can be catastrophic if a vessel is torn.
7. Give minimal maintenance fluids. These patients are often overhydrated preoperatively and do not have third-space losses.
8. Manual ventilation is often useful as the ductus is approached. Many of these infants have congested lungs and poor compliance. Watch for surgical retraction compromising the heart; if the infant becomes hypotensive, ask the surgeons to remove all retractors.

9. Careful intercostal nerve blocks by the surgeons are to be encouraged.

Postoperative

1. Continued ventilation is necessary for most patients, with increased attention to respiratory care in view of possible post-thoracotomy complications (e.g., atelectasis).
2. Improvement in respiratory status after ligation of PDA is dictated by the relative contributions of pulmonary vascular congestion and pulmonary disease (respiratory distress syndrome or bronchopulmonary dysplasia) to the preoperative status.

Aortopulmonary Window

This anomaly presents a clinical picture much like that of PDA but represents a failure of the aorta and PA to completely septate during development. The shunt is usually larger than with PDA, and consequently most patients develop pulmonary vascular changes and CHF earlier. Repair on CPB is usually required, and pulmonary hypertension may be a problem postoperatively.

Division of Vascular Rings and Suspension of Anomalous Innominate Artery

Abnormalities of the great vessels may encircle or compress the trachea, bronchi, and esophagus. There may be a double aortic arch, a vascular ring that is completed by a PDA or ligamentum arteriosum, or an abnormal course of the subclavian artery. Severe compression by vascular rings leads to stridor and difficulty with feeding during early infancy.

The infant with a vascular ring often assumes a characteristic opisthotonic position. A chest radiograph with barium swallow is often diagnostic. Anomalous vessels may compress the bronchi and lead to gas trapping in an individual lobe of the lung, with compression of the adjacent lung by the resultant emphysematous lobe. Infants with vascular compression are prone to sudden cardiorespiratory arrest.

Patients with repaired tracheoesophageal fistula are particularly prone to develop tracheal compression between the aorta and esophagus during feeding. The onset of symptoms of dyspnea and "dying spells" during feeding is usually seen between 2 and 4 months of age. This condition is caused when an abnormally soft trachea becomes compressed against the aorta by a dilated esophagus. Aortopexy usually relieves symptoms, but in some patients insertion of an external stent to reinforce the trachea may be necessary.

Special Anesthesia Problems

1. Respiratory failure may exist.
   a. Chronic or recurrent respiratory infection may have impaired pulmonary function.

   b. Vascular compression may have resulted in emphysema of one or more lobes, compressing other lung tissue.

2. Airway compression may be at the level of the carina or main bronchi; if so, a normally situated endotracheal tube will not relieve the obstruction.
3. Endotracheal intubation may be required preoperatively to relieve serious symptoms. Air trapping in a lobe as a result of vascular compression can often be alleviated by the application of PEEP.
4. The use of an esophageal stethoscope in infants with vascular rings has been reported to cause acute airway obstruction.

Anesthesia Management

Preoperative

1. Order intensive respiratory care to achieve optimal pulmonary status. The infant should be allowed to remain in a position that permits optimal ventilation.
2. Bronchoscopy may be required to evaluate the site of airway compression and is useful for endobronchial suction.

Perioperative

1. For intubation, use a method that ensures a good airway past the obstructing lesion. If the obstruction is low, do one of the following:
   a. Pass a long endotracheal tube into a main bronchus and add side holes for ventilation of the other bronchus.
   b. Ventilate the patient via a rigid bronchoscope (which can be placed accurately under direct vision and adjusted perioperatively if necessary).
2. Monitor the BP via an arterial line placed in the right radial artery. Operations on the great vessels can cause serious bleeding; establish a reliable, large-bore intravenous infusion route.
3. For aortopexy, a bronchoscope should be used to ensure that the compression is relieved. Compression of the trachea should always be assessed during spontaneous ventilation and coughing. If controlled ventilation is used, the trachea is held open and always appears widely patent.
4. If it is necessary to assess the airway during operation, use general anesthesia and spray the larynx with lidocaine before inserting the bronchoscope. During the remainder of the operation, ventilation can be assisted or controlled. Do not give relaxants.

Postoperative

1. Order constant care with added humidified oxygen for at least the first 24 hours.
2. If residual obstruction persists, continue nasotracheal intubation for 24 hours, then reassess.
3. Partial obstruction may be improved by placing a small bolster, 1 to 2 inches thick, below the shoulders.

4. Racemic epinephrine and/or dexamethasone may be required for postinstrumentation croup.

Resection of Aortic Coarctation

Aortic coarctation is classified according to its site in relation to the ductus arteriosus (i.e., preductal, juxtaductal, or postductal). The preductal (infantile) type is usually accompanied by other anomalies (e.g., VSD, PDA) and manifests as cardiac failure in an infant under 6 months of age. The juxtaductal or postductal (adult) type may be asymptomatic; it is usually diagnosed during investigation of hypertension in the upper limbs in preschoolers.

Preductal (Infantile Type)

Special Problems

1. Most of these infants have severe cardiac failure and are already being treated with digoxin and diuretics. Assisted ventilation is essential for some, and it benefits many others.
2. Severe associated cardiovascular anomalies are common.
3. Blood flow to the lower portion of the body is dependent on the ductus arteriosus. Therefore, it must be maintained patent by infusion of prostaglandin until surgical repair is performed.
4. Hypoplasia of the arch of the aorta may be present and, if significant, may require repair with CPB (*see below*).

Anesthesia Management

Preoperative

1. Blood gases should be determined and abnormalities corrected. Maintain prostaglandin infusion.
2. Ensure that supportive drugs are at hand (e.g., epinephrine, dopamine); they may be needed during surgery.

Perioperative

1. Carefully maintain normothermia.
2. While the aorta is clamped, do not allow the systolic pressure to exceed 100 mmHg. In the (rare) event that a drug is necessary to lower the BP, administer low concentrations of isoflurane and titrate this against the BP. A small dose of heparin (1 mg/kg) usually is given before clamping.
3. Be prepared to support the circulation when the clamps are removed; infusion of fluid and/or cardiotonic drugs may be required.
4. Prostaglandin may be discontinued once the ductus is ligated and the aorta repaired.

Postoperative

The course is sometimes stormy. Therefore:

1. Transfer the patient to the ICU with a nasotracheal tube in place.
2. Controlled ventilation is usually necessary for at least 48–72 hours.

Postductal (Adult Type)

Special Considerations

1. Clamping the aorta could compromise the blood supply to the spinal cord; hence the need to maintain an optimal BP in the distal aorta ($\pm$45 mmHg).
2. While the aorta is clamped, severe proximal hypertension may occur and require treatment.
3. Hypertension can be troublesome postoperatively; this may be controlled by the use of β-blockers over the perioperative period, but it may also require the use of SNP.
4. Although blood must (of course) be available for transfusion, surprisingly few children require it. (Bleeding from chest wall collateral vessels is much less profuse than in adults.)
5. In the very rare event that severe proximal hypertension cannot be controlled after aortic clamping or if the distal pressure is very low, a temporary shunt must be placed to bypass the site of anastomosis, or left heart bypass must be used.

Anesthesia Management

Preoperative

1. Monitor BP and saturation in the right arm. Place a second oximeter probe on a foot.
2. Establish reliable intravenous infusions at sites other than in the left arm. Place a right radial artery line and a central venous line; the latter may be used to infuse drugs as necessary to control hypertension.
3. Consider the use of an epidural catheter for administration of morphine and/or bupivacaine for postoperative pain management.

Perioperative

1. Maintain anesthesia with N_2O and isoflurane; use vecuronium or rocuronium for relaxation.
2. Place an arterial line into the right radial artery.
3. During the period of aortic clamping, control the BP if necessary, by increasing the inspired concentration of isoflurane. The BP should not be allowed to exceed 140 mmHg, but do not attempt to reduce the pressure if it remains below that level. Distal aortic pressure during clamp-off varies directly with the proximal pressure; distal

pressure should be maintained at or above a mean of 45 mmHg, to ensure perfusion of the spinal cord.

4. The surgeon first removes the distal clamp and then (slowly) the proximal clamp. Watch the BP continuously. If hypotension develops, infuse fluids; if this is unsuccessful, ask the surgeon to partly reapply the proximal clamp briefly. The BP may remain slightly lower for a while, but usually it is back to above-normal levels by the end of the operation. Anticipate the need to treat postoperative hypertension: prepare
   a. SNP, which should be used to immediately control hypertension if necessary
   b. Esmolol—a loading dose 500 μg/kg over 1 minute followed by an infusion of 100–250 μg/kg/min greatly facilitates the management of hypertension.

5. Blood loss is usually minimal and transfusion unnecessary.

6. In most cases, controlled ventilation is not required postoperatively and the patient can be extubated at the end of the operation.

Postoperative

1. The patient should be monitored continuously in the ICU, special attention being paid to signs of blood loss. Measure the chest drainage and observe the clinical indices.

2. Hypertension usually persists for several days postoperatively; if severe, it may necessitate therapy with SNP and/or esmolol. Prevention of hypertension is essential to prevent arteritis (*see below*). The cause of this postoperative hypertension has been linked to multiple factors: carotid baroreceptor function, plasma norepinephrine levels, and the renin-angiotensin system.

3. Very rarely, the postoperative course is complicated by intestinal ileus caused by mesenteric arteritis. In extreme cases, bowel resection may be required.

4. Other serious postoperative complications include recurrent laryngeal nerve palsy, phrenic nerve palsy, chylothorax, and paraplegia due to spinal cord ischemia during repair (very rare).

5. Recoarctation may occur in later years, particularly after repair in infancy. Repeat operation may be technically much more difficult and may involve major blood losses.

N.B. Coarctation and/or recoarctation of the aorta is sometimes managed by balloon dilatation (*see* Interventional Cardiology). The merits of this approach compared with open operation are at present controversial.

Interrupted Aortic Arch

This lesion, which is frequently associated with VSD and often also with DiGeorge syndrome, requires repair using CPB with profoundly hypothermic circulatory arrest. The patency of the ductus arteriosus must be maintained with a prostaglandin infusion until the operation.

Palliative Surgery to Increase Pulmonary Blood Flow

The operations that may be used include the following:

1. Blalock-Taussig procedure (systemic artery anastomosed to PA). A modified Blalock procedure using a synthetic graft between the aorta or innominate artery and the central portion of the PA is now the most commonly performed procedure.
2. The Potts operation (PA anastomosed to descending aorta) and the Waterston procedure (PA anastomosed to ascending aorta) are now rarely performed because they tend to become too large and may also cause unilateral pulmonary edema.

The operation is performed for infants and children with tetralogy of Fallot, tricuspid atresia, and other conditions in whom right-sided cardiac lesions have decreased the pulmonary blood flow. They are usually performed during infancy to increase pulmonary blood flow and stimulate growth of the PAs; they may then be followed by total correction of the defect at an older age.

Special Anesthesia Problems

1. Many of these patients are severely hypoxemic and polycythemic.
2. During surgery, one PA is partly occluded so that the anastomosis can be completed; this causes a further temporary decrease in pulmonary blood flow.
3. Patients with polycythemia may have a coagulation defect, although this is rarely a problem.
4. In small infants, the narrow lumen of the new shunt is prone to thrombose. This may be avoided by using a small dose of heparin and appropriate fluid therapy.

Anesthesia Management

Preoperative

1. Ensure that the respiratory system is in an optimal state for that patient, with no active infection or recent history of upper respiratory tract infection.
2. If the patient is taking digoxin, order the morning dose for the day of operation to be given at 6:00 AM.
3. Order adequate sedation for older infants to prevent them from crying and becoming further desaturated.
4. If the patient is taking β-blocking agents, they should be continued up to the evening before surgery.
5. Allow liberal fluids up to 3 hours before operation. Otherwise, order intravenous maintenance fluids during any prolonged preoperative fasting period for patients with an Hb greater than 16 g/dl.

Perioperative

1. Follow routine management, as on page 342.
2. Induce anesthesia intravenously (most of these patients have a right-

to-left shunt); a small dose of thiopental followed by fentanyl and vecuronium is preferred.

3. An arterial line should be placed either in the radial artery—*in the rare event that the subclavian artery will be used, place the line in the opposite side!*—or in the femoral artery.

4. Maintain anesthesia with 0.5%–0.75% halothane in at least 50% O_2.
   a. Halothane is useful for patients with tetralogy, because it tends to decrease the RV contractility and hence obstruction to outflow.
   b. If desaturation occurs intraoperatively, it may be treated with esmolol (500 μg/kg IV slowly) and/or small doses of phenylephrine (100 μg/kg IV).
   c. If excessive hypotension occurs with halothane (rare), it will be necessary to substitute fentanyl.

5. Immediately before the PA is clamped, switch to 100% O_2, inflate the lungs well, and give a further dose of relaxant.

6. Once the clamps are in place and if the patient's oxygenation appears stable, allow the surgeon to proceed with the anastomosis. (Once this is commenced, the PA will be open and the clamps cannot come off until the anastomosis is completed.)

7. While the anastomosis is being performed: if there is a serious decline in BP or bradycardia occurs, infuse cardiotonic drugs (e.g., epinephrine 1–5 μg/kg, calcium chloride 10 mg/kg) until the anastomosis is completed and the clamps are removed.

8. A "modified" Blalock anastomosis is usually performed using a synthetic graft. In small infants, it is usual to give a small dose of heparin (100 units/kg) to prevent thrombosis of the shunt. A bolus of fluid after the clamps are released may enhance flow through the shunt.

9. Throughout the surgery, give albumin as necessary to replace blood loss and decrease the Hct.

Postoperative

1. Check that a new murmur is audible (this indicates that the shunt is functioning).

2. Extubation in the OR is preferred. IPPV is seldom necessary, and spontaneous ventilation with low intrathoracic pressure may improve flow through the new shunt.

3. Review the digitalis dosage; the child may require a larger dose than previously (RV work is now increased, myocardial perfusion may be compromised by the lower diastolic pressure, and RV failure could ensue).

4. If the anastomosis is small and considered likely to be blocked by thrombosis, order heparin in suitable dosage for several days postoperatively.

Palliative Surgery to Decrease Pulmonary Blood Flow

PA banding is performed to diminish blood flow to the lungs in infants who have a large left-to-right shunt, thereby improving systemic perfusion, decreasing pulmonary vascular congestion, and averting the development of fixed pulmonary hypertension. This is usually performed as an emergency procedure in the newborn.

Special Anesthesia Problems

Many of these patients are in severe CHF.

Anesthesia Management

Preoperative

1. Follow routine management, as on page 340.
2. Check that the CHF is under optimal control.
3. Employ all necessary measures to improve the infant's general status (e.g., IPPV for several hours can be very beneficial).

Perioperative

1. Do not administer myocardial depressants (e.g., halothane).
2. Give a muscle relaxant, such as vecuronium or rocuronium plus fentanyl.
3. Monitor the patient closely as the band is applied. With an optimal band tightness:
   a. The systemic BP should rise, and the saturation may fall very slightly.
   b. The distal PA pressure should fall to approximately 30%–50% of systemic pressure.
   c. The end-tidal carbon dioxide value may fall very slightly. (A large decline indicates that the band is too tight.)

Postoperative

1. Controlled ventilation may be required for several days.

SPECIFIC OPEN HEART PROCEDURES

The considerations discussed here are a supplement to all the other important general principles outlined previously.

Atrial Septal Defect (Secundum Type)

ASD may be associated with partial anomalous pulmonary venous drainage, in which case a baffle is required to redirect this flow to the left atrium. This may complicate and prolong the simple ASD closure procedure slightly.

1. Plan to extubate the patient at the end of surgery. A single dose of caudal morphine (75–100 µg/kg of Duramorph) given after induction before surgery provides for early postoperative analgesia and lasts up to 24 hours.
2. Closure of the ASD is performed either with cardioplegia or with

induced ventricular fibrillation, so as to avoid the possibility that air may enter the LV and be pumped into the circulation. Ensure that the patient is very well paralyzed during CPB to avoid the possibility that the patient might take a breath while the atrium is open, which could draw air into the left side of the heart; give a suitable additional dose of relaxant as the patient is being cannulated.

3. As the last suture is being tightened to close the defect, the surgeon may request sustained inflation of the lungs to promote flow of blood via the pulmonary veins into the left atrium to remove any residual air from the left side of the heart.
4. Bypass is short and post-CPB inotropic therapy is unlikely to be needed.

Total Anomalous Pulmonary Venous Drainage

The pulmonary veins drain into the right atrium or its venous connections. There are three common types:

1. *Supracardiac (50% of cases):* Pulmonary veins drain into the left SVC.
2. *Cardiac (30% of cases):* Pulmonary veins drain into the coronary sinus or right atrium.
3. *Infracardiac (10% of cases):* Pulmonary veins drain into the inferior vena cava via a common trunk below the diaphragm.

Total anomalous pulmonary venous drainage manifests in early neonatal life with severe cyanosis and acidosis. Obstruction of the pulmonary veins may be present and may cause pulmonary edema and cardiac failure. Survival depends on a right-to-left, usually via an ASD or patent foramen ovale, which may need enlarging by balloon dilatation. The presence of obstruction to the pulmonary veins exacerbates the symptoms.

Special Considerations

1. If the pulmonary veins are obstructed, pulmonary edema, pulmonary hypertension, and cardiac failure may be present.
2. Preoperative ventilation may be required to treat pulmonary edema and improve oxygenation.
3. The left atrium and LV may be small and the LV compliance reduced; aggressive inotropic therapy may be required after bypass.
4. The pulmonary vasculature may have a thick medial layer, and PVR may remain high after repair.

Anesthesia Plan

1. Maintain controlled ventilation and PEEP; monitor acid-base status frequently.
2. High-dose narcotic anesthesia technique is preferred.
3. After repair, the LV may require generous inotropic support and afterload reduction to maintain cardiac output. High left atrial pressures should be avoided to prevent fluid overload.

4. Active measures to reduce PVR and prevent pulmonary hypertensive crisis must be instituted. The PA pressure should be monitored. Prepare to administer NO if it becomes necessary.

Cor Triatriatum

This lesion consists of a membrane within the left atrium that obstructs pulmonary venous return and requires surgical excision on CPB.

Ventricular Septal Defect

VSD is the most common single defect (20% of CHD cases). The position of the VSD is used to classify the disease and also may predict complications:

1. *Type I (supracristal, 5%):* under the annulus of the aorta; may affect the adjacent cusp and cause aortic incompetence; also associated with narrow aortic isthmus
2. *Type II (infracristal, most common, 80%):* in the membranous septum—often large with a big shunt
3. *Type III (AV canal type, 11%):* beneath the tricuspid valve
4. *Type IV (muscular 4%):* may be multiple ("Swiss cheese" defect)

The physiologic effects of the VSD depend on its size. If it is large (nonrestrictive), the left-to-right shunt is similarly large, resulting in early CHF and subsequent pulmonary vascular obstructive disease (PVOD). Small defects (restrictive) allow only a small shunt, which may be physiologically insignificant. Early operation is performed for large defects to prevent the onset of PVOD.

Special Considerations

1. Infants with severe CHF may benefit from intubation and ventilation preoperatively.
2. Infants with CHF cannot tolerate myocardial depressant drugs (e.g., halothane).
3. Postoperative conduction disturbances, which may be temporary (possibly due to edema around a stitch), should be anticipated.
4. Pulmonary vascular crisis may occur in small infants postoperatively.

Anesthesia Plan

1. Avoid myocardial depressants; high-dose narcotics are preferred. Titrate drugs slowly.
2. Bidirectional shunts are common; be careful to avoid air bubbles in intravenous lines.
3. Maintain PVR to avoid increasing left-to-right shunting; avoid hyperventilation. Minor reductions in SVR (perhaps minimal isoflurane) may be beneficial.
4. Be prepared to institute pacing if conduction is abnormal after repair.

5. In the case of large defects, postbypass therapy to reduce PVR and to prevent pulmonary vascular crisis may be required.

Atrioventricular Canal

AV canal is frequently associated with Down syndrome and may be complete (ASD, VSD, and cleft AV valve) or partial (ostium primum ASD plus cleft mitral valve). The most significant hemodynamic changes are a large left-to-right shunt, leading to pulmonary hypertension, and mitral incompetence. Early surgical repair in infancy is preferred.

Special Considerations

1. Down syndrome often present (*see* page 171).
2. Pulmonary hypertension may be a problem postoperatively; prepare to measure PA and institute therapy. Aggressive inotropic therapy may be required.
3. Disturbances of conduction are relatively common after repair and may persist; chronic pacemaker therapy may be required.
4. Mitral valve malfunction may occur in the early or late postoperative period, and reoperation to repair the valve may be required.

Tetralogy of Fallot

The clinical picture results from the large VSD in the presence of RV outflow obstruction, which together produce a large right-to-left shunt; the other features of tetralogy are overriding of the aorta and RV hypertrophy. RV obstruction may be infundibular (50%), valvular (10%), PA (10%), or combined (30%). Acute dynamic increases in infundibular obstruction may result in severe desaturation episodes ("tet" spells). Most patients are now treated by complete repair in infancy, except those with small PAs, who are treated initially with a systemic-to-pulmonary shunt.

Special Considerations

1. Adequate preoperative sedation and sufficient anesthesia and analgesia to suppress any response to surgical stimulation are important to prevent tet spells. Avoid drugs that reduce SVR significantly (e.g., isoflurane); high-dose narcotic technique is preferred. Titrate the drug carefully.
2. Halothane in low concentrations may be useful to depress the muscle of the RV infundibulum and prevent tet spells.
3. Otherwise, intraoperative tet spells should be treated with oxygen, fluid infusion, and esmolol 0.5 mg/kg slowly and/or phenylephrine 10 μg/kg.
4. After CPB, a high filling pressure may be required owing to the thickened, poorly compliant right ventricle. Rarely, conduction defects require AV pacing.

5. The use of LV afterload reduction may be poorly tolerated, because the RV output is the limiting factor on overall cardiac output.

Transposition of the Great Arteries

The most common cause of cyanotic CHD in the neonate is transposition of the great arteries, whereby the aorta arises from the RV and the PA arises from the LV. The pulmonary and systemic circulations are thus separate and in parallel; survival depends on mixing via the patent foramen ovale (PFO), ASD, VSD, or PDA. Without treatment, 90% of infants with transposition of the great arteries die within 12 months. Current surgical treatment is to perform an arterial switch procedure; this must be performed in the neonatal period for infants with an intact septum but may be performed later in those with a large VSD.

Special Considerations

1. The neonate with an intact septum, dependent on mixing via the PFO and PDA, will become desperately hypoxic when the latter closes. Balloon atrial septostomy has been used to improve mixing, or, if the neonate is having early surgery, PGE_1 may be used to maintain the PDA.
2. The effective pulmonary or systemic blood flow is limited to that volume of blood that shunts between the circulations.

Anesthesia Plan

1. A technique that maintains myocardial function and cardiac output should be used; a high-dose narcotic technique is preferred.
2. Hyperventilation with a high FIO_2 may reduce PVR and thereby increase pulmonary blood flow, mixing, and arterial saturation.
3. PGE_1 infusion must be continued and may be useful after CPB for neonates at risk for pulmonary vascular crises.
4. Post-CPB measures to optimize blood flow in the reimplanted coronary arteries are required. An infusion of nitroglycerine (1 μg/kg/min) should be commenced before weaning from CPB. Maintain an optimal preload; the arterial BP should not be allowed to decline!
5. Bleeding from multiple suture lines is to be expected. Order blood components to correct the coagulopathy that is common after CPB in newborns. Platelet suspensions, fresh-frozen plasma, and cryoprecipitate are required.

Aortic Stenosis

Critical aortic stenosis can cause severe CHF in the neonate. Older children with aortic stenosis may be asymptomatic, but they are at increasing risk for angina, syncope, and sudden death. Aortic stenosis may be subvalvular, valvular—usually with a bicuspid valve (80% of cases), or supravalvular (often associated with Williams' syndrome [*see* page 495]).

Special Considerations

1. Infants with critical aortic stenosis are hypotensive, poorly perfused, and acidotic, with respiratory distress and hepatomegaly. The disease often becomes apparent as the ductus arteriosus closes. The thickened LV is prone to ischemia and arrhythmias. Subendocardial fibroelastosis may also be present. These infants require aggressive resuscitation and early operation; even so, the mortality rate is high.
2. Older children with valvular aortic stenosis commonly have a bicuspid valve, and cardiac function is usually quite good despite a high gradient across the stenosed valve.

Anesthesia Plan—Infants

1. The infant will be receiving an infusion of prostaglandin to maintain the ductus arteriosus; this must be carefully continued.
2. A high-dose narcotic technique with vecuronium is preferred.
3. Maintain body temperature carefully.
4. Serious arrhythmias—including ventricular fibrillation—may occur as the heart is manipulated, especially if any cooling has occurred. A very small dose of propranolol (10 μg/kg) may reduce this danger.

Anesthesia Plan—Older Children

1. The aim is to maintain the heart rate constant, avoid tachycardia or bradycardia, and prevent any major decline in SVR and aortic root pressure. Narcotic plus vecuronium with low concentrations of halothane is usually satisfactory.
2. Halothane may be useful to reduce dynamic LV outflow tract obstruction in those with subvalvular aortic stenosis.
3. Beware that patients with supravalvular aortic stenosis and Williams' syndrome may be difficult to intubate.
4. Hypertension is not uncommon postoperatively after aortic valvotomy, and SNP infusion may be required.

Hypoplastic Left Heart Syndrome

In hypoplastic left heart syndrome, the LV and ascending aorta are hypoplastic and the LV is nonfunctional. Immediate survival depends on the pumping action of the RV and systemic flow via the PDA with retrograde flow in the aortic arch. Blood mixes in the right atrium (via an ASD or PFO), and pulmonary-to-systemic flow ratio depends on the size of the intra-atrial communication, the PVR, and the SVR. Treatment of this condition is either by heart transplantation or by conversion to a univentricular series-type circulation by means of a staged repair:

1. *Stage 1:* Norwood procedure. Division of the PA, connection of the RV to a reconstructed aortic arch, atrial septectomy, and a modified Blalock-Taussig shunt.
2. *Stage 2:* Bidirectional Glenn (SVC-PA) anastomosis or hemi-Fontan

procedure. This procedure is designed to direct some of the blood flow directly to the lungs and so reduce the load on the RV.

3. *Stage 3:* Completion of the Fontan procedure, which places the systemic and pulmonary circulations in series.

Special Considerations

1. Preoperative management is aimed at maintaining the ratio of pulmonary to systemic blood flow (Qp:Qs) close to 1. The ease with which this can be achieved depends first on the patient's anatomy; patients fall into groups depending on the size of the interatrial communication:
   a. If it is large and unrestrictive, pulmonary blood flow is excessive and systemic hypoperfusion with metabolic acidosis occurs.
   b. Those patients with relative restriction (a high percentage) may achieve Qp:Qs near 1 when breathing room air.
   c. Patients with a very small or absent ASD have pulmonary hypoperfusion and are profoundly hypoxic at birth.

Infants in the first group must be treated by intubation and IPPV to raise the PCO_2 to a higher level and thereby increase PVR. The FIO_2 must also be strictly limited, possibly to below 21%. It may not be possible to achieve the desired PCO_2 and maintain oxygen saturation if ventilation is simply reduced; it may be necessary to add CO_2 to the inspired gases. Infants in the second group must be managed to maintain the status quo (i.e., to avoid changes in ventilation or oxygenation). The last group of patients require immediate surgery to survive.

2. All patients require a continuous infusion of PGE_1 to maintain patency of the ductus arteriosus.
3. Some patients may require inotropic agents to increase cardiac output and systemic perfusion; these must be used with caution to avoid adverse changes in SVR.

Anesthesia Plan—Norwood Stage 1

1. Take great care to maintain FIO_2 and ventilation unchanged during transport to and from the OR. It is preferred to use a transport ventilator. It is very easy to overventilate the patient accidentally and cause a disastrous fall in PVR!
2. Care during the prebypass stage is similar for those undergoing either the Norwood procedure or transplantation. Carefully maintain the level of ventilation and oxygenation to balance the PVR:SVR ratio. The arterial saturation should be ±80%. In some cases it may be necessary to add N_2 to the inspired gases to achieve an FIO_2 of less than 21%. CO_2 may be cautiously added if necessary to rapidly increase PVR.
3. High-dose narcotic anesthesia is preferred, but fentanyl must be titrated slowly, balancing surgical stimulation, to avoid hypotension. Pancuronium is the relaxant of choice.
4. Post-CPB after a Norwood procedure and measures to maintain the

PVR and limit pulmonary blood flow may still be required, depending on the size of the shunt. Expect the saturation to be 70%–80%. Inotropic therapy with standard doses of dopamine and dobutamine is usually adequate.

5. Rarely, if pulmonary blood flow is inadequate and the infant is severely hypoxic, measures to reduce PVR may be needed (e.g., NO). In some such cases, a larger shunt may be needed.

For post-transplantation care, see page 377.

Tricuspid Atresia

Tricuspid atresia is a condition in which there is no communication between the right atrium and the RV, which is usually hypoplastic. Survival depends on the presence of an adequate atrial communication (PFO or ASD) and a systemic-to-pulmonary shunt (VSD or PDA). Palliation in the neonate is required, and the ASD may have to be enlarged by balloon septostomy. For those patients with diminished pulmonary blood flow, a systemic-to-PA shunt (i.e., modified Blalock operation) is performed. Those with increased pulmonary blood flow, CHF, and systemic hypoperfusion need a PA band. Later in life, when PVR falls, other procedures are possible. The Glenn procedure (SVC-PA anastomosis) was commonly used for these patients but has now been superseded by the Fontan repair (right artery-to-PA anastomosis). The Fontan procedure and its modifications are now also used to treat other forms of CHD in which there is a single functional ventricle. After this operation, the right atrial pressure must serve to perfuse the lungs. A low PVR is obviously crucial.

Fontan Procedure

Special Considerations

1. After the operation, the total cardiac output supplies the systemic circulation. There is no shunting, so there is improved saturation and less load on the ventricle. The pulmonary circulation is passive and in series.
2. PVR must be demonstrated not to be increased if the operation is to succeed (PVR less than 4 units/m²). However, in some patients with mildly elevated PVR, a Fontan operation is performed but a fenestration is left in the vena cava–to-PA baffle. This allows for some right-to-left shunting and limits the right arterial pressure; cyanosis may occur, but ventricular filling and cardiac output are maintained.
3. Pleural and pericardial effusions are very common after the Fontan procedure and may require drainage for a prolonged period.

Anesthesia Plan

1. Establish several reliable intravenous routes before the operation; postoperative edema may make venous access difficult.
2. A very reliable CVP line is essential for postoperative monitoring.

3. Before terminating bypass, ensure that sinus rhythm is present or institute sequential pacing. Commence an infusion of SNP to reduce PVR and SVR. Establish hyperventilation; use a short inspiratory phase, minimal peak inspiratory pressure, and PEEP just adequate to maintain optimal lung volume.
4. After bypass, maintain the CVP at 14–16 mmHg to maintain pulmonary blood flow. It is hoped that this will provide a left atrial pressure of 4–8 mmHg. The gradient across the pulmonary bed should be less than 10 mmHg.
5. Early return to spontaneous ventilation and extubation are considered beneficial to pulmonary blood flow.
6. Fluid retention with peripheral edema, pleural and pericardial effusions, and ascites is common. Protein-losing enteropathy may occur in some patients.

Truncus Arteriosus

There are several types:

1. *Type I:* PA arises from truncus and then divides
2. *Type II:* separate PAs arise from posterior to truncus
3. *Type III:* separate PAs arise from sides of truncus

The optimal time for repair is now considered to be in the first month of life.

Special Considerations

1. DiGeorge syndrome is present in 25% of cases. Monitor the Ca^{++} level. Immune deficiency: use washed red blood cells (*see* page 456).
2. High pulmonary blood flow predisposes to pulmonary vascular hypertensive crises.
3. Low aortic diastolic pressure may result in inadequate coronary flow and myocardial ischemia.
4. The truncal valve is semilunar and commonly is incompetent.

Anesthesia Plan

1. Patients may require preoperative ventilation and inotropic support.
2. SVR and PVR should be maintained to support aortic diastolic pressure and coronary flow. Therefore, avoid hyperventilation, excess O_2, or vasodilating drugs.
3. High-dose narcotic technique is preferred.
4. After CPB and postoperatively, institute measures to protect against pulmonary vascular crisis.

Suggested Additional Reading

Textbook

Lake CL: Pediatric Cardiac Anesthesia, 3rd ed. Appleton & Lange, Norwalk, CT, 1998.

General

Baum VC and Palmisano BW: The immature heart and anesthesia. Anesthesiology 87:1529–1548, 1997.

Driscoll DJ: Evaluation of the cyanotic newborn. Pediatr Clin North Am 37:1–23, 1990.

Anesthesia Management

Anand KJS and Hickey PR: Halothane-morphine compared with high dose sufentanil for anesthesia and postoperative analgesia in neonatal cardiac surgery. N Engl J Med 326:1–9, 1992.

Burrows FA: Physiologic dead space, venous admixture, and the arterial to end-tidal carbon dioxide difference in infants and children undergoing cardiac surgery. Anesthesiology 70:219–225, 1989.

Daley MD, Roy WL, and Burrows FA: Hypoxaemia produced by an oesophageal stethoscope: a case report. Can J Anaesth 35:500–502, 1988.

Drop LJ: Ionised calcium, the heart, and hemodynamic function. Anesth Analg 64:432–451, 1985.

Hickey PR and Hansen DD: Fentanyl and sufentanil-oxygen-pancuronium anesthesia for cardiac surgery in infants. Anesth Analg 63:117–124, 1984.

Hickey PR, Hansen DD, and Strafford M: Pulmonary and systemic effects of nitrous oxide in infants with normal and elevated pulmonary vascular resistance. Anesthesiology 65:374–378, 1986.

Hickey PR, Hansen DD, Cramolini GM, et al.: Pulmonary and systemic hemodynamic responses to ketamine in infants with normal and elevated pulmonary vascular resistance. Anesthesiology 62:287–293, 1985.

Hickey PR, Hansen DD, Wessel DL, et al.: Blunting of stress responses in the pulmonary circulation of infants with fentanyl. Anesth Analg 64:1137–1142, 1985.

Jonmarker C, Larsson A, and Werner O: Changes in lung volume and lung-thorax compliance during cardiac surgery in children 11 days to 4 years of age. Anesthesiology 65:259–265, 1986.

Laishley RS, Burrows FA, Lerman J, and Roy WL: Effect of anesthetic induction regimens on oxygen saturation in cyanotic congenital heart disease. Anesthesiology 65:673–677, 1986.

Lucero VM, Lerman J, and Burrows FA: Onset of neuromuscular blockade in children with congenital heart disease. Anesth Analg 66:788–790, 1987.

Nicholson SC, Jobes DR, Zucker HA, et al.: The effect of administering or withholding dextrose in prebypass intravenous fluids on intraoperative blood glucose concentrations in infants undergoing hypothermic circulatory arrest. J Cardiothorac Vasc Anesth 6:316–318, 1992.

Stow PJ, Burrows FA, Lerman J, and Roy WL: Arterial oxygen saturation following premedication in children with cyanotic congenital heart disease. Can J Anaesth 35:63–66, 1988.

Warnecke I, Bein G, and Bucherl ES: The relevance of intraoperative pressure and oxygen saturation monitoring during pulmonary artery banding in infancy. J Cardiothorac Vasc Anesth 3:31–36, 1989.

Yates AP, Lindahl SGE, and Hatch DJ: Pulmonary ventilation and gas exchange before and after correction of congenital cardiac malformations. Br J Anaesth 59:170–178, 1987.

Cardiopulmonary Bypass and Myocardial Protection

D'Errico C, Shayevitz JR, and Martindale SJ: Age-related differences in heparin sensitivity and heparin-protamine interactions in cardiac surgery patients. J Cardiothorac Vasc Anaesth 10:451–457, 1996.

Horrow JC: Protamine: a review of its toxicity. Anesth Analg 64:348–361, 1985.

Jonas RA: Hypothermia, circulatory arrest, and the pediatric brain. J Cardiothorác Vasc Anesth 10:66–74, 1996.

Journois D, Pouard P, Greeley WJ, et al.: Hemofiltration during cardiopulmonary bypass in pediatric cardiac surgery. Anesthesiology 81:1181–1189, 1994.

Mattox KL, Guinn GA, Rubio PA, et al.: Use of the activated coagulation time in intraoperative heparin reversal for cardiopulmonary operations. Ann Thorac Surg 19:634, 1975.

Murkin JM, Farrar JK, Tweed WA, et al.: Cerebral autoregulation and flow/metabolism coupling during cardiopulmonary bypass: the influence of $PaCO_2$. Anesth Analg 66:825–832, 1987.

Naik SR and Elliott MJ: Ultrafiltration and pediatric cardiopulmonary bypass. Cardiol Young 3:331–339, 1993.

Shin'oka T, Shum-Tim D, Jonas RA, et al.: Higher hematocrit improves cerebral outcome after deep hypothermic circulatory arrest. J Thorac Cardiovasc Surg 112:1610–1621, 1996.

Yamashita M, Wakayama S, Matsuki A, et al.: Plasma catecholamine levels during extracorporeal circulation in children. Can Anaesth Soc J 29:126–129, 1982.

Transesophageal Echocardiography

Gilbert TB, Panico FG, McGill WA, et al.: Bronchial obstruction by transesophageal echocardiography probe in a pediatric cardiac patient. Anesth Analg 74:156–158, 1992.

Lunn RJ, Oliver WC, Hagler DJ, and Danielson GK: Aortic compression by transesophageal echocardiographic probe in infants and children undergoing cardiac surgery. Anesthesiology 77:587–590, 1992.

Muhiudeen IA, Roberson DA, Silverman NH, et al.: Intraoperative echocardiography for evaluation of congenital heart defects in infants and children. Anesthesiology 76:165–172, 1992.

HEART TRANSPLANTATION

The indications for heart transplantation in infants and children are as follows:

1. Severe congenital malformations (e.g., hypoplastic left heart syndrome)
2. Cardiomyopathy
3. Myocardial tumors (rare)

General Principles

1. The preoperative PVR is the most important determinant of the suitability of the infant or child for transplantation. Neonates have a high PVR, but a neonatal donor heart should be able to cope with this, and PVR may be expected to decrease over the first weeks of life. Otherwise, for older patients, strategies must be used to reduce PVR or, failing this, heart-lung transplantation must be considered.
2. Other contraindications to transplantation include serious hepatic, renal, or central nervous system disease and chronic infections (e.g., hepatitis, cytomegalovirus, human immunodeficiency virus).

3. A stable family and social environment is most desirable to ensure the continued care that will be required after transplantation.

Care of the Donor

Care of the donor patient during the harvesting procedures is discussed on page 320.

Anesthesia Management of the Recipient—Special Considerations

1. The basic management is similar to that for other open heart procedures. However, the patient may have been urgently admitted and may not have been fasted. Precautions for dealing with the full stomach may be necessary. If a rapid-sequence induction is planned, drugs and doses should be carefully worked out to avoid excessive cardiovascular effects. Ketamine is useful for the patient with minimal reserve.
2. Very strict attention to aseptic technique is required. All intravascular lines should be inserted with full sterile precautions. The puncture site should be treated with povidone-iodine ointment and covered with a clear adhesive dressing.
3. Do not aspirate the stomach after induction if oral cyclosporin may have recently been given as a component of the antirejection therapy.
4. Most patients have very poor cardiac function and a dilated heart; therefore, take care to avoid inducing bradycardia or any additional myocardial depression. Fentanyl-O_2 anesthesia plus pancuronium is usually preferred. Carefully continue solutions of inotropic agents and/or PGE_1. Some patients may need additional inotropic support as surgery commences.
5. Patients who have had previous cardiac surgery should be given aprotinin to reduce postoperative bleeding.
6. Increased PVR should be managed to prevent any further pulmonary vasoconstriction.
7. Neonates with hypoplastic left heart syndrome should be treated as for the Norwood procedure before CPB.
8. While the patient is on CPB and before weaning, prepare solutions of dopamine and dobutamine, isoproterenol, SNP, and PGE_1 for neonates.
9. On weaning from CPB, immediately give methylprednisolone (Solu-Medrol) 15 mg/kg and other antirejection drugs as indicated. Sinus tachycardia is often present at this stage, and the action of two atrial pacemakers may be observed (one from the remains of the patient's native atrium and one from the implanted atrium). In the absence of sinus rhythm, AV pacing should be commenced. A slow sinus rhythm usually responds well to an isoproterenol infusion. Infuse other inotropic solutions (e.g., dopamine) as necessary to maintain good cardiac action (*see below*).
10. Measures to minimize PVR should be continued.

11. Remember the special properties of the newly implanted but denervated heart:
    a. Cardiac drugs will exert only their direct effects; atropine will have no chronotropic effect; anticholinesterases will not affect heart rate. Epinephrine, isoproterenol, and norepinephrine will all cause an increase in heart rate. Dopamine and dobutamine are effective inotropic agents.
    b. Increased filling pressure will, through the Frank-Starling mechanism, result in increased stroke volume. A CVP of 10–12 mmHg is usually optimal. Hypovolemia is poorly tolerated.
    c. There is no change in heart rate with the respiratory cycle or with a Valsalva maneuver.
    d. Arrhythmias are not common in children, but the response to those antiarrhythmic drugs that have both direct and indirect effects on the heart will be altered:
        i. Digoxin, bretylium, and procainamide normally exert a mixture of direct and indirect effects on the heart and will have a less predictable effect on the denervated heart.
        ii. The effects of lidocaine, phenytoin, β-adrenergic blocking drugs, and calcium channel–blocking drugs are direct and similar to those in the intact heart.

Suggested Additional Reading

Martin RD, Parisi F, Robinson TW, and Bailey L: Anesthetic management of neonatal cardiac transplantation. J Cardiothorac Anesth 3:465–469, 1989.

Zickmann B, Boldt J, and Hempelmann G: Anesthesia in pediatric heart transplantation. J Heart Lung Transplant 11:S272–S276, 1992.

HEART-LUNG OR LUNG TRANSPLANTATION

Lung transplantation in children is usually performed with the aid of CPB; the considerations are similar to those for heart-lung transplantation.

Indications

1. The indications for heart-lung transplantation are
   a. Eisenmenger syndrome
   b. Other congenital defects with pulmonary vascular disease
   c. Complex CHD, inadequate pulmonary vessels not amenable to further repair
2. The indications for lung transplantation are
   a. Primary pulmonary hypertension
   b. Pulmonary fibrosis
   c. Cystic fibrosis

Care of the Donor

The general principles are outlined on page 319. Selection of a donor for lung transplantation is more difficult:

1. Significant lung disease, infection, or damage from recent aspiration or pulmonary edema associated with resuscitative interventions and artificial ventilation must be excluded. It is suggested that a PO_2 of 100 mmHg or more with an FiO_2 of 0.4, and peak inflating pressures of 30 cmH_2O or less with a tidal volume of 15 ml/kg and PEEP of 5 cmH_2O, indicate acceptability for transplantation.
2. The lungs must be an appropriate size to fit the thorax of the recipient; if they are too large, atelectasis will result. Perfect match or slightly smaller donor lungs are accepted; otherwise, lobar transplantation or tailoring of the donor lung may be required.
3. Before harvesting the lungs, the donor should receive 30 mg/kg of methylprednisolone and an infusion of PGE_1 (25 ng/kg/min) increased until the systemic arterial pressure decreases by 10%–20%. This produces maximal pulmonary vasodilation before infusion of the pulmoplegic solution.
4. Cardioplegia and pulmoplegia are induced, and the lungs are held inflated prior to tracheal clamping.
5. In selected cases, donor lung tissue may be obtained from living related donors (e.g., one lobe from each parent may be transplanted into a child).

Anesthesia Management of the Recipient: Special Considerations

1. Older children with critical respiratory disease may be very apprehensive; consider the use of well-monitored preoperative sedation (e.g., midazolam intravenously or lorazepam intravenously and/or orally with pulse oximetry in place and constant attention).
2. Maintain meticulous aseptic technique for all procedures; remove all existing intravenous lines and replace them with new lines using strict asepsis.
3. Before induction, verify administration of immunosuppressants and antibiotics as ordered.
4. Induction and maintenance of anesthesia should be planned as for CPB, bearing in mind the advanced respiratory disease.
5. Intubation: Use a cuffed tube and place the cuff just below the cords. For patients with cystic fibrosis, suction the tube frequently during dissection of the native lungs.
6. Fluid therapy should be limited to basal rates.
7. Aprotinin (protease inhibitor) infusions should be commenced after induction to decrease postoperative bleeding. These may represent most of the fluid infusion allowed.
8. Plan for optimal postoperative pain management—early extubation may be possible.
9. During bypass, be prepared to reintubate with a new sterile endotracheal tube, using appropriate aseptic technique. For patients with pulmonary infections (e.g., those with cystic fibrosis), change the entire breathing circuit. In addition, once the native lungs are removed, the proximal trachea and bronchi should be lavaged with a solution of tobramycin.

10. Prepare solutions of dopamine, dobutamine, and PGE₁. For patients with pulmonary infections, prepare a Neo-Synephrine infusion.
11. Immediately on weaning from CPB, administer methylprednisolone 15 mg/kg IV and furosemide 0.5–0.75 mg/kg. Give inotropic agents as required. Pulmonary function may be improved by albuterol inhalations and aggressive diuretic therapy.
12. Adjust the FIO_2 to maintain oxygen saturation at $\pm 93\%$ and to avoid hyperoxic damage to lungs. Hyperventilate slightly to maintain pulmonary flow using tidal volumes of 15 ml/kg. PEEP to 6–10 cmH_2O should be added to maintain optimal lung volume, minimize PVR, and prevent pulmonary edema.
13. Patients with a history of severe lung infections (e.g., cystic fibrosis) may demonstrate signs of sepsis: low BP despite good cardiac action. In such cases, an infusion of Neo-Synephrine may be required.
14. Extensive bleeding is to be expected, especially if the patient had previous thoracotomy. Order appropriate supplies of replacement factors.
15. Postoperative problems may be related to damage to the phrenic, vagus, or recurrent laryngeal nerves.

CARDIOLOGIC PROCEDURES

Cardiac Catheterization

This is usually an elective procedure, and older children will benefit from preoperative teaching, a visit to the catheter laboratory, and familiarization with the procedures to be performed. Cardiac catheterization may be performed under general anesthesia or with a combination of sedation plus local or regional analgesia. The important prerequisites for gathering reliable catheter data are as follows:

1. Hemodynamic parameters should be maintained as constant and unchanged as possible.
2. The inspired O_2 concentration should remain constant throughout the procedure. Room air is preferred if safe for the patient. Otherwise, a constant optimum inspired O_2 concentration should be selected.
3. Spontaneous ventilation is preferred when appropriate; controlled ventilation may lead to changes in intracardiac shunts and modification of intracardiac pressure measurements.
4. The patient should be maintained in an optimal physiologic state (normothermic, well hydrated, euglycemic, and so on).

Special Anesthesia Problems

1. The patient may be seriously ill and in cardiac failure.
2. The condition may further deteriorate during cardiac catheterization, especially if arrhythmias occur.
3. Contrast media used for angiograms may cause adverse effects.

When the procedure is to be performed under sedation, the following technique has proved satisfactory:

1. Establish an intravenous route using local analgesia.
2. Apply monitors (ECG, pulse oximeter, BP cuff and Doppler, temperature probe). Means to maintain body temperature of small infants (e.g., overhead warmer) should be positioned.
3. Administer intravenous sedation. An infusion of propofol with or without small doses of midazolam has been found to be most useful. When combined with good local or regional analgesia, only very small doses of drugs are required to ensure sleep, and very stable cardiovascular parameters are maintained.
4. Small infants may be offered a "sucrose soother" and often settle with this alone.
5. Caudal analgesia may be useful for some children, especially if bilateral femoral catheterization is necessary or if large catheters are to be inserted (e.g., for balloon dilatation).
6. Angiography requires that the patient be absolutely still; therefore, augment the sedation if necessary. Contrast media are hyperosmolar (although new nonionic agents are less so); they can cause aggregation of erythrocytes and, rarely, anaphylaxis. The total dose administered should be carefully recorded, especially in small infants; 5 ml/kg is usually considered a safe limit.
7. When it is considered advisable to ventilate the patient during the procedure, the same technique (propofol infusion) may be used with the addition of a suitable muscle relaxant (e.g., vecuronium) and endotracheal intubation. Normocapnia should be maintained.
8. In some patients the response of the pulmonary circulation to hyperventilation, hyperoxia, or the inhalation of NO may be studied.
9. Postcatheterization care: The patient should be carefully monitored until the effects of sedation resolve and smooth awakening occurs. It is necessary that the child lie quietly to avoid bleeding and bruising at the catheter site; additional mild sedation may be necessary to achieve this state. The catheterization site should be examined for bleeding, and the pulses distal to arterial cannulation should be evaluated regularly. The patient should be discharged when awake, with stable vital signs, and with no evidence of vascular complications.

Interventional Cardiology

Sedation and/or general anesthesia are now quite frequently required for complex interventional techniques. These include

1. Balloon dilatation of pulmonary or aortic valves, or recoarctation of the aorta
2. Occlusion of the ductus arteriosus
3. Closure of septal defects or other fistulas

Special Problems

1. The patient may be critically ill.
2. Absolute immobility is essential during the critical stages.
3. An urgent call for open operation if complications occur is a real possibility. The heart may be perforated, vessels may be ruptured, or the occlusive device may become displaced. Complications are most likely during valve dilation procedures.
4. The procedure may be carried out in a darkened room.
5. A steady hemodynamic state is required for measurements to be made.
6. Simultaneous TEE may be required to monitor results.

Anesthesia Management

1. The patient should be carefully prepared and monitored as for an open procedure. A large-bore, reliable intravenous route should be established.
2. For some very simple procedures in older children, sedation with propofol with spontaneous ventilation and local analgesia may be suitable.
3. For more complex procedures (e.g., balloon dilatation of a stenotic valve, "umbrella" closure of a septal defect), endotracheal intubation with neuromuscular block and controlled ventilation is preferred. Anesthesia may be maintained with a propofol infusion.
4. Plans must be made for transfer to the OR should a complication occur. Supplies of blood for rapid transfusion should be immediately available.
5. During the procedure, the anesthesiologist must constantly monitor for signs of blood loss or cardiac tamponade.
   a. Cardiac perforation manifests with hypotension, tachycardia with ectopic beats.
   b. Cardiac tamponade leads to hypotension, with reduced cardiac motion on fluoroscopy. Confirm by echocardiogram.

Pericardiocentesis should be performed in either case. Continued bleeding from a cardiac perforation requires thoracotomy.

ELECTROPHYSIOLOGIC STUDIES

Children may require anesthesia or sedation for electrophysiologic studies and radiofrequency catheter ablation of accessory conduction pathways in the treatment of dysrhythmias. These procedures are not painful but may be prolonged (consider inserting a urinary catheter!), and absolute immobility is essential. Hence, general endotracheal anesthesia with controlled ventilation is recommended for all small children.

Isoproterenol may be infused during the procedure in order to elicit dysrhythmias. Facilities for defibrillation and antiarrhythmic drugs should be immediately at hand.

An important consideration is the possible effect of anesthesia or sedative drugs on cardiac conduction. It has been demonstrated that neither isoflurane nor propofol in usual doses has a significant effect on cardiac conduction. Pancuronium also has no effect. Therefore, these agents would be acceptable during electrophysiologic studies.

CARDIOVERSION

Cardioversion is usually an emergency. The arrhythmia may be severe, markedly reducing cardiac output and producing shock.

Anesthesia Management

Preoperative

1. Give 100% O_2 by mask until cardioversion can be performed.
2. Ascertain whether the child has eaten recently (*see below*).
3. Prepare and check all equipment.
4. Apply monitors:
   a. Precordial stethoscope
   b. Pulse oximeter and BP cuff
   c. ECG

Perioperative

1. Ensure that there is a free-flowing, reliable intravenous route.
2. Continue 100% O_2 by mask.
3. When ready to cardiovert, induce anesthesia using a sleep dose of propofol.
4. If it is suspected that the patient has a full stomach:
   a. Continue 100% O_2.
   b. Give atropine 0.015 mg/kg IV.
   c. Inject propofol 2.5–3.5 mg/kg and succinylcholine 1–2 mg/kg.
   d. Have an assistant apply cricoid pressure until intubation is complete.
5. As soon as anesthesia has been induced and good oxygenation achieved, countershock may be applied. Repeat propofol doses if necessary.

Postoperative

1. The period of recovery is short, but the patient should be closely monitored (including ECG) for several hours afterward.
2. If the patient was intubated, remove the endotracheal tube after the patient is fully conscious.

Suggested Additional Reading

Friedrich SP, Berman AD, Baim DS, and Diver DJ: Myocardial perforation in the cardiac catheterization laboratory: incidence, presentation, diagnosis and management. Cathet Cardiovasc Diagn 32:99–107, 1994.

Hickey PR, Wessel DL, Streitz SL, et al.: Transcatheter closure of atrial septal defects: hemodynamic complications and anesthetic management. Anesth Analg 74:44–50, 1992.

Lavoie J, Walsh EP, Burrows FA, et al.: Effects of propofol or isoflurane anesthesia on cardiac conduction in children undergoing radiofrequency catheter ablation for tachydysrhythmias. Anesthesiology 82:884–887, 1995.

Lebovic S, Reich DL, Steinberg LG, et al.: Comparison of propofol versus ketamine for anesthesia in pediatric patients undergoing cardiac catheterization. Anesth Analg 74:490–494, 1991.

Malviya S, Burrows FA, Johnston AE, and Benson LN: Anaesthetic experience with paediatric interventional cardiology. Can J Anaesth 36:320–324, 1989.

Meretoja OA and Rautiainen P: Alfentanil and fentanyl sedation in infants and small children during cardiac catheterization. Can J Anaesth 37:624–628, 1990.

Rautiainen P: Alfentanil infusion for sedation in infants and small children during cardiac catheterisation. Can J Anaesth 38:980–984, 1991.

Vitiello R, McCrindle BW, Nykanen D, et al.: Complications associated with pediatric cardiac catheterization. J Am Coll Cardiol 32:1433–1440, 1998.

Williams GD, Jones TK, Hanson KA, and Morray JP: The hemodynamic effects of propofol in children with congenital heart disease. Anesth Analg 89:1411–1416, 1999.

ANESTHESIA FOR NONCARDIAC SURGERY IN INFANTS AND CHILDREN WITH CONGENITAL HEART DISEASE

CHD often occurs in association with other congenital defects, some of which may require surgery in the neonate or infant. Older children with CHD frequently require anesthesia for noncardiac procedures (e.g., dental surgery). Therefore, the anesthesiologist may be called on to provide care for children with CHD for other types of surgery. Some of these patients have uncorrected cardiac lesions, others have undergone partial (palliation) procedures, and others have had complete repair of their defect. However, even after "complete repair" there may be important considerations, such as the need for prophylactic antibiotics, the presence of a pacemaker for heart block, or other residual defects.

Diagnosis of Congenital Heart Disease

The first problem may be to decide whether the child presented for anesthesia does indeed have CHD. In neonates the diagnosis of CHD can be quite difficult:

1. Cardiac murmurs are not uncommon in the perinatal period and may not be indicative of significant heart disease.
2. Serious cardiac lesions may be present in the absence of a loud murmur.
3. The transitional circulation of the neonate may obscure the diagnosis: high PVR limits left-to-right shunts, and the patency of the ductus arteriosus provides flow to the lower body (e.g., in patients with coarctation).

Signs suggesting CHD in the neonate include murmurs, cyanosis, tachypnea, prominent precordial pulsations, bounding peripheral pulses, hepatomegaly, and large heart on radiography. The definitive diagnosis, however, is most likely to be confirmed by echocardiography. Therefore, all neonates with lesions that are commonly associated with CHD (e.g., tracheoesophageal fistula, diaphragmatic hernia, omphalocele) and those with the signs just listed should be screened by a cardiologist with the use of echocardiography.

Older children may be found to have a previously undetected and undiagnosed murmur when examined before anesthesia. The problem is to determine whether significant heart disease is present and whether it is necessary to refer the child to a cardiologist. First, it is important to determine whether the child has normal exercise tolerance. It is very unlikely that a child with unlimited activity has a lesion that will cause problems during anesthesia. On physical examination, the characteristics of the murmur should be analyzed:

1. *Innocent murmurs* are soft, systolic, and not radiated; they may vary with position, may disappear on exercise, are not characteristic of any lesion, and are heard in healthy children.
2. *Noninnocent murmurs* include all diastolic murmurs, all pansystolic and late systolic murmurs, all loud murmurs, all continuous murmurs (except venous hum), and all transmitted murmurs.

If a soft and presumably innocent murmur is heard in a healthy child, surgery usually is not delayed. If a murmur suggestive of a definite, previously undiagnosed cardiac lesion is heard, delay elective surgery and refer to a cardiologist. Emergency surgery must proceed, and the child should be managed with due regard for the cardiac disease; prophylactic antibiotics should be administered and appropriate monitoring established.

Anesthesia Management

Preoperative

1. Many of the potential problems during noncardiac surgery are similar to those associated with cardiac surgery, and the same considerations for each specific lesion apply. For any major surgery, the patient should be monitored as for cardiac surgery.
2. The anesthesiologist must clearly understand the pathophysiology of the patient's disease and carefully assess the current physical status.
3. The patient's current medication schedule must be reviewed and discussed with the parents. All cardiac medications should be continued up to the day of surgery. For patients taking digoxin, a recent blood level should be available (therapeutic range, 0.8–2 ng/ml).
4. Care must be taken to avoid excessive fluid restriction, especially in children with cyanotic CHD. The parents should be instructed to encourage clear fluids until 2 hours before the operation. If oral fluids cannot be taken, intravenous fluid therapy must be established.

5. Anesthesia must be very carefully planned to minimize the possibility of adversely affecting the cardiovascular status of the patient.
   a. Use extreme care with potent inhalational agents, especially in those with a history of or predisposition to CHF.
   b. Avoid causing major alterations in PVR or SVR.
6. Ensure that suitable antibiotic prophylaxis is ordered (Table 14–2). All children with a history of CHD require prophylactic antibiotics except those who have had a simple ligation of PDA or a suture closure of ASD. Patients with a history of ASD may have mitral valve prolapse, in which case they also need antibiotics.
7. Order appropriate preoperative sedation, but avoid producing respiratory depression. The child should be sedated but not depressed. Oral midazolam is ideal, but the child should be monitored with a pulse oximeter once sedation is achieved. Apply a topical analgesic cream to a likely intravenous site.
8. Ensure that equipment for cardiopulmonary resuscitation (including a defibrillator with paddles of suitable size) is available in the OR suite.

Table 14–2. Antibiotic Routine for Patients with Cardiac Disease

---

Dental Procedures, Oropharyngeal Surgery, Instrumentation of the Respiratory Tract Including Nasotracheal Intubation

Standard oral regimen for children includes those having prosthetic heart valves and other high-risk factors*
  Amoxicillin 50 mg/kg PO 1 hr preoperatively to a maximum of 2 g
Regimen for children allergic to amoxicillin/penicillin
  Clindamycin 20 mg/kg PO 1 hr preoperatively
Alternative regimen for children unable to take oral medications
  Ampicillin 50 mg/kg IV or IM 30 min preoperatively
Regimen for children allergic to ampicillin/penicillin and unable to take oral medications
  Clindamycin 20 mg/kg IV 30 min preoperatively
Regimen for children with methicillin sodium–resistant staphylococcal infections
  Vancomycin 20 mg/kg (maximum, 1 g) IV given over 1 hr, starting 1 hr preoperatively

Gastrointestinal or Genitourinary Procedures or Instrumentation

Standard regimen for children at high risk
  Ampicillin 50 mg/kg (up to 2 g) plus gentamicin 1.5 mg/kg (up to 120 mg), IV/IM, 30 min preoperatively and repeat ampicillin 25 mg/kg IV/IM 6 hr later, or amoxicillin 25 mg/kg PO
Regimen for high-risk children allergic to ampicillin
  Vancomycin 20 mg/kg (maximum, 1 g) IV plus gentamicin 1.5 mg/kg (maximum 80 mg) IV 1 hr preoperatively
Alternative regimen for children at moderate risk
  Amoxicillin 50 mg/kg PO 1 hr preoperatively or ampicillin 50 mg/kg IV/IM 30 min preoperatively

---

*High-risk factors for subacute bacterial endocarditis include the presence of prosthetic valves or materials (e.g., Gore-Tex shunts), cyanotic lesions, and especially tetralogy of Fallot.

9. Check coagulation status in those patients with cyanotic heart disease; coagulopathy is a common complication of polycythemia.

Perioperative

1. Attach all monitors before inducing anesthesia.
2. Establish a reliable intravenous route, but be aware of the risk of paradoxic emboli. Be careful to remove all bubbles from intravenous lines, especially in patients with right-to-left shunts, but remember that others also may have bidirectional shunts.
3. Give 100% O_2 by mask.
4. Induce anesthesia with intravenous thiopental; use a small dose (3–4 mg/kg) injected slowly. Otherwise, inhalation induction with sevoflurane may be acceptable in some patients, but beware of producing unacceptable myocardial depression or allowing any ventilatory obstruction.
5. Intubate the patient for all but the most minor procedure (e.g., myringotomy). Give a suitable relaxant, but remember that if the circulation time is prolonged, there will be a longer delay before muscle paralysis is complete.
6. Children with less severe disease tolerate low concentrations of volatile agents well; for minor procedures, maintain anesthesia with N_2O and sevoflurane or isoflurane with spontaneous or assisted ventilation. Patients with more severe disease and those with any history of CHF cannot tolerate the use of myocardial depressant potent volatile agents. These patients should be managed with a high-dose narcotic and relaxant (pancuronium or vecuronium) technique, with controlled ventilation.
7. Maintain an adequate inspired concentration of oxygen, and monitor the oxygen saturation carefully. Oximeters are less accurate at lower saturations; therefore, err on the safe side.
8. For major noncardiac surgery, insert arterial and other lines and monitor the patient as for cardiac surgery. Consider the effects of previous surgery (e.g., systemic-to-pulmonary shunts) in choosing where to place the BP cuff.
9. End-tidal carbon dioxide values do not correlate well and tend to underestimate arterial tension in those patients with right-to-left shunts. They do, however, give valuable information about pulmonary blood flow. For example, a fall in end-tidal carbon dioxide concentration in the child with tetralogy indicates a fall in pulmonary blood flow and impending cyanotic spell!

Postoperative

1. Continue to monitor the patient (including ECG and oximeter) until the patient is fully recovered from all effects of anesthesia.
2. Give O_2 by mask until recovery is complete. Patients with cyanotic CHD have a reduced ventilatory response to hypoxemia.
3. Provide good pain relief. Pain and restlessness increase oxygen demand.

4. Give maintenance fluids intravenously until oral intake is adequate, but avoid inducing a fluid overload.

Suggested Additional Reading

Burrows FA: Anesthetic management of the child with congenital heart disease for noncardiac surgery. Can J Anaesth 39:R60–R65, 1992.

Dajani AS, Taubert KA, Wilson W, et al.: Prevention of bacterial endocarditis: recommendations of the American Heart Association. JAMA 277:1794–1801, 1997.

Litman RS: Anesthetic considerations for children with congenital heart disease undergoing noncardiac surgery. Anesthesiol Clin North Am 15:93–103, 1997.

Orthopaedic Surgery

A considerable proportion of children who undergo elective orthopaedic surgery have multiple congenital anomalies and/or neuromuscular disease (*see* Appendix I). Underlying disease, particularly with muscle weakness, requires special anesthesia care, and minor surgery may be fraught with major anesthesia complications.

GENERAL PRINCIPLES

1. Children with orthopaedic deformities may require repeated surgery and may spend much time in the hospital. Their sympathetic management is particularly important, and preoperative sedation should be chosen carefully.
2. Drug selection is influenced by the underlying disease; therefore, check the history carefully. Neuromuscular disease is particularly relevant; in general, muscle relaxants should be avoided if possible for patients with myopathies (*see* Appendix I). Succinylcholine, particularly, should not be given to patients with muscle disease.
3. Major surgery of the vertebral column deserves special consideration; the operations are extensive and may involve massive blood loss.
4. Malignant hyperthermia, though very rare, is more common in patients with orthopaedic diseases. Maintain vigilance for the early signs.
5. Many surgical procedures are performed with the use of a tourniquet. Be especially cautious in monitoring when a tourniquet

is in use; the surgeon is not able to report on the color of the blood!

6. When a tourniquet is used, blood loss is negligible. In other cases, surgery involving bone may result in significant losses (e.g., innominate osteotomy). Therefore, establish a reliable intravenous route and check that blood is available.

7. When a tourniquet is inflated, there usually follows a progressive increase in the heart rate and the blood pressure (BP). The exact cause is unknown, but it has been attributed to stimulation of sympathetic nerves. The danger is that, on release of the tourniquet, the blood pressure may decrease precipitously. If the anesthesiologist has been "chasing" the tourniquet-induced hypertension by giving higher levels of volatile agents, serious hypotension may then ensue. Therefore, use caution with dosages of potent volatile agents while the tourniquet is being used, and reduce the concentration in anticipation of tourniquet release.

8. Hemodynamic responses to tourniquet release in children are usually not clinically significant. A transient decrease in arterial pH associated with an increase in base deficit and carbon dioxide tension (PCO_2) does occur; this is most marked after long tourniquet times (more than 75 minutes) or with the use of double tourniquets. General recommendations include the following:

   a. Attempt to limit tourniquet times to less than 75 minutes.
   b. Do not release bilateral tourniquets simultaneously.
   c. Use controlled ventilation before and after tourniquet release to remove the respiratory component of the acidosis.
   d. In children who might have difficulty compensating for the metabolic or respiratory acidosis (e.g., those with renal disease or pulmonary disease), consider measuring blood gases 5 minutes after tourniquet release to check their status.

9. Orthopaedic surgery is associated with high levels of postoperative pain. Plan for optimal management, using regional analgesia whenever possible.

KYPHOSCOLIOSIS

Kyphoscoliosis may be congenital (15% of cases), but more commonly it is acquired. It is idiopathic in 65% of cases and occurs secondary to neuromuscular disease in 20%. More than 80% of patients with idiopathic scoliosis are female. Pulmonary function may be impaired.

Pulmonary Function

Changes in pulmonary function are related to the underlying cause, the speed of development of the scoliosis, and the severity of the curvature. The cardiorespiratory effects of scoliosis are summarized in Figure 15–1.

The pulmonary abnormality is restrictive rather than obstructive. Lung compliance is reduced. The vital capacity and the total lung capac-

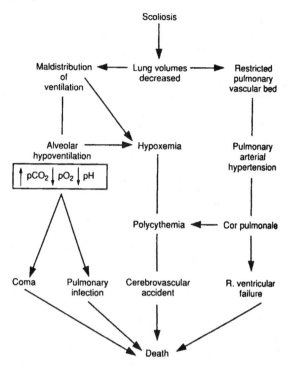

Figure 15–1. Pathophysiology of the cardiorespiratory effects of kyphoscoliosis. Progressive alveolar hypoventilation, leading to hypoxia, may be accompanied by pulmonary hypertension and right ventricular failure. (Courtesy of Henry Levison, M.D., F.R.C.P.C., Director of Respiratory Physiology, The Hospital for Sick Children, Toronto.)

ity may be greatly reduced, and the functional residual capacity somewhat less so. The respiratory volume tends to be maintained. The elastic resistance of the chest wall may be high, increasing the work and energy cost of breathing. Severe and prolonged lung compression impairs gas exchange, but that becomes evident only in later stages of the disease in the untreated patient.

The principal concern for young patients with idiopathic scoliosis is the cosmetic effect of the spinal and pelvic or chest wall deformity, especially when the curvature increases during the years of rapid body growth. At this stage, respiratory symptoms are uncommon, but pulmonary function studies may reveal an abnormality. Although lung volumes can be normal, exercise tolerance may be reduced. In severe cases the mechanical effects of scoliosis on respiratory function are apparent even at rest.

Pulmonary function is relatively normal in most children who present for correction of idiopathic scoliosis with a curvature of less than 65%.

Respiratory disability is more likely to occur in association with congenital scoliosis or curvature of paralytic etiology.

Surgical Procedures

1. Posterior spinal fusion may be performed using contoured metal rods to stabilize the spine postoperatively until bony fusion occurs. In some patients with a flexible spine, the deformity is corrected solely by a posterior fusion.
2. In some patients an anterior thoracoabdominal approach may be used to remove the intervertebral discs or a hemivertebra to correct a lateral curve.
3. In many patients the two procedures are combined: an anterior release followed by a posterior fusion. This makes for a long operation, often associated with significant blood loss: a challenge for the anesthesiologist.
4. Anterior release procedures may be carried out endoscopically, in which case the special considerations for endoscopic surgery apply.

Special Anesthesia Problems

1. Anesthesia management must take into account the following:
   a. Cause and severity of the curvature
   b. Degree of respiratory and cardiovascular impairment
   c. Type of corrective procedure proposed
2. If the scoliosis is secondary to neuromuscular disease:
   a. Special consideration of drug selection may be necessary.
   b. Pulmonary function impairment caused by the mechanical effects of the spinal curvature may be compounded by involvement of respiratory muscles in the disease process. Postoperative respiratory insufficiency is more likely.
   c. Increased bleeding may be expected. This may be a result of altered vascular responses associated with myopathy.
3. Preoperative assessment must include the following:
   a. Detailed history and examination for an indication of abilities and stamina
   b. Pulmonary function studies, including blood gas analysis. (These studies may not be possible in very young patients due to lack of cooperation.)
   c. Echocardiogram to assess myocardial function for all patients with very severe curves or associated myopathy
4. Be alert for signs of significant respiratory impairment (e.g., tachypnea at rest, severely reduced vital capacity, abnormal blood gas values, inability to cough effectively). Postoperatively, hypoventilation, secretion retention, and atelectasis are likely in response to pain, analgesic drugs, and immobilization.
5. Severe impairment of respiratory function is not a contraindication to surgery, provided that resources are available for postoperative intensive respiratory care (including controlled ventilation if necessary). Fixation of the spinal deformity is essential to prevent

further deterioration of respiratory function (but usually does not result in significant improvement).
6. Children with a vital capacity less than 35% of normal may develop major respiratory complications postoperatively; those with a vital capacity less than 30%–40% of normal will probably require postoperative ventilation.

N.B. A combined anterior and posterior approach to the correction of spinal deformity is now often used to achieve optimal correction and fixation. The two operations may be performed concurrently (usually a very long procedure), or they may be separated by a period of approximately 1 week.

Corrective Surgery by the Posterior Approach

Special Anesthesia Problems

1. Because the patient must be prone, very careful fixation of the endotracheal tube is essential. If preoperative correction of the spinal curvature has been achieved with an exoskeletal apparatus, intubation will probably be difficult; fixation of the head and neck may render adequate direct laryngoscopy impossible, and the use of a fiberoptic technique is required.
2. Blood loss may be severe (in excess of 50% of the estimated blood volume [EBV]). Most bleeding originates from the vertebral veins, which become engorged if there is any pressure on the anterior abdomen. Blood loss is also related to the extent of the surgery (length of spine to be fused) and to the surgeon's speed and expertise. Patients with scoliosis secondary to a recognized neuromuscular disorder usually have a larger blood loss than those with idiopathic scoliosis. Alternatives to homologous transfusion should be considered:
   a. Autologous predeposit programs are very suitable for these patients.
   b. Acute normovolemic hemodilution may be used intraoperatively. This may be optimized by giving oral ferrous sulfate daily, beginning 4 weeks before surgery, and then administering twice-weekly intramuscular injections of erythropoietin commencing 2 weeks before surgery. The hematocrit (Hct) should not exceed 55% preoperatively.
   c. The cell saver may be used to salvage erythrocytes from suctioned blood. However, transfusion of large volumes of cell saver blood may lead to coagulopathy due to dilution of coagulation factors.
3. Spinal cord function should be monitored during the operation: the use of somatosensory evoked potentials (SSEPs) from the posterior tibial nerve has become a standard technique. However, SSEPs monitor only sensory pathways in the spinal cord, and, in fact, the anterior cord may be more at risk. Motor evoked potentials (MEPs), stimulating the cord above the level of the surgery and recording the electromyogram from the lower limb, may also be performed.

Alternatively, the "wake-up test" has been used, but it is not without risk; it mainly tests the motor pathways. It is common to monitor SSEPs routinely and MEPs sometimes, but also to use a wake-up test for very severe deformities. Anesthesia techniques to permit the monitoring of evoked potentials should avoid high concentrations of volatile agents; 0.5% isoflurane is acceptable, and large doses of narcotics may be given. During the testing of MEPs, better results are obtained with minimal neuromuscular blockade; an infusion of an intermediate-acting nondepolarizing relaxant may be used to achieve a controllable level of neuromuscular blockade. Every patient should be awake at the end of the operation, so that both sensory and motor function can be tested immediately.

4. Pulmonary function may be severely impaired. The anesthesiologist must check that the present state is optimal and exclude any superimposed acute respiratory disease.

5. Postoperative pain is considerable; intrathecal opioids administered intraoperatively have been effective for postoperative analgesia and may also facilitate intraoperative BP control and reduce blood loss.

Anesthesia Management

Preoperative

1. Premedication with oral midazolam is usually adequate if combined with reassurance and a full explanation of procedures to be performed.

2. Do not give respiratory depressant drugs to patients whose respiratory function is impaired.

3. Ensure that all equipment and drugs are at hand in case of emergency.

4. Check that an adequate supply of blood and other fluid replacements is at hand.

5. If the patient is to be wakened intraoperatively (*see* item 7, page 396), explain that this will happen and give reassurance that no pain will be felt at that time—and, in fact, the event probably will not be remembered postoperatively.

Perioperative

1. If halo-loop traction is in place, check that instruments to release the connecting rods are at hand.

2. Intubation:
   a. In uncomplicated cases, induce anesthesia with thiopental followed by succinylcholine or a short-acting nondepolarizing relaxant* and intubate. If monitoring of SSEPs is planned, it is necessary to allow the patient to recover from the succinylcholine and to check the positioning of the stimulating electrodes over the posterior tibial nerve before giving further relaxants.

---

*Do not use succinylcholine for patients with Duchenne-type muscular dystrophy.

  b. If the exoskeletal apparatus is present, direct laryngoscopy may not be possible.

   i. Do not give muscle relaxant drugs until airway control by intubation has been accomplished.

   ii. Select a suitable intubation technique (e.g., fiberoptic intubation under general anesthesia).

3. Maintenance: Use nitrous oxide and oxygen (N_2O/O_2) controlled hyperventilation and a long-acting muscle relaxant. Either of the following narcotic infusions may be used:

   a. Fentanyl-loading dose of 5 μg/kg; infusion at 2 μg/kg/hr

   b. Morphine-loading dose of 100 μg/kg; infusion at 10–30 μg/kg/hr

   Low concentrations of isoflurane (0.5%–1%) or desflurane (3%–5%) may be added to control the BP as necessary. This technique does not interfere with SSEP monitoring and does allow for the possibility of a wake-up test. If MEPs are to be measured, total neuromuscular block is contraindicated; a controlled mivacurium infusion permits recording of MEPs and provides some relaxation.

4. Position the patient on a scoliosis operating frame that avoids any external pressure on the anterior abdominal wall (e.g., the Relton frame). Maintenance of the correct prone-suspended position is essential to ensure minimal blood loss. (If the patient is malpositioned so that pressure on the abdomen results in vertebral venous engorgement, heavy blood loss is inevitable.)

5. Monitor the following:

   a. Ventilation—esophageal stethoscope, airway pressure

   b. Circulation—ECG, pulse oximeter, arterial line, and central venous pressure (CVP)

   c. Temperature—rectal or esophageal probe

   d. Neuromuscular blockade—peripheral nerve stimulator

   e. Blood loss—gravimetric method

   f. Urine output—indwelling catheter

   g. SSEPs and/or MEPs—before, during, and after correction

   h. Hematology and biochemistry—acid-base and blood gas status, Hct and coagulation status as indicated by the duration and severity of the procedure.

6. Blood loss is minimized by

   a. Proper posture (*see* item 5, *above*) and complete muscle relaxation

   b. Deep infiltration of the wound site (by the surgeon) with a large volume of dilute epinephrine/saline solution (up to 500 ml of 1:500,000 solution may be used)

   c. Controlled ventilation, maintaining PCO_2 at 30–35 mmHg to avoid hypercarbia and vasodilation

   d. Surgical technique (firm packing and meticulous subperiosteal plane dissection)

   e. Use of a propofol infusion to avoid high concentrations of anesthetic agents that cause vasodilation (e.g., isoflurane)

   f. Hypotensive anesthesia—sodium nitroprusside infusions or other techniques may be used, but the mean BP should be kept at 60 mmHg or higher. In the prone patient, the spinal cord is elevated above the heart and, with hypotension, ischemia of the spinal cord may result, especially while it is being manipulated or stretched, thus leading to paraplegia.

g. Acute normovolemic hemodilution (i.e., an alternative blood conservation method) is carried out as follows:

i. A calculated volume of blood is withdrawn to reduce the Hct to 30%. Use the preoperative Hct and the EBV (in milliliters) to calculate the volume to be withdrawn:

$$\text{Volume withdrawn} = (\text{Hct} - 30) \times \text{EBV}/\text{Hct}$$

ii. When the patient is anesthetized and lines have been inserted, a weighed volume of blood is withdrawn into citrate phosphate dextrose bags for storage via the arterial line.

iii. During blood withdrawal, a volume of warmed lactated Ringer's solution equal to three times the blood volume withdrawn is infused.

iv. As surgery progresses, the blood that has been withdrawn is reinfused. This method results in loss of lower-Hct blood during surgery and conservation of the patient's cells for reinfusion.

v. Monitor the oxygen tension (PO_2), pH, and plasma lactate levels to ensure an adequate tissue supply of oxygen.

7. If the evoked potential recordings show any changes, or if the surgeon requests confirmation of spinal cord integrity after application of the distraction and compression apparatus, perform a wake-up test.

a. Anticipate this request by withholding relaxant increments for 1 hour before the patient awakens, if possible. Discontinue isoflurane. Consider using a propofol and remifentanil infusion.

b. Discontinue N_2O. Decrease ventilation or administer 5% CO_2 in O_2 for 3 minutes to return the PCO_2 to normal levels. Ask the patient to move the toes. (Voluntary movement of the feet confirms spinal cord integrity.) Reanesthetize the patient using midazolam (0.1 mg/kg) and propofol (3–5 mg/kg) IV. Beware of allowing the patient to awaken too much; excessive movements may result in dangerous loss of position on the frame, and attempts to breathe spontaneously against the ventilator have been reported to result in air embolism.

Postoperative

1. Insert a nasogastric suction tube.
2. The patient must be awake before leaving the operating room.
   a. Check for movement of legs and feet.
   b. Check air entry throughout the lungs. (Pneumothorax is a possible complication of spinal surgery.)

3. On arrival in the postanesthetic care unit:
   a. Give 40% O_2 by mask.
   b. Supplement analgesia as necessary (e.g., morphine infusion, patient-controlled analgesia).
   c. Obtain plain radiographs of the chest and vertebral column. Check the lung fields, looking especially for pneumothorax.
   d. Obtain hemoglobin and Hct values; order blood transfusion accordingly.
4. The patient must remain supine for at least 12 hours. Order physiotherapy; encourage breathing exercises.
5. Ensure that the patient is nursed in a warm environment. (Body temperature usually falls 1°–2°C during surgery because of large wound exposure, air-conditioning, and so on.)

Postoperative Pulmonary Insufficiency

Clinical observation and serial blood gas analyses during the early postoperative period indicate the patient's ability to ventilate adequately. Pulmonary insufficiency postoperatively may result from

1. Severe pulmonary neuromuscular disease
2. Pneumothorax, hemothorax, pleural effusion
3. Retention of secretions and atelectasis (due to pain, analgesics, and/or immobilization, especially in patients with neuromuscular disease)
4. Aspiration of gastric contents
5. Fat embolism syndrome
6. Alteration in thoracic mechanics and/or persistent effects of muscle relaxants

Pulmonary Management

1. Continue to monitor arterial blood gases.
2. Insert a nasotracheal tube, and institute intermittent positive-pressure ventilation.
3. Bear in mind that weaning from assisted ventilation may take days or weeks.
4. A decision to establish a tracheotomy can be deferred depending on the patient's progress.

Corrective Surgery by the Anterior Approach

Zielke Instrumentation

For treatment of a curve in the lumbar region, the vertebral column is approached laterally on the convex side of the curvature. Thoracotomy is performed, and the diaphragm may be divided at its peripheral attachments to provide access to the vertebrae.

N.B. This surgical trauma to the diaphragm and chest wall increases the risk of postoperative respiratory insufficiency.

Anesthesia management is the same as for the posterior approach—N_2O, controlled hyperventilation, muscle relaxation, and supplementary analgesia, with the following modifications:

1. Selective endobronchial intubation of the dependent lung may be advantageous, permitting easier access to upper thoracic curvatures. (Serial blood gas measurements dictate the feasibility of continuing this technique throughout the procedure, but it is usually well tolerated.)
2. If bilateral ventilation is selected, ventilation of the exposed lung will be impeded by surgical packing and retractors. Periodically, expand the lung fully (to avoid prolonged atelectasis).

Spinal Osteotomy

Spinal osteotomy with wedge excision consists of local resection of deformed vertebrae. This procedure may result in excessive blood loss owing to the proximity of the vertebral and epidural venous plexuses. It may be difficult to control the hemorrhage.

Monitor blood loss by

1. Gravimetric method (weigh sponges and measure suction losses)
2. Continuous CVP measurement and direct BP readings via an arterial line
3. Clinical observation (e.g., skin temperature, urine output)

If massive transfusion is required:

1. Use packed cells in recently thawed fresh-frozen plasma.
2. Warm all blood to 40°C.
3. Monitor coagulation indices, especially platelets.
4. Order platelet concentrates (1 unit/5 kg) if the platelet count is less than $100,000/mm^3$.
5. Monitor the acid-base status and correct acidosis.
6. If citrate toxicity is suspected (hypotension despite volume replacement), inject calcium gluconate intravenously (2 ml 10% solution slowly; repeat as indicated).

FRACTURES

See Trauma (page 413).

See also Plastic and Reconstructive Surgery (page 270) for mandibular fractures.

Suggested Additional Reading

Goodarzi M, Shier NH, and Ogsen JA: Physiologic changes during tourniquet use in children. J Pediatr Orthop 12:510–513, 1988.

Grundy BL, Nelson PB, Doyle E, and Procopio PT: Intraoperative loss of somatosensory evoked potentials predicts loss of spinal cord function. Anesthesiology 57:321–322, 1982.

Jenkins JD, Bohn D, Edmonds JF, Levison H, et al.: Evaluation of pulmonary function in muscular dystrophy patients requiring spinal surgery. Crit Care Med 10:645, 1982.

Lynn AM, Fischer T, Brandford HG, and Pendergrass TW: Systemic responses to tourniquet release in children. Anesth Analg 65:865–872, 1986.

Relton JES: Anesthesia in the surgical correction of scoliosis. In Riseborough EJ and Herndon JH (eds.): Scoliosis and Other Deformities of the Axial Skeleton. Little, Brown, Boston, 1975, p 309.

Relton JES and Hall JE: An operation frame for spinal fusion: a new apparatus designed to reduce hemorrhage during operation. J Bone Joint Surg Br 49:327, 1967.

Rosenberg H and Heiman-Patterson T: Duchenne's muscular dystrophy and malignant hyperthermia: another warning. Anesthesiology 59:362, 1983.

Shannon DC, Riseborough EJ, and Kazemi H: Ventilation perfusion relationships following correction of kyphoscoliosis. JAMA 217:579, 1971.

Chapter 16

Urologic Investigation and Surgery

GENERAL PRINCIPLES

The anesthesia risk depends on the state of the patient's renal function.
1. Most children who come for investigation or surgery of the lower urinary tract have good renal function.
2. Many of those who require renal biopsy have mild renal dysfunction (usually insufficient to influence anesthesia risk).
3. All children in renal failure are seriously ill and present multiple problems for the anesthesiologist (as well as the nephrologist).
4. Renal disease may be part of a syndrome and therefore requires consideration of all aspects of the condition (*see* Appendix I).
5. Surgery of the genitalia may have significant psychological effects on small children; one thing that can be done to help minimize these effects is to provide good postoperative pain relief.

CHILDREN WITH GOOD RENAL FUNCTION

Anesthesia Management—Minor Procedures

For minor procedures, such as cystoscopy, retrograde pyelography, circumcision, or hypospadias repair, children almost always require general anesthesia, using agents appropriate for the procedure. Healthy children undergoing short investigative procedures or operations are almost all treated as day cases.

Preoperative

1. Sedatives are useful for some patients, especially those who require repeated surgery. Oral midazolam is appropriate for most patients.

Perioperative

1. Induce anesthesia with intravenous or inhalational agents.
2. Maintain anesthesia with nitrous oxide (N_2O), oxygen (O_2), and sevoflurane or halothane by mask.
3. Provide regional analgesia for postoperative pain control whenever possible.

Postoperative

1. Give supplementary analgesia as required; those patients with a successful block will require little else. Day patients are usually discharged after 1 hour. Anticipate the need for additional analgesia at home as the block wears off. Instruct parents to administer a suitable analgesic (e.g., acetaminophen) before pain occurs.

Anesthesia Management—Major Genitourinary Surgical Procedures

Apply anesthesia management as for minor procedures (*see above*), plus the following:

1. Use general endotracheal anesthesia with muscle relaxants and controlled ventilation.
2. Be prepared for major hemorrhage: Insert a reliable large-bore intravenous line, measure blood losses carefully, and replace as indicated.
3. Use regional analgesia when possible to provide for postoperative pain relief. For example, for reimplantation of ureters, a single caudal shot provides analgesia for the first few hours. Intercostal nerve blocks or, preferably, a lumbar epidural block provides good analgesia after renal surgery.
4. Children who have dilated ureters may develop hypertension postoperatively. This may require treatment with hydralazine.

CHILDREN WITH POOR RENAL FUNCTION OR IN RENAL FAILURE

These children may have many physiologic and psychological disturbances and deserve very careful consideration.

Special Anesthesia Problems

1. Anemia (usually normochromic, normocytic), caused by
   a. Decreased erythropoietin production. If erythropoietin is absent, the hemoglobin concentration (Hb) will not rise above 7–9 g/dl. Recombinant human erythropoietin therapy may not be effective if severe uremia is present.
   b. Decreased erythrocyte survival and increased hemolysis
   c. Increased bruising and bleeding from increased capillary fragility

    d. Iron and/or folic acid deficiency
    e. Bone marrow depression due to an increase in blood urea nitrogen (BUN)

The anemia leads to compensatory changes; that is, increased cardiac output and increased red blood cell (RBC) 2,3-diphosphoglycerate (2,3-DPG), although the latter is minimal. The P_{50} values are not different from those of normal children.

After successful renal transplantation, the Hb rises rapidly.

N.B. Arterial oxygen desaturation (cyanosis) cannot be detected clinically in the very anemic patient. The pulse oximeter will measure the saturation level, though slightly less accurately; hence, it remains an invaluable monitor. Blood transfusions, once thought to be contraindicated in the pretransplantation patient, are now recognized to improve posttransplantation graft survival.

  2. Coagulopathies, caused by
    a. Increased capillary fragility
    b. Functional platelet defect (decreased adhesiveness), possibly due to elevation of guanidinosuccinic acid
    c. Thrombocytopenia due to bone marrow depression
    d. Drugs (e.g., heparin, acetylsalicylic acid)
  3. Acid-base imbalance:
    a. Children produce even more acid than adults; when urinary ammonia production decreases, a metabolic acidosis predominates and plasma bicarbonate falls to 12–15 mEq/L. This is compensated to a variable degree by respiratory alkalosis.
    b. In long-standing stable renal failure, H^+ displaces Ca^{++} from bone and K^+ from intracellular fluid.
  4. Fluid and electrolyte changes. Children undergoing dialysis (particularly hemodialysis) are likely to be hypovolemic.
    a. "Sodium losers" are those children with polycystic kidneys or severe pyelonephritis (tubular damage is disproportionately greater than glomerular injury):
      i. Normotension or slight hypotension is present.
      ii. Edema is present uncommonly.
      iii. Hypokalemia is present in some.
      iv. Renal function is improved by increasing intake of sodium and water; sodium restriction may lead rapidly to severe hyponatremia.
    b. "Sodium retainers" are children with glomerulonephritis; salt retention, hypertension, and edema predispose them to cardiac failure.
    c. Potassium shifts, due to displacement of K^+ from the cells by H^+:
      i. High serum K^+ levels
      ii. Depressed excitability of muscles and nerves. This is particularly significant if cardiac muscle is affected—further sudden rises in K^+ (e.g., with succinylcholine or increased acidosis) may precipitate cardiac arrest.

    d. Calcium shifts:
       i. If displacement of Ca^{++} by H^+ is prolonged, osteoporosis may develop.
    e. Anion changes:
       i. Plasma bicarbonate (HCO_3^-) is decreased.
       ii. Plasma (SO_4^{--}) is increased.
       iii. Plasma (HPO_4^{--}) is increased.
       iv. Plasma chloride (Cl^-) is increased.

5. Cardiovascular problems:
    a. Hypertension may result from abnormalities of extracellular fluid regulation, fluid overload, and derangement of the renin-angiotensin-aldosterone system:
       i. In many patients (those with hypertension secondary to sodium and water retention), this can be controlled conservatively (e.g., by careful moderate salt restriction).
       ii. In some patients, the BP can be titrated against sodium and water content during dialysis.
       iii. In others, drug therapy with diuretics and vasodilators is necessary.
       iv. In a few, even large doses of antihypertensive agents fail to control the hypertension (which is probably caused by overproduction of renin). Retinopathy and/or encephalopathy may develop, and bilateral nephrectomy may become necessary.
       v. Hypertensive crisis may occur, occasionally in the perioperative period. Diazoxide (5 mg/kg) has commonly been used for this indication, but a labetalol infusion may now be the therapy of choice.
    b. Congestive heart failure may occur with advanced renal failure, as a result of hypertension, volume overload, anemia, electrolyte imbalance, and the effects of an arteriovenous (AV) fistula:
       i. Digitalis therapy is difficult to control.
       ii. Pericardial effusion and tamponade may occur.
    c. Fatty degeneration of the myocardium may occur secondary to chronic renal failure.

6. Pulmonary congestion:
    a. The alveolar-arterial partial oxygen pressure difference ($A\text{-}aDO_2$) may be large.
    b. Sodium and water retention, left ventricular failure, and hypoproteinemia contribute to the development of "uremic lung."
    c. Pleural effusions may develop.

7. Gastrointestinal disturbances:
    a. Anorexia, nausea, and vomiting (due to bacterial breakdown of urea to ammonia in the gastrointestinal tract) may aggravate the water, electrolyte, and acid-base imbalance. Gastric emptying may be delayed.

8. Multiple medications:
    a. Many of these patients are receiving long-term steroid therapy with resultant osteodystrophy, cushingoid state, and glycosuria:

      i. Continue steroid therapy perioperatively.
      ii. Observe aseptic techniques meticulously.
   b. Antihypertensive polypharmacy: potential cardiovascular instability under anesthesia must be anticipated. (The drugs should not be discontinued before surgery.)
   c. Digitalis and diuretic therapy may lead to K^+ depletion and thus to increased susceptibility to cardiac arrhythmias.
   d. Antibiotics (e.g., gentamicin) may prolong the effect of nondepolarizing muscle relaxants.
   e. Antimetabolites (e.g., azathioprine) that are highly protein-bound may increase the bioavailability of other protein-bound drugs by displacing them on the protein molecule.

9. Reduced immunity (risk of infection): it is vital to practice very careful asepsis.
10. Poor quality of life and potentially major psychological disturbances:
   a. Resulting from chronic debilitating disease
   b. Heightened by the uremic state and knowledge of a life-threatening condition

In summary, these children have:
1. Reduced O_2 carrying capacity, which is dependent on a stressed cardiovascular system
2. Increased tendency to bleed (in an already anemic state)
3. Incipient or apparent cardiac failure:
   a. Left ventricular failure if hypertensive, hypervolemic, and anemic
   b. Right ventricular failure (late)
4. Higher risk of cardiac arrest (e.g., due to increased K^+ and acidosis)
5. Intolerance of inaccurate administration of blood, other fluids, and electrolytes
6. Cardiovascular instability due to long-term administration of antihypertensive drugs
7. Low resistance to infection
8. Very low tolerance to further discomfort, however minor (e.g., finger prick, movement from one bed to another)

N.B. Many children with disturbed renal function are undergoing hemodialysis regularly and therefore have an AV shunt or fistula inserted, usually in the arm. Special care must be taken to ensure that this shunt is kept functioning throughout the perioperative period. The patient must not be allowed to lie on that limb at any time, and it should not be used for blood pressure determinations. The function of the AV fistula should be monitored with the use of a Doppler flowmeter.

Preoperative Assessment and Preparation

Pay careful attention to the following physical and psychological aspects:

1. Patients in a dialysis program are usually dialyzed 12–18 hours before surgery. Check postdialysis fluid and electrolyte status.

2. Plan ahead so that the child's discomfort is not increased and any necessary disturbances are minimized.
3. Psychological preparation and support are of special benefit to these patients—and are safer than depressant medication. Some sedation may help.
4. Check results of laboratory tests:
   a. Hb: chronic anemia is surprisingly well tolerated by these patients.
      i. Take into account the patient's usual Hb level and what the patient can do at that level. (Some children are quite active even at 4 g/dl.)
      ii. A level of 5 g/dl is acceptable for anesthesia if there has been no recent or sudden decline.
      iii. Transfusions may be given if deemed essential and may help the pretransplantation patient. Packed RBCs are preferable. However, transfusion is of temporary benefit only.
   b. Serum potassium: values lower than 5 mEq/L are acceptable—even in an emergency, levels higher than 6 mEq/L are unacceptable. (But remember that slightly higher levels are normal in very small preterm infants.)
      i. If the serum K^+ level is elevated, surgery is usually delayed until hemodialysis has been performed.
      ii. In an emergency, K^+ can be lowered rapidly by giving 0.5 g/kg glucose as a 10% solution with 1 unit of regular insulin added for each 5 g of glucose.
   c. Acid-base balance:
      i. A pH higher than 7.32 is acceptable. If necessary, administer sodium bicarbonate ($NaHCO_3^-$) for correction of acidosis, even if sodium (Na^+) levels are elevated.
      ii. Correction must be cautious and gradual. If the serum calcium (Ca^{++}) level is low, sudden correction may precipitate tetany or convulsions.

Anesthesia Management

1. Pay meticulous attention to details of asepsis.
2. For short procedures (e.g., insertion of a peritoneal catheter) in a poor-risk patient who is cooperative and emotionally stable, use local anesthesia (1%–2% lidocaine without epinephrine; maximum, 3 mg/kg).
3. For all other cases and if in doubt, use general anesthesia.
4. Anesthesia drugs and renal failure:
   a. Patients with renal failure are sensitive to narcotics; use these with caution. Fentanyl, alfentanil, and sufentanil are relatively safe, because their elimination is little changed. Morphine and meperidine may have prolonged effects owing to failure to excrete active metabolites.
   b. Thiopental should be used cautiously in reduced doses; less protein binding results in an increased free active fraction.
   c. Volatile inhalation agents are eliminated via the lungs and hence

are most useful. Fluoride nephrotoxicity is not a problem associated with halothane, isoflurane, sevoflurane, or desflurane. Enflurane causes higher fluoride levels, which may have been associated with renal failure; therefore, it should not be used.

d. Succinylcholine may be used as a single dose provided that the serum potassium (K^+) concentration is 5.5 mEq/L or less. It should be preceded by a small dose of a nondepolarizing relaxant.

e. Muscle relaxants, nondepolarizing: *cis*-atracurium and vecuronium are drugs of choice. Pancuronium, metocurine, gallamine, pipecuronium, and doxacurium are partially or completely excreted by the kidneys and should not be used. *d*-Tubocurarine is excreted via the kidneys, but biliary excretion is an alternate pathway and the drug has been used successfully in patients with renal failure.

f. Local anesthesia drugs have not been extensively studied in patients with renal failure; they may be used in normal doses for "single-shot" techniques. Repeat doses or infusions might be dangerous if clearance of the drug is delayed.

Preoperative

1. Use smaller doses of drugs than for "healthy" patients.
2. Do not discontinue antihypertensive drugs.
3. Premedicate when required, using one-third to one-half the standard dose of sedative (e.g., midazolam by mouth or intravenously).
4. Check all medications that have been given and note their last dose before surgery.
5. Check the location of a shunt or fistula. Avoid any pressure to this area, and monitor function with a Doppler flowmeter.
6. Ensure that all supportive drugs are available in the operating room.
7. Ensure that adequate supplies of blood and other fluids are available (including washed cells if and when indicated).

Perioperative

1. Give 100% O_2 by mask.
2. Apply monitors:
   a. Precordial stethoscope
   b. Electrocardiogram and pulse oximeter
   c. Automated blood pressure—do not use a limb with a shunt or fistula
3. Ensure that the limb with the shunt or fistula is easily accessible. Monitor function continually throughout the procedure.
4. Induce anesthesia with thiopental 2–3 mg/kg (more may be required), followed by N_2O/O_2 + sevoflurane or halothane.
5. For intubation:
   a. Do not give succinylcholine unless the serum K^+ concentration is less than 5.5 mEq/L—and always pretreat with curare (0.05 mg/kg). Always limit succinylcholine to a single dose.
   b. Otherwise give atracurium or vecuronium for intubation.

6. Maintain anesthesia with N_2O/O_2 and isoflurane with atracurium or vecuronium.
7. Control the ventilation in all procedures that last longer than 15 minutes. Use moderate hyperventilation to compensate for metabolic acidosis and to encourage K^+ movement back into the cells. In general it is advised to control ventilation to maintain the arterial carbon dioxide pressure ($PaCO_2$) at the usual level for that particular patient.
8. Administer fluids to ensure adequate blood volume for satisfactory BP, good peripheral perfusion, and function of an AV fistula or shunt.
   a. Give intravenous fluids to replace the preoperative deficit and for perioperative maintenance.
   b. For small blood losses, replace with maintenance solution.
   c. For significant blood losses, replace with washed RBCs and salt-poor albumin.
      i. Check Hb and hematocrit (Hct); keep Hct below 30%.
      ii. Avoid overtransfusion.
9. Reverse muscle relaxants at end of surgery.

Postoperative

1. Ensure good ventilation and oxygenation.
2. Order analgesics in one-third to one-half the usual doses; monitor the effect and give supplements if necessary.
3. Ensure that the shunt or fistula is functioning; record this fact.
4. Check Hb, Hct, electrolytes, and blood gases.
5. Consult a nephrologist for continuing care.

RENAL TRANSPLANTATION

Transplantation offers the chance of a relatively normal life for the child with chronic renal failure. Organs for transplantation are in very limited supply. The anesthesiologist, by paying careful attention to the details of intraoperative management, can make a real difference in the probability that the graft will survive. An aggressive approach to attaining conditions that optimize graft survival should be taken.

Anesthesia Management

Preoperative

1. General management is the same as for patients in renal failure.
2. Discuss with the nephrologist and urologist to ascertain the patient's exact present status (state of hydration, electrolyte and acid-base status, renal function, cardiopulmonary state).
3. If the patient is not in optimal condition (e.g., volume overload), surgery should be postponed until after dialysis. The basic objective is to implant the kidney within 24 hours.
4. Review the immunosuppressive therapy plan for the child (e.g., drug dosage, timing). A typical plan includes administration of

cyclosporin, methylprednisolone succinate (Solu-Medrol), and azathioprine; an antibiotic is also given.

The Donor Kidney

1. If the kidney has already been removed from the donor, it will arrive in the operating room perfused or cooled and ready for implantation.
2. If the donor is brought to the operating room for removal of a kidney:
   a. In the case of a "brain-dead" donor, maintain full respiratory and cardiovascular support to ensure good urinary output until the kidneys have been removed.
   b. Ensure that preservation of the kidney (cooling, perfusion) is started immediately and continued until implantation into the recipient.

Perioperative

1. General management is the same as for patients in renal failure.
2. After induction of anesthesia:
   a. Insert a central venous line.
   b. Check its position with a pressure tracing and/or radiograph.
   c. Maintain the central venous pressure (CVP) at an acceptably high level to ensure diuresis (8–12 mmHg). Normal saline is the preferred initial maintenance fluid. (Compare lactated Ringer's solution, which contains K^+.)
   d. The objective is to adequately replace any existing deficit and ongoing losses. This may require infusions at four to five times normal maintenance rates (i.e., at 10–20 ml/kg/hr).
3. Insert an arterial line (to monitor blood gases, Hb, Hct, and electrolytes):
   a. If an external (Scribner) shunt is available, the arterial end may be used for monitoring and the venous end as an infusion route. (Use very careful aseptic technique.)
   b. Do not interfere with a subcutaneous fistula—insert an arterial line in the other arm.
   c. If a new radial artery catheter is inserted, do not use a cannula larger than a 22 gauge, and arrange to have the catheter removed as soon as possible postoperatively. The artery should then be available if required in the future for a shunt or AV fistula.
4. Transfuse with packed RBCs to obtain an Hct value in the 35%–40% range at the end of the operation. Patients with chronic renal failure tend to lose third-space fluid extensively; a higher Hct and colloid administration may limit this effect and improve graft perfusion.
5. During vascular anastomosis and before clamp release, give 1 mg/kg of furosemide and 1 g/kg of mannitol. Anticipate a decline in

blood pressure as the clamps are removed, and prepare for fluid infusions.

6. Increase the blood pressure to 140 mmHg systolic, if possible, as the clamps are removed. Lighten anesthesia and use dopamine 5 μg/kg/min if necessary. A high pressure at this time increases the perfusion of the graft and improves the chances for early good function and graft survival.

7. The solution used to preserve the kidney has a high potassium level; hyperkalemia and acidosis after release of the clamps has on rare occasions resulted in cardiac arrest. This may be a greater danger in small patients.

8. Placement of a large adult kidney in a small infant introduces some problems. The kidney should be well flushed by the surgeon before it is implanted. Blood must be rapidly infused as the clamps are released in order to fill the vascular space of the graft. The CVP should be raised to 15–20 mmHg in anticipation of unclamping. The danger of hyperkalemia (due to preservative fluid) and acidosis (due to clamping of the aorta or iliac artery) is increased. Check acid-base status and give calcium chloride and sodium bicarbonate as necessary.

9. Maintain the CVP at a level that produces a good urine output (i.e., up to 15–18 mmHg). If the CVP is adequate but urine flow is still low:
   a. Give furosemide 2–4 mg/kg IV.
   b. If necessary, add 20% mannitol 1 g/kg.

10. Anticipate the need to infuse large volumes of fluid (three to five times the normal) to compensate for third-space losses.

11. At the end of surgery, determine serum electrolytes:
   a. If urine output is adequate, serum K^+ should be within the normal range.
   b. If the serum K^+ is greater than 6 mEq/L and urine output is poor, continue to hyperventilate the patient and plan to arrange for dialysis or therapy with glucose and insulin.

12. With such an aggressive approach to fluid management, pulmonary edema may threaten. In such cases, continue with controlled ventilation into the postoperative period.

Postoperative

1. General management is the same as for patients in renal failure.

2. The pulmonary status of all patients should be monitored by pulse oximetry, blood gases, and periodic chest radiography. Small infants with large implanted kidneys may be predisposed to pulmonary complications (especially atelectasis). This may be a combined result of the abdominal surgery, the mass of the implanted kidney, and aggressive fluid therapy. The need to "push fluids" to ensure diuresis may result in pulmonary edema; occasionally treatment may be required.

3. Renal function in the transplanted kidney is as follows:
   a. Glomerular function is initially normal but falls during the first

48 hours as the kidney swells. Increased intravenous fluids are required to maintain diuresis at that time.

b. Some degree of tubular damage is always present. Diuresis and loss of sodium result, and replacement of sodium and water is required. Other electrolytes must be infused as indicated by serum studies.

c. Declining urine flow after 48 hours despite fluid loading is indicative of mechanical problems (vascular) or rejection of the transplant.

4. Hypoglycemia has been described as a late complication after renal transplantation in small children. This may have been associated with the use of β-blocking drugs.

Suggested Additional Reading

Beebe DS, Belani KG, and Mergens P, et al.: Anesthesia management of infants receiving an adult kidney transplant. Anesth Analg 73:725–730, 1991.

Don HF, Dieppa RA, and Taylor P: Narcotic analgesics in anuric patients. Anesthesiology 42:745, 1975.

Geha DG, Blitt DC, and Moon BJ: Prolonged neuromuscular blockade with pancuronium in the presence of acute renal failure: a case report. Anesth Analg 55:343, 1976.

Ghoneim MM and Pandya H: Plasma protein binding of thiopental in patients with impaired renal or hepatic function. Anesthesiology 42:545, 1975.

Gradus D and Ettenger RB: Renal transplantation in children. Pediatr Clin North Am 29:1013, 1982.

Hunter JM, Jones RS, and Utting JE: Use of atracurium in patients with no renal function. Br J Anaesth 54:1251, 1982.

Koide M and Waud BE: Serum potassium concentrations after succinylcholine in patients with renal failure. Anesthesiology 36:142, 1972.

Miller RD, Way WL, Hamilton WK, and Layzer RB: Succinylcholine-induced hyperkalemia in patients with renal failure? Anesthesiology 36:138, 1972.

Chapter 17

Trauma, Including Acute Burns and Scalds

Children are commonly involved in accidents; trauma is the leading cause of death between the ages of 1 and 14 years. Even if the injury is relatively minor, some patients require emergency anesthesia, the potential dangers of which may overshadow the injury.

Most children injured in accidents were previously healthy. Therefore, considerations of past health are usually less significant in them than in an adult. However, a complete medical history must be obtained as soon as possible.

From the time of arrival of the child with major trauma in the emergency department, the anesthesiologist must be included in the treatment team. The anesthesiologist can contribute to immediate care while evaluating the patient's condition for anesthesia and the need for further continuing care.

MAJOR TRAUMA

Diagnosis and treatment must proceed rapidly and simultaneously. Vigorous resuscitative measures must be continued without interruption during anesthesia. The common major problems for the anesthesiologist are

1. To secure and maintain a safe, reliable airway and to optimize ventilation
2. To achieve adequate blood and fluid replacement
3. To maintain body temperature

N.B. Injuries are often multiple. Although injuries may appear to be limited to a single anatomic site or body system, the possibility of serious injuries elsewhere must constantly be kept in mind. The fractured femur may be the obvious injury, but the as yet undiagnosed ruptured liver could be the greater threat to life.

Initial Urgent Procedures

1. Ensure a safe and protected airway, and optimize ventilation and oxygenation.
2. The cardiovascular status must be determined:
   a. If hypovolemia is present, it must be corrected.
   b. Effective cardiac action must be maintained or restored.
3. Blood is withdrawn without delay for typing and cross-matching. The blood bank should be advised immediately if massive transfusion is likely to be necessary.

Establishing the Airway

Airway obstruction is common in head and facial injuries and can have a disastrous effect on the outcome.

1. All children with head injury should be given oxygen by mask immediately on admission.
2. For patients with depressed consciousness, if simple positioning does not provide a clear airway, perform endotracheal intubation without delay.
3. Do not use an oropharyngeal airway for unconscious patients. It has more resistance to ventilation than an endotracheal tube and does not protect against aspiration of gastric contents. Indeed, if the patient can tolerate an oropharyngeal airway, an endotracheal tube is indicated.
4. If injury of the cervical spine is suspected, do not move the child's neck. Immobilize the neck with the use of sandbags, a plaster shell, or a bean bag.* Note that cervical spine injury may occur without any radiologic evidence. Optimal airway management must be the

---

*Vac-Pac surgical positioning system, VenTech Healthcare Inc., Toronto, Canada.

first priority, but caution concerning cervical spine injury is required.

5. Be alert to the possibility of foreign bodies (e.g., teeth, bone fragments) in the mouth, pharynx, or trachea, especially if there are facial injuries.

6. "Awake" laryngoscopy and intubation causes a marked increase in intracranial pressure (ICP), which may be detrimental in the head-injured child. Such children should preferably be given intravenous lidocaine 1–2 mg/kg, thiopentone 5 mg/kg, atropine 0.02 mg/kg, and succinylcholine 1–2 mg/kg before intubation. This procedure cannot, however, be safely followed if the patient is also hypovolemic; in such instances, either ketamine should be substituted for thiopental or intravenous lidocaine alone should be given. All trauma patients must be assumed to have a full stomach, and cricoid pressure should be used to prevent regurgitation during induction. Succinylcholine does not increase intragastric pressure in young children and therefore does not increase the risk of regurgitation. Succinylcholine increases ICP only insignificantly, and the advantages of rapidly securing a safe and clear airway and instituting controlled hyperventilation are considered to be more important.

7. Vomiting and aspiration commonly occur after an accident. Immediately after intubation, check air entry to all lung regions and suction via the endotracheal tube if necessary. Examine chest radiographs for endotracheal tube position and evidence of pathology.

8. A gastric tube should be passed in all children to decompress the stomach, especially in those with chest or abdominal injuries, in whom acute gastric dilation is common. Even children with relatively minor injuries may swallow enough air to cause significant gastric distention that interferes with ventilation and predisposes to vomiting and aspiration. Do not pass a tube through the nose in children who may have a basal skull fracture.

9. Be alert to the possibility of pneumothorax or hemothorax.

Intravenous Therapy

Large-bore intravenous lines must be established. These must be placed in the upper limbs or neck in children with injuries at the level of the thorax and below, because flow through the inferior vena cava may be (or may become) compromised. *All intravenous fluids should be warmed to 37°C.*

Percutaneous cannulation of large veins, using at least 20-gauge cannulas, is preferable. Alternatively, a cutdown or an intraosseous needle may be required. Those with much experience and skill in placing internal jugular or subclavian lines may insert these immediately if no other routes are available; beware, however, of the possibility of compounding the problems if a pneumothorax or hemothorax results! A central venous catheter will be useful during the further management of the patient, but it may be inserted after the initial acute fluid resuscitation.

Clues to blood volume status are as follows:

1. Cardiovascular indices:
   a. Tachycardia suggests hypovolemia in patients of all ages. A heart rate in excess of 140 beats/min in infants or 100 beats/min in older children is suggestive.
   b. In infants, the systolic blood pressure (BP) varies in parallel with the intravascular volume and is a very good guide to volume status.
   c. In older children, as in adults, hypovolemia stimulates early constriction of venous capacitance vessels. Therefore, the systolic BP may remain near normal, despite a loss of up to 20% of the blood volume. The central venous pressure (CVP) may also be maintained initially. When such vasoconstriction can no longer compensate and maintain the venous return to the heart, rapid decompensation may occur. At this point the CVP falls and becomes a more reliable guide to the adequacy of replacement of the blood volume.
2. General appearance: Pallor, mottling, sweating, and coolness of the skin, especially over the extremities, are signs of hypovolemia. The latter can be quantified by simultaneous measurement of skin and body core temperatures: a large difference indicates vasoconstriction, and lessening of the difference indicates improving skin perfusion as blood volume increases toward normal.
3. Confusion and irrational behavior are common signs of hypovolemia in children.
4. Urine output: The severely injured child should be catheterized and the urine output should be monitored. A urine flow of more than 1 ml/kg/hr indicates adequate renal perfusion and may indicate adequate volume replacement.
5. Biochemical studies: Metabolic acidosis (lactic acidosis) may result from impaired organ perfusion and is a confirmatory sign of a low circulating blood volume. This acidosis may be corrected by adequate volume replacement. Sodium bicarbonate administration is not recommended except for severe acidosis that may compromise cardiac action (e.g., pH less than 7.2 despite normocapnia or hypocapnia).

Selection of Fluids for Infusion

The types of fluid given depend on (1) what is indicated and (2) what is available.

Frequently, initial replacement is necessarily with fluids other than blood. If at all possible, do not transfuse non–cross-matched universal donor blood. (A rapid cross-match can be performed in 20 minutes.) If blood loss is massive, consider the possibility of autotransfusion.

A balanced salt solution (e.g., lactated Ringer's solution) can be used initially to expand the circulating blood volume, but, if used to excess (more than 100 ml/kg), it may contribute to pulmonary insufficiency later. An initial rapid infusion of 20 ml/kg is appropriate for the hypotensive patient and may have to be repeated.

Other plasma substitutes may be used (e.g., dextran 70, pentastarch). Note that dextrans may impair coagulability and interfere with cross-matching: do not exceed 7 ml/kg. Pentastarch does not impair coagulation, and it may be used in volumes up to 25 ml/kg.

Dextrose-containing solutions should not be given (except, very rarely, to treat documented hypoglycemia); hyperglycemia may occur and may increase the extent of neurologic damage should cerebral hypoxia/ischemia occur.

Expansion of the blood volume with albumin may be very effective in the immediate treatment of hypovolemic shock, but there is a concern that, if large quantities of infused albumin are given, some may "leak" into the lungs and lead to impaired pulmonary function later.

Indications for Blood Transfusion

It is seldom possible to measure the volume of blood lost after trauma. Large amounts may be lost from the intravascular volume but remain within hematomas (e.g., after fracture of the femur) or body cavities. Volume replacement must therefore be judged on the basis of the clues listed previously. I recommend that the fluid replacement be sufficient to correct clinical signs of hypovolemia and that blood be given in volumes sufficient to maintain the hematocrit (Hct) at 30% or higher.

The young child who is showing obvious signs of hypovolemia (pallor, sweating, hypotension) must be assumed to have lost at least 25% of the blood volume. Estimate the weight of the child and assume the normal blood volume to be 70–80 ml/kg; 25% of this total is the initial volume to be replaced rapidly. The situation can then be reassessed. The need for continuous infusion to maintain the BP, or deterioration after an apparently stable period, indicates persistent bleeding.

Children who have lost large volumes of blood require transfusion of whole blood. The trend toward blood component therapy has made it difficult to obtain whole blood. Packed cells resuspended in plasma (preferably recently thawed fresh-frozen plasma) must be substituted.

Massive Blood Transfusion

Loss of an amount of blood that would be negligible in an adult (500 ml) may constitute a major loss in a child. Therefore, massive blood transfusion is required for many severely injured children. For example, after thoracoabdominal injury, it may be necessary to replace more than 250% of the estimated blood volume.

Serious problems may be expected after the rapid infusion of 150% of the estimated blood volume (i.e., transfusion of 120 ml/kg). These problems include

1. Hypothermia and accompanying cardiac arrhythmias. Warm all blood and fluids to 40°C.
2. Coagulation problems

    a. Thrombocytopenia and impaired platelet function
       i. Check platelet count after each 50% blood volume replacement.
      ii. If the platelet count is lower than 100,000/mm^3, order platelet concentrates (1 unit/5 kg).
    b. Deficiency of coagulation factors
       i. Measure prothrombin time (PT) and partial thromboplastin time (PTT) or International Normalized Ratio.
      ii. If these times are prolonged, give recently thawed fresh-frozen plasma (20 ml/kg).
    c. Disseminated intravascular coagulation (DIC).
       i. Bleeding increases at all sites (e.g., old venipuncture sites).
      ii. Measure PT, PTT, clot lysis time, fibrinogen, and fibrin split product levels.
     iii. Prolonged PT and PTT, low fibrinogen level, and presence of fibrin split products suggest DIC.
     iv. If DIC is suspected, enlist the aid of a hematologist if possible. Treatment must include removal of the cause (e.g., correction of hypovolemic shock), replacement of coagulation factors, and possibly heparinization.
3. Acidosis
    a. Check acid-base determinations frequently.
    b. Correct metabolic acidosis with sodium bicarbonate.
4. Citrate toxicity (due to infusion of citrated blood or plasma)
    a. May cause more problems in infants and small children than in adults.
    b. Results in hypotension that persists despite adequate volume replacement. Remember that fresh-frozen plasma and platelet suspensions contain more citrate per unit volume than whole blood does.
    c. May be diagnosed by measuring the ionized Ca^{++} concentration or clinically by observing a prolonged rate-corrected Q-T interval on the electrocardiogram (ECG). But, in practice, if hypotension appears unresponsive to volume replacement, a therapeutic test using intravenous calcium chloride (10 mg/kg) is justified.
    d. Correct by administering 10% calcium chloride 10–30 mg/kg slowly under ECG control.
5. Serum potassium disturbances: Monitor serum K^+ levels periodically. Contrary to expectation, hypokalemia may sometimes be found after massive transfusion. However, serious hyperkalemia may also occur, especially in the presence of a low cardiac output, and may lead to serious cardiac arrhythmias. The effects of hyperkalemia may be treated acutely by slow administration of intravenous calcium chloride 10–30 mg/kg, sodium bicarbonate 1–2 mmol/kg, and hyperventilation.
6. Post-traumatic pulmonary insufficiency. This is characterized by falling compliance, impaired gas exchange, and radiographic findings of diffuse infiltrates. The following factors may contribute:
    a. Too liberal use of clear fluids and/or albumin
       i. Give diuretics (furosemide 1 mg/kg) if indicated.

   b. Microembolization of the pulmonary vessels by infused
     particulate matter (platelet or leukocyte clumps)
      i. Filter all blood given through a micropore (20–40 μm) filter.
   c. Damage to alveolar-capillary membrane
      i. This results in low-pressure pulmonary edema.
      ii. Large doses of steroids may help to prevent it.

Autotransfusion

Autotransfusion can be life-saving for some trauma patients. Advantages
are the ready availability of absolutely compatible warm blood and the
possible prevention of some coagulation problems. In the extreme emergency, autotransfusion can be performed using only a large syringe and
an in-line filter in the intravenous line. A collection of freshly shed
uncontaminated blood in an accessible body cavity (e.g., the pleural
cavity) is the main requirement.

Head Injury

Head injury is extremely common during childhood, and it is a cause of
very significant mortality and morbidity, much of which might be reduced by early and efficient medical intervention. Children with head
injury are less likely than adults to develop a mass lesion but are more
likely to develop intracranial hypertension, secondary to diffuse hyper-
emia and edema. Early aggressive treatment to ensure oxygenation and
to control ICP and cerebral perfusion pressure (CPP) and prevent a
secondary brain insult is essential if optimal recovery is to be obtained.

If consciousness is depressed, airway obstruction is very common and
seriously compromises the prognosis. The first priority of the anesthesiologist must be to ensure an absolutely clear airway, excellent oxygenation,
and optimal ventilation. Therefore, in serious head injury:

1. Give oxygen and intubate the patient without delay; use an oral
   tube. Nasal tubes (and nasogastric tubes) are contraindicated in
   patients with fractures of the base of the skull; perforation of the
   cribriform plate may occur.
2. Apply controlled ventilation to produce normocapnia—ending
   further evaluation of the patient's injuries. Aggressive
   hyperventilation should be avoided because it may precipitate
   cerebral ischemia.
3. Continue anesthesia (if required) with nitrous oxide (N_2O), oxygen
   (O_2), fentanyl, and relaxant drugs. Avoid sufentanil, which increases
   ICP in head-injured patients.
4. Stabilize the hemodynamic state to ensure an optimal CPP. Glucose-
   free, isotonic fluids should be infused.

The use of computed tomography and magnetic resonance imaging
permits accurate anatomic mapping of traumatic lesions and removes
the need for exploratory burr holes. The characteristic appearance of
diffuse cerebral damage on the scan can obviate the need for craniotomy

and permit early specific monitoring and therapeutic measures, such as the following:

1. Intracranial pressure monitoring—most commonly with the use of an extradural bolt connected to an external transducer
2. Jugular bulb oxygen saturation and cerebral oxygen extraction monitoring via a retrograde venous catheter
3. Treatment to control ICP:
   a. Optimal positioning, 35°–45° head-up and face central
   b. Diuretics—mannitol and/or furosemide
   c. Hypertonic saline infusions
   d. Barbiturates (thiopental 2–4 mg/kg), which may be more effective in controlling ICP in children than in adults and may also be useful to control seizures
   e. Controlled ventilation, preferably adjusted on the basis of measurements of ICP, CPP, and cerebral metabolic rate for oxygen ($CMRO_2$). Excessive hyperventilation may be detrimental.
4. Maintenance of optimal CPP (more than 70 mmHg), hemoglobin level, and arterial oxygenation: Glucose-free isotonic or hypertonic fluids should be used for volume expansion. Dopamine may be required to treat hypotension (but see caution, *below*). Hyperglycemia should be avoided because it may exacerbate secondary brain injury.
5. Control of seizure activity, as evidenced by electroencephalographic monitoring
6. Control of body temperature: Prevent hyperthermia; mild hypothermia may be beneficial.

N.B. Head injuries do not normally cause shock. When anesthetizing or caring for the child with a head injury, be alert for evidence of other injuries. Do not ascribe signs of hypovolemic shock (e.g., tachycardia, hypotension) to the head injury. If such signs are present, an exhaustive search must be made for bleeding from wounds in the scalp and/or other sites (intra-abdominal, intrathoracic, or in the limbs). Be constantly aware that hemorrhage at another site may have been overlooked. While anesthetizing a patient for emergency neurosurgery, monitor the cardiovascular system closely and continue measurements (e.g., abdominal girth) to detect hemorrhage.

Cervical Spine Injury

It was previously thought that cervical spine injury was rare in pediatric trauma patients. This was probably incorrect; it is now recognized that spinal cord injury without radiologic abnormality (SCIWORA) may occur. This means that many such injuries may have been overlooked in the past.

A pattern of high cervical spine injury occurs in children, often as a result of motor vehicle accidents. This is in contrast to the involvement of the lower cervical and upper thoracic spine in older patients. Severe high cervical spinal cord injury may result in apnea and cardiac arrest, and such children may be admitted to the hospital with absent vital signs.

The concern for the anesthesiologist is to achieve rapid, safe intubation of the injured child but to avoid causing injury to the spinal cord. Early relief of an obstructed airway and controlled hyperventilation are essential for optimal recovery from severe head injury. Current opinion suggests that some children may experience immediate damage to the spinal cord at the time of their accident; the outcome from such established injuries will not be altered by the technique of intubation chosen.

Techniques of intubation other than by direct vision are more difficult in children, and it has been demonstrated that careful direct oral intubation can be performed without causing damage to the cord. Hence, it is recommended that careful direct laryngoscopy and intubation be performed in injured children. Unnecessary head and neck movement should be avoided by using gentle manual in-line stabilization. Appropriate steps to prevent aspiration should be taken.

Thoracoabdominal Injury

Blunt abdominal trauma is most commonly managed conservatively in children. Bleeding from the spleen or liver can be assessed by scanning techniques and usually resolves spontaneously; blood transfusion requirements are not increased beyond those for operation. Operation is necessary for penetrating wounds and if continued excessive bleeding causes hemodynamic instability.

During initial assessment of the child with thoracoabdominal trauma, one must consider possible physiologic consequences of the injury and the additional effect of anesthesia on the patient's condition. In patients with intra-abdominal injuries, the anesthesiologist's prime concerns are the amount of blood lost and the problem of securing a safe endotracheal airway.

Special Anesthesia Problems

1. Major hemorrhage requiring massive blood transfusion
2. The possibility of a full stomach (food or blood)
3. Impaired cardiorespiratory function (in patients with diaphragmatic or thoracic trauma)

Immediate Management

1. Prepare for transfusion:
   a. Insert a wide-bore plastic cannula into an upper limb or neck vein, by cutdown if necessary.
   b. Send a blood sample for typing and cross-matching.
   c. Insert a central venous cannula via a second upper limb or neck vein for measurement of CVP and to provide an alternative route for transfusion if necessary.
2. Assess the extent of hypovolemic shock.
3. Infuse appropriate solutions with the use of a blood warmer.
4. Never infuse large volumes of cold fluids via a central vein.

Anesthesia Management

During anesthesia, the anesthesiologist is responsible for continuing vigorous blood volume replacement and other resuscitative measures.

Preoperative

1. Before induction, make every effort to restore the blood volume to near-normal levels. (This may not be possible until the source of bleeding has been controlled surgically.)
2. Order adequate supplies of blood for transfusion and have them immediately available in the operating room (OR).
3. Premedication usually is not required.
4. If the patient is hypovolemic, give any necessary drugs in minimal dose, slowly, and only by the intravenous route.

Perioperative

Induction

1. Prepare and check all necessary equipment and drugs.
2. In the OR, reexamine the patient rapidly to ascertain the exact current status.
3. Give 100% O_2 by mask for at least 4 minutes.
4. Check intravenous lines.
5. Connect monitoring equipment.
6. Consider the possibility of persisting hypovolemia:
   a. If hypovolemia has been corrected, induce anesthesia intravenously with thiopental (up to 4 mg/kg), atropine (20 μg/kg), and succinylcholine 1–2 mg/kg or rocuronium 1 mg/kg. Inject these agents directly into a wide-bore venous cannula (to avoid the delayed transit through intravenous lines).
   b. If the hypovolemia cannot be corrected and anesthesia is urgently required, give ketamine 2 mg/kg IV in place of thiopental.
7. Position the patient supine and horizontally for intubation (to facilitate rapid insertion of the tube).
8. Do not inflate the lungs before intubation (ventilation may precipitate vomiting). Have an assistant apply cricoid pressure until an endotracheal tube of suitable size is in place and the cuff (if any) is inflated.
9. Do not give any drugs (except atropine and midazolam) to moribund patients before intubation.

Maintenance

1. Give O_2, fentanyl, and a nondepolarizing neuromuscular blocking agent (vecuronium or rocuronium preferred). N_2O may cause distention of air-containing spaces (e.g., bowel, pneumothorax) and should be avoided. Low concentrations of volatile agents may be appropriate.
2. Control the ventilation to produce a near-normal arterial carbon

dioxide tension ($PaCO_2$). If the hypovolemia is still uncorrected, avoid positive end-expiratory pressure and adjust the inspiratory:expiratory ratio to give a low mean intrathoracic pressure. Use a heated humidifier.
3. Monitor ventilation, heart rate and rhythm, temperature, BP, CVP, pulse oximeter, end-tidal carbon dioxide, and urine output.
4. Insert an arterial cannula for direct BP monitoring and for repeated blood sampling for serial determination of the acid-base status, blood gases, Hct, and coagulation studies.
5. Insert a double-lumen CVP line. This provides for monitoring and drug infusions.
6. Maintain body temperature carefully—use a forced air heater (e.g., Bair Hugger).
7. Be alert to the possibility of sudden hypotension as the abdomen is opened in the patient who has intra-abdominal bleeding requiring vigorous fluid resuscitation.

Postoperative

1. In the absence of chest injury or significant impairment of pulmonary function, remove the endotracheal tube after full reversal of relaxant drugs and with the patient awake, responding, and in a lateral position.
2. In the patient who has thoracic injuries or impaired pulmonary function, who remains unconsciousness, or whose condition is otherwise labile, continue ventilatory support and reevaluate later in the intensive care unit.
3. Plan for good postoperative pain relief.

Special Considerations

1. Overt or suspected hepatic injury: Do not give large doses of drugs that are metabolized by the liver (e.g., barbiturates, narcotic analgesics). Substitute those that are excreted relatively unchanged by the lungs or kidneys (e.g., isoflurane or desflurane, pancuronium or rocuronium).
2. Overt or suspected renal injury or likely acute renal failure as a complication of prolonged hypovolemia and hypotension: Do not give drugs that are excreted through the kidneys (e.g., pancuronium).
3. Ruptured diaphragm: Rupture of the diaphragm, as a consequence of blunt abdominal trauma, is more common in children than in adults and may be overlooked, because respiratory distress is usually not severe. This condition requires thoracoabdominal repair.
   a. Insert a gastric tube to decompress the upper gastrointestinal tract.
   b. N_2O is contraindicated if the chest cavity contains a large volume of bowel.
4. Injury to chest wall and lungs:
   a. In young children, the ribs are relatively soft and less likely to

fracture; however, the injury may separate the costochondral junctions, and this, in association with fractures of posterior ribs, may lead to "flail chest." If this results in hypoventilation, intubate the patient and control the ventilation without delay.

b. Trauma to the chest wall is usually accompanied by contusion of underlying lung, even when there are no rib fractures. This results in shunting of blood through damaged lung tissue and the need for O_2 therapy and possibly positive-pressure ventilation to maintain arterial saturation levels.

    i. Pneumothorax, hemothorax, or both may be present. If these are suspected, request insertion of a chest drain with a suitable valve or underwater seal before the patient is anesthetized. Pneumothorax should be suspected in the patient with grunting respiration and may occur without rib fracture in children.

5. Overt or suspected tracheal or bronchial injury:

  a. If there is any evidence to suggest such injury, or if there is subcutaneous emphysema of the face, neck, or chest, bronchoscopy is required to define the extent of damage.

  b. Induce anesthesia with sevoflurane or halothane in O_2 (very smoothly and deeply, avoiding coughing and straining). Maintain spontaneous ventilation and avoid positive pressure, which may increase any air leak. Do not use N_2O. In the case of a penetrating wound, cover the wound with a sterile polyethylene dressing (e.g., Opsite).

  c. Give lidocaine 1.5 mg/kg IV, wait 3 minutes, then perform laryngoscopy and spray the larynx with lidocaine. The bronchoscope may then be inserted.

  d. During bronchoscopy, give halothane in O_2 via the bronchoscope.

  e. If thoracotomy is required and damage is limited to one bronchus, intubate the uninjured main bronchus with a long endotracheal tube. During one-lung ventilation, add O_2 in high concentration.

  f. If a tracheal injury is present, tracheostomy may be required, although immediate surgical repair is sometimes possible. During such repair, the endotracheal tube may be passed almost to the carina. Check bilateral ventilation and allow spontaneous respiration.

6. Injury to the heart and pericardium is rare in children but may occur in association with severe thoracic trauma. Cardiac contusion may result in changes in ventricular function that are detectable by echocardiography and scanning techniques; the ECG usually is not abnormal. The clinical significance of such changes is not yet fully understood.

7. Injuries to the great vessels are less common than in adults, owing to the greater elasticity and mobility of the mediastinal structures. However, rarely, a widened mediastinum indicates the need for immediate exploration.

  a. If cardiac tamponade develops secondary to hemopericardium, induction of anesthesia may be very hazardous, because the fixed low cardiac output cannot compensate for any drug-induced alterations in systemic vascular resistance.

b. In hypotensive patients with hemopericardium, the surgeon should drain the pericardium (under local analgesia) before inducing general anesthesia. If tamponade is less severe, induction with ketamine may be possible. (**Note:** Until the pericardium is open, maintain spontaneous ventilation to augment venous return.)

Suggested Additional Reading

Birch AA Jr, Mitchell GD, Playford GA, and Lang CA: Changes in serum potassium response to succinylcholine following trauma. JAMA 210:490, 1969.

Bricker SWR, McLuckie A, and Nightingale DA: Gastric aspirates after trauma in children. Anaesthesia 44:721–724, 1989.

Bohn D, Armstrong D, Becker L, and Humphries RP: Cervical spine injuries in children. J Trauma 30:463–469, 1990.

Cosentino CM, Luck SR, Barthel MJ, et al.: Transfusion requirements in conservative nonoperative management of blunt splenic and hepatic injuries during childhood. J Pediatr Surg 25:950–954, 1990.

Dykes EH. Paediatric trauma. Br J Anaesth 83:130–138, 1999.

Hamilton Farrell MR, Edmondson L, and Cantrell WDJ: Penetrating tracheal injury in a child. Anaesthesia 43:123–125, 1988.

Ilstad ST, Tollerud DJ, Weiss RG, et al.: Cardiac contusion in pediatric patients with blunt thoracic trauma. J Pediatr Surg 25:287–289, 1990.

Kissoon N, Dreyer J, and Walia M: Pediatric trauma: differences in pathophysiology, injury patterns and treatment compared with adult trauma. Can Med Assoc J 142:27–39, 1990.

Lam WH and Mackersie A: Paediatric head injury: incidence, aetiology and management. Paediatr Anaesth 9:377–385, 1999.

Meyer P, Legros C, and Orliaguet G: Critical care management of neurotrauma in children: new trends and perspectives. Childs Nerv Syst 15:732–739, 1999.

Olsson GK and Hallen B: Pharmacological evacuation of the stomach with metoclopramide. Acta Anaesth Scand 26:417, 1982.

Peclet MH, Newman KD, Eichelberger MR, et al.: Thoracic trauma in children: an indicator of increased mortality. J Pediatr Surg 25:961–966, 1990.

Rasmussen GE, Fiscus MD, and Tobias JD: Perioperative anesthetic management of pediatric trauma. Anesthesiol Clin North Am 17:251–262, 1999.

Salem MR, Wong AY, and Collins VJ: The pediatric patient with a full stomach. Anesthesiology 39:435, 1973.

Sanchez JI and Paidas CN: Childhood trauma: now and in the new millennium. Surg Clin North Am 79:1503–1535, 1999.

Acute Burns and Scalds

Children are often the victims of burns and scalds. Extensive burns have widespread systemic effects: massive fluid shifts occur, plasma protein is lost, and all the major organ systems are affected.

1. The upper airway and lungs may be directly damaged, leading to obstruction secondary to edema, bronchospasm, or sloughed tissue. Later, pulmonary function may be affected by infection (pneumonia) or pulmonary vascular changes.

2. The cardiovascular system is affected by changes in blood volume and also possibly by a circulating myocardial depressant factor.
3. The kidneys are subject to direct damage from myoglobin and hemoglobin, and acute tubular damage may occur as a result of hypovolemia.
4. The liver may be damaged as a result of hypotension, hypoxemia, inhaled toxins, or sepsis.
5. Anemia and thrombocytopenia occur, and a consumptive coagulopathy may develop.
6. Gastric distention, intestinal ileus, and bleeding secondary to stress ulcers may develop.

The anesthesiologist may become involved in the early treatment, consisting of

1. Airway management and fluid resuscitation
2. Fasciotomy
3. Early debridement and grafting

Special Anesthesia Problems

1. Airway and pulmonary involvement, leading to airway obstruction and respiratory failure: Edema of the tissues surrounding the upper airway may occur very rapidly and make intubation extremely difficult. Airway burns must be suspected in all patients involved in enclosed-space fires and whenever singeing of facial hair and/or eyebrows is present.
2. Maintenance of fluid balance and renal function: Several formulas are used to calculate fluid regimens for the burned patient; these are based on the burn area (excluding erythema). The Parkland formula prescribes that 4 ml/kg of lactated Ringer's solution for each 1% of burn area be added to normal maintenance requirements. One-half of this amount is given in the first 8 hours and the other half over the next 16 hours. In practice, fluid therapy should frequently be adjusted as dictated by the clinical and biochemical status of the patient. The urine output is an essential guide.
3. Acute gastric dilation: This commonly occurs and adds to the danger of regurgitation. The stomach should be decompressed, and special care should be taken during induction and emergence from anesthesia.
4. Management of body temperature: Loss of normal skin severely impairs the patient's ability to conserve heat.
5. In patients with extensive burns:
   a. Monitoring may be difficult.
   b. Sites for intravenous infusions may be limited.
6. Possibility of carbon monoxide (CO) and/or other gaseous poisoning (e.g., cyanide) caused by burning plastics: Toxic gases may damage epithelium and result in lower airway obstruction, bronchial and pulmonary edema, and loss of surfactant. Large areas of the airway mucosa may slough and cause obstruction.

7. Circumferential thoracic burns: These may lead to severely compromised ventilation requiring multiple escharotomy to restore chest wall compliance.

8. Danger of infection: Extreme care must be taken to observe strict asepsis with invasive procedures.

Anesthesia Management

Preoperative

1. If the fire occurred in a closed space or involved burning hydrocarbons, suspect respiratory tract burns.
   a. Look for burning around the face (e.g., singed eyebrows).
   b. Assess the airway very carefully. (Patients with airway burns may have considerable swelling of the pharyngeal and laryngeal tissues, making intubation difficult.)
   c. In the child with airway burns, early endotracheal intubation should be performed before massive upper airway edema forms. Tracheostomy is contraindicated because of the very high risk of local infection leading to generalized sepsis and death.

2. Give all patients with extensive burns humidified O_2 by mask. This is especially important if there are signs of possible CO poisoning (impaired consciousness). Severe respiratory impairment dictates immediate intubation and ventilation.

3. Check the blood CO level if indicated. Suspect CO poisoning in the child who has unexplained confusion or coma plus cherry-red discoloration of the mucosa.

4. Check the adequacy of fluid and blood replacement:
   a. The Hct should be greater than 25%–30%, and the serum albumin concentration should be greater than 2 g/dl.
   b. The patient should be catheterized, and urine output should be at least 1 ml/kg/hr.
   c. Fresh-frozen plasma or platelets may be required to correct documented deficiency resulting in coagulopathy.

   Beware of the use of excessive glucose-containing solutions for fluid resuscitation. Hyperosmolar, hyperglycemic nonketotic coma may occur in association with burns.

5. Ensure that the OR temperature is at least 24°C and that heating blankets and lamps are ready for use. Humidify all anesthetic gases. All blood and intravenous fluids should be warmed.

6. Check whether the child has been given narcotic analgesics. (In many cases these are not necessary in the early stages of severe burns.) Analgesics should be given to prevent pain during transportation to the OR.

Perioperative

General endotracheal anesthesia may be required, but remember:

1. The dose requirement for thiopental may be increased by 40% in

children with burns. However, use caution with this drug if the patient's volume status is uncertain; ketamine may be useful in severe burns.

2. Succinylcholine is contraindicated because it may cause cardiac arrest secondary to massive potassium release from muscle.

3. The dose requirements for nondepolarizing muscle relaxant drugs are increased in proportion to the burn area. The drug must be titrated to achieve the desired effect. Reversal of high doses is not a problem.

4. Potent volatile agents may not be tolerated by the patient with extensive burns. However, fentanyl in high doses is usually satisfactory. Alternatively, ketamine has been used to greatly simplify the anesthetic management of burned or scalded children; for example,
    a. Give atropine 0.02 mg/kg IV followed by ketamine 2 mg/kg IV.
    b. Maintain anesthesia with ketamine 8 mg/kg IM or incremental doses of 2 mg/kg IV.

For all patients:

1. Carefully monitor the following:
    a. Cardiac rate—via an esophageal stethoscope and the ECG (peripheral or esophageal leads) plus pulse oximeter. The probe may be placed on the tongue if no other site is available.
    b. BP—if possible, place a BP cuff at any available site; for severe burns, insert an arterial line.
    c. Temperature—esophageal and/or rectal.
    d. Blood loss—it is often difficult to estimate losses. Replacement must then be dictated by cardiovascular parameters and urine output.
    e. CVP—consider necessity versus danger of introducing infection. (If BP can be measured, CVP measurement may be unnecessary.)

2. Replace blood losses carefully; large volumes may be required. Anticipate coagulation problems with massive transfusions.

3. Beware of hypocalcemia. Chronic low levels of ionized calcium have been described in burn patients. Plasma and platelet suspensions contain more citrate per unit volume than whole blood does. Give calcium chloride if unexpected hypotension occurs. If large volumes of blood or plasma are given, give calcium chloride prophylactically (100–150 mg/unit).

Postoperative

1. Order maintenance fluids:
    a. Clear fluids to maintain urine output at more than 1 ml/kg/hr
    b. Blood to maintain Hct at greater than 30%
    c. Plasma to maintain total serum protein at greater than 3 g/dl
    d. Electrolyte supplements as indicated by serial determinations

2. Order analgesics as required. Burn patients should be provided with

constant nursing supervision so that a generous dosage of analgesics can be safely administered.

3. Watch closely for developing respiratory insufficiency. (This may occur during the first 24 hours, even if the chest appears clear initially.) Rhonchi and a falling level of arterial oxygenation are the usual first signs of trouble. In severe airway burns, beware of the possibility of sudden airway obstruction due to sloughed mucosa.

4. Ranitidine and antacids should be administered to protect against stress ulcer. Burn patients may require larger than usual doses to reduce acid secretion.

5. Children with facial burns who have been intubated for a period in the intensive care unit are at high risk for development of postextubation stridor, especially if there was no detectable leak around the tube before extubation. Such children require careful monitoring for 24–48 hours after extubation; treatment with racemic epinephrine, helium O_2, or even reintubation may be required.

Suggested Additional Reading

Belin RP and Karleen CI: Cardiac arrest in the burned patient following succinylcholine administration. Anesthesiology 27:516, 1966.

Charnock EL and Meehan JJ: Postburn respiratory injuries in children. Pediatr Clin North Am 27:661–676, 1980.

Cote CJ and Petkau AJ: Thiopental requirements may be increased in children reanesthetized at least one year after recovery from extensive thermal injury. Anesth Analg 64:1156–1160, 1985.

Hickerson W, Morrell M, and Cicala RS: Glossal pulse oximetry. Anesth Analg 69:73, 1989.

Kemper KJ, Benson MS, and Bishop MJ: Predictors of postextubation stridor in pediatric trauma patients. Crit Care Med 19:352–355, 1991.

Martyn JAJ, Szyfelbein SK, and Ali HH: Increased *d*-tubocurarine requirement following major thermal injury. Anesthesiology 52:352–355, 1980.

Moncrief JA: Burns. N Engl J Med 288:444–454, 1973.

Overton JH and Kilham HA: Aspects of management of the burned child. Anaesth Intensive Care 1:535, 1973.

Peters WJ: Inhalation injury caused by the products of combustion. Can Med Assoc J 125:249–251, 1981.

Raine PA and Azmy A: A review of thermal injuries in young children. J Pediatr Surg 18:21–26, 1983.

Szyfelbein SK, Drop LJ, and Martyn JAJ: Persistent ionized hypocalcemia during resuscitation and recovery phases of body burns. Crit Care Med 9:454–458, 1981.

Tredget EE, Shankowsky HA, and Taerum TV: The role of inhalation injury in burn trauma. Ann Surg 212:720–727, 1990.

Gunshot Wounds

Children frequently become victims of gunshot wounds, especially in the United States. The free access to military-style weapons in the United

States and the wide access that many children have to guns in the home contribute to this toll.

Anesthesiologists should be particularly aware of the tissue damage that is caused by modern high-velocity bullets. Tissue over an extensive area surrounding the path of the bullet is damaged or destroyed by the energy of the projectile. This is of particular importance when such wounds occur in the upper chest or neck region. Tissue swelling can be expected to spread to involve a wide surrounding area, possibly jeopardizing the airway. The airway should be secured as early as possible, before distortion of the anatomy progresses further.

Very aggressive fluid resuscitation (guided by invasive monitoring) is required for any major wound.

MINOR TRAUMA

Children with minor trauma must be provided with anesthesia that is safe, as pleasant as possible, and suitable for a young patient who may be ready to go home in an hour or so. Usually there is no extreme urgency in these cases, permitting a considered approach to the selection of both the anesthetic and the optimal time for surgery. However, fractures with vascular compression may require immediate intervention.

Keep in mind the full stomach: gastric emptying may be considerably delayed after even minor injury. Some children starved for well over 8 hours after an accident still have a large volume of acid stomach contents. A safe period between oral intake, injury, and induction of anesthesia cannot be predicted. Hence, even if one can wait for a full normal fasting period, it is still advisable to use a regional technique or to induce general anesthesia using a rapid-sequence induction with cricoid pressure.

Although metoclopramide (Maxeran) may help to speed gastric emptying, neither regional analgesia nor general anesthesia should be administered without fasting unless surgery is needed urgently. The need to convert unsatisfactory regional anesthesia to general anesthesia arises more frequently in children than in adults.

Limb Fractures

Closed Limb Fractures

Injuries to upper limbs constitute the largest group for emergency anesthesia. Many of these patients are older children; therefore, regional analgesia can be used. If so:

1. Use sufficient local analgesic drug to produce a profound block.
2. Perform the block well in advance of the scheduled surgery so that it has plenty of time to become well established.
3. If supplementary analgesia or sedation is required, midazolam is usually very satisfactory.

Fractures of the Forearm

1. Perform a block of the brachial plexus via the axillary route, using 1% lidocaine (maximum 5 mg/kg).
2. Intravenous blocks are not satisfactory for reduction of fractures. It is more difficult to apply an optimally tight cast to an exsanguinated limb.

Fractures of the Femur

1. A block of the femoral nerve with lidocaine is easy to perform and relieves pain and muscle spasm as traction apparatus is being applied.
2. A catheter may be introduced to the femoral sheath and a continuous femoral nerve block maintained with 0.5% bupivacaine (*see* page 145).

Anesthesia Management When General Anesthesia Is Required

Do not give general anesthesia in an emergency room unless the room is fully equipped and is staffed with nurses experienced in the care of anesthetized patients. An adequately staffed recovery area must also be available.

Every child with a recent fracture must be considered to have a full stomach and should be intubated using a rapid-sequence induction of anesthesia. Vomiting frequently occurs during emergence from anesthesia; therefore, the child should be fully awake and in a lateral position before extubation.

Chapter 18

Remote Anesthesia for Pediatric Patients

REMOTE ANESTHESIA

In recent years there has been an increased demand for the pediatric anesthesiologist to travel outside the operating room to provide general anesthesia or monitored sedation for a variety of medical investigations or procedures in infants and children of all ages. The concept that treatment in a pediatric hospital should be a pain- and stress-free experience for all the patients is now well accepted, and this has placed additional responsibilities on the anesthesia service.

Equipment for the Remote Location

Each area should be fully equipped to provide for the anesthesia care of the patient and for any resuscitation that might be required; much of this may be provided by means of a travel cart. Each area should be provided with

1. Primary and back-up oxygen supply
2. Facilities for gas scavenging if inhalation agents are used
3. Wall suction and suction apparatus
4. Adequate lighting
5. Electrical outlets (operating room standards)
6. Means of immediate communication to the operating room
7. Facilities and staff for preparation and recovery of patients
8. Resuscitation cart and defibrillator (immediately available)

In addition, all drugs and equipment for patient management during the procedure must be provided:

1. Monitoring for pulse oximetry, electrocardiography (ECG), end-tidal carbon dioxide, blood pressure, and body temperature
2. Airway supplies—laryngoscopes, endotracheal tubes, oropharyngeal airways, laryngeal mask airways, and so on
3. Appropriate anesthesia equipment, infusion pumps, etc.
4. Drugs for anesthesia and sedation
5. Emergency resuscitation drugs
6. In addition—where indicated: equipment to maintain body temperature (e.g., Bair Hugger for cardiac catheter laboratory).

Administrative Procedure for Remote Anesthesia

For patients anesthetized in remote locations, the following steps should be taken:
1. A preanesthesia evaluation should be performed and recorded.
2. Informed consent should be obtained.
3. An anesthesia record should be completed.
4. A recovery record should be completed.
5. The patient should be checked by the anesthesiologist when recovered and signed out of the unit.

General Principles

1. The technique chosen should result in minimal (if any) postanesthesia sequelae.
   a. Use short-acting drugs that will not delay recovery and are not associated with postoperative nausea and vomiting. (Therefore, avoid narcotic analgesics, barbiturates, and ketamine.) Propofol is ideal.
   b. Avoid endotracheal intubation if possible. The laryngeal mask airway may be a useful alternative. Many children can be managed with an oxygen mask or nasal prongs.
   c. When repeated anesthetics will be needed, a chronic intravenous line should be maintained—either a central line or a "Hep-Locked" peripheral line.
   d. Monitor every patient as you would in the operating room.

Suggested Additional Reading

Martin LD, Pasternak LR, and Pudimat MA: Total intravenous anesthesia with propofol in pediatric patients outside the operating room. Anesth Analg 74:609–612, 1992.

Roy WL: Anaesthetizing children in remote locations: necessary expeditions or anaesthetic misadventures. Can J Anaesth 43:764–768, 1996.

DIAGNOSTIC AND THERAPEUTIC MEDICAL PROCEDURES

Computed Tomography

1. Computed tomography (CT) scans require absolute immobility of the patient throughout. For this reason, it is often necessary to sedate infants (except the very small), young children, and mentally handicapped patients. Rarely, a general anesthetic may be required. Older children of normal intelligence can cooperate and do not require any form of sedation or anesthetic, and small infants can be bundled and restrained during the procedure.
2. If general anesthesia is required, use only plastic materials in the breathing circuit; metal components distort the image.
3. Intravenous sedation alone is suitable for many patients:
   a. A propofol infusion may be used.
   b. Intravenous pentobarbital is an alternative; an initial dose of 3 mg/kg of pentobarbital may be given. After 3 minutes, further doses of 1 mg/kg may be titrated up to a maximum of 7 mg/kg.
   c. The patient should be monitored with a pulse oximeter, and all equipment required to establish an airway and ventilate the patient should be on hand.
4. Contrast media may be injected intravenously to enhance the images obtained; very rarely, reactions may occur (*see below*).

Magnetic Resonance Imaging

Magnetic resonance imaging (MRI) scans are commonly used to secure accurate anatomic diagnoses, but they may also provide valuable information on the physiologic changes associated with disease. The basic component of the system is a powerful superconducting magnet into which the patient must be placed. This presents some problems:

1. The patient is placed in a very confined space, which is frightening to children, may cause claustrophobia, and also limits access.
2. There may be a high noise level within the magnet (approximately 95 decibels).

Because of these considerations, deep sedation or general anesthesia may be required for infants and children having MRI scans.

3. Ferrous metal objects are attracted to the magnet and become dangerous projectiles.

4. The magnetic field may induce currents in wire leads, cables, and temperature probes used for monitoring, especially if they form loops; this can lead to heat production and burns to the patient.
5. The powerful magnetic field may affect the performance of anesthesia delivery systems; syringe pumps may be unreliable, and vaporizers become inaccurate.
6. MRI is very motion sensitive; if the patient moves at any stage, a whole scan sequence must be repeated.

Monitoring During Magnetic Resonance Imaging Scans

Monitoring during the scan is essential; a plastic precordial or esophageal stethoscope may be used, and equipment that is compatible with the MRI machine has been developed:

1. Pulse oximetry may be used continuously, and various suitable machines are available. For example, the Nonin series 8604D portable machine* may be used, but caution must be taken that there are no loops in the cable leads to the patient—otherwise currents may be induced and the patient may be burned. The Nonin 8600FO* has fiberoptic sensors and cables that contain no magnetic or electrically conductive features, eliminating the possibility of burns in the MRI unit.
2. Blood pressure may be measured with a Dinamap† 1846 SX machine fitted with nylon connections.
3. The ECG may be monitored using the Hewlett-Packard HP 78352A machine‡ with nonferromagnetic fasteners, cables, and electrodes (e.g., NDM 01-5010§). Great care must be taken to avoid looping any leads. An ECG is also available that uses fiberoptic cables, thus eliminating the danger of burns (Magnetic Resonance Equipment Corp—*see below*).
4. Alternatively and more optimally, very satisfactory combined units are available for the MRI suite.
   a. The Omni Trak 3100 MRI vital signs monitoring system‖ provides for continuous monitoring of all of the above parameters.
   b. The Magnetic Resonance Equipment Corporation Model 9500¶ provides for pulse oximetry, ECG, noninvasive blood pressure, invasive pressures, end-tidal carbon dioxide, minimum inspired carbon dioxide, nitrous oxide (N_2O), and inspired and expired anesthetic agent. This incorporates a fiberoptic pulse oximetry and ECG system.

Management for Magnetic Resonance Imaging

Satisfactory immobilization of the child during the scanning process may be achieved by intravenous sedation/anesthesia or general endotracheal

---

*Nonin Medical Inc., Plymouth, MN.
†Criticon Inc., Tampa, FL.
‡Agilent Technologies, Andover, MA.
§NDM Corp., Dayton, OH.
‖Invivo Research, Inc., Orlando, FL.
¶Magnetic Resonance Equipment Corporation. Bay Shore, NY.

anesthesia. The former is suitable for relatively healthy patients; the latter is required for the critically ill child.

Intravenous Sedation/Anesthesia

An intravenous propofol infusion has been demonstrated to be a safe and reliable method.

1. The patient should be fasted as for general anesthesia.
2. Monitors are placed and sedation is initiated with a bolus dose of propofol 2–3 mg/kg followed by an infusion of propofol at a rate of 250 µg/kg/min. The infusion pump should be MRI-compatible (e.g., Medfusion syringe pump #2010*) or be placed as far from the magnet as possible (we have used a 25-foot low-volume line for this purpose†).
3. If the patient moves, an additional bolus of 1 mg/kg of propofol is given.
4. After 15–20 minutes the infusion rate is reduced to 200 µg/kg/min, and after a further 15–20 minutes to a rate of 150 µg/kg/min.
5. A mask or nasal prongs may be used to administer oxygen during the procedure. Samples of expired gas to monitor ventilation by end-tidal carbon dioxide may be obtained from a gently inserted small-diameter nasal catheter.
6. The airway is usually well maintained during propofol sedation, but
   a. If obstruction occurs, reposition the head and place a small bolster under the shoulders and neck.
   b. If obstruction persists, insert an oropharyngeal airway or a laryngeal mask airway.
7. At the end of the scan, the infusion is discontinued; the patient usually recovers fully within 20–30 minutes.

General Anesthesia

General anesthesia with endotracheal intubation and controlled ventilation may be required for more seriously ill patients, especially those with central nervous system disease or multiple injuries. In such patients, a propofol infusion can be combined with a muscle relaxant, endotracheal intubation, and controlled ventilation.

N.B. MRI scans are contraindicated for patients with

1. Cardiac pacemakers
2. Transthoracic or transvenous pacing wires
3. Metal (ferrous) implanted prostheses, wire, or clips
4. Metallic foreign bodies
5. Any other condition in which ferrous metals are essential within or near the patient

---

*Medfusion Inc., Duluth, GA.
†Luer-Lok Microbore extension set (240″); Walrus Medical Inc., Woburn MA.

Equipment

Monitoring equipment can be employed as outlined previously. In addition, if invasive arterial and/or central venous monitoring is to be employed, a long low-compliance extension tubing should be used to connect to transducers, which are placed at a distance from the magnet.

An anesthesia machine and vaporizers built of nonferrous metals and with aluminum gas cylinders are available but expensive (Ohmeda Excel MRI compatible*). Alternatively, the mixture of anesthetic gases can be delivered via a long fresh gas flow line from outside the MRI suite. Vaporizers may deliver unpredictable concentrations if placed within the magnetic field; this is presumed to be a result of effects on the bimetallic strip, an essential component of the temperature-compensating mechanism.

An ultralong Mapleson D anesthetic circuit prepared with rubber and plastic components can be used to deliver anesthetic gases and ventilate the patient. Manual ventilation may be used or, alternatively, the Narco Airshield Ventimeter II ventilator† may be used in the MRI suite. The Siemens 900C ventilator‡ can be readily modified to make it compatible with the MRI Suite.

Once the equipment has been assembled, conduct of anesthesia may be chosen to suit the individual patient. Endotracheal intubation can be performed outside the suite. (Even plastic laryngoscopes may have batteries with ferromagnetic components.) The patient can then be moved into the suite for scanning.

Suggested Additional Reading

Kross J and Drummond JC: Successful use of a Fortec II vaporizer in the MRI suite: a case report with observations regarding magnetic field-induced vaporizer aberrancy. Can J Anaesth 38:1065–1069, 1991.

Patteson SK and Chesney JT: Anesthetic management for magnetic resonance imaging: problems and solutions. Anesth Analg 74:121–128, 1992.

Pope KS: An infusion pump that works in MRI. Anesth Analg 77:645, 1993.

Tobin JR, Spurrier EA, and Wetzel RC: Anaesthesia for critically ill children during magnetic resonance imaging. Br J Anaesth 69:482–486, 1992.

Vangerven M, Van Hemelrijck J, Wouters P, et al.: Light anaesthesia with propofol for paediatric MRI. Anaesthesia 47:706–707, 1992.

Other Radiologic Procedures

General anesthesia is often necessary for arteriography in pediatric patients, because the procedure may be long and uncomfortable and the patient must be immobile.

---

*Ohmeda Inc. Madison, WI.
†Air Shield, Hatboro, PA.
‡Siemens Medical Systems, Inc. Danvers, MA.

Special Anesthesia Problems

1. Intracranial pressure (ICP) may be increased.
2. The radiologic examination may require special positioning and tilting of the patient.
3. It may be difficult to maintain body temperature in infants.
4. Reactions to contrast media may occur; this is now quite rare with the use of nonionic agents.
5. Patients must recover rapidly so that their neurologic status can be checked.

Anesthesia Management

Preoperative

1. Assess the patient's neurologic status carefully.
2. Check for a history of allergy, asthma, or previous reactions to radiologic contrast media.
3. Do not give sedatives or narcotics.

Perioperative

1. An intravenous induction is preferred. Give thiopental (3–5 mg/kg) followed by relaxant.
2. For patients with increased ICP, give lidocaine 1.5 mg/kg IV to attenuate the hypertensive response to laryngoscopy and intubation.
3. Insert an endotracheal tube. A nasal or armored tube should be used if the positioning or movement of the patient might result in kinking of an oral tube.

Cerebral Arteriography

1. If a tumor or arteriovenous malformation is suspected, maintain anesthesia with N_2O and a low concentration of a volatile agent plus a relaxant. Ventilation should be controlled to produce a carbon dioxide partial pressure (PCO_2) of 30 mmHg (confirm by sampling from the arterial catheter). This degree of hypocapnia may improve radiographic definition by constricting the normal vessels while abnormal vessels remain dilated.

   N.B. If an arteriovenous malformation is suspected, preoperative management and induction of anesthesia should be as outlined on page 215.

2. Chart the total volume of contrast medium and flush fluid carefully, especially in small infants. Beware of fluid overload, especially in small infants with arteriovenous malformations.
3. A transient bradycardia with hypotension may occur at the time of injection into the carotid artery owing to baroreceptor activity; atropine prevents this.

Postoperative

1. The patient must be awake before being moved to the postanesthesia care unit. After angiography, it is necessary to

maintain pressure over the catheterization site to prevent hematoma formation; this is easier to achieve if the child is quiet and immobile.
2. Narcotic analgesic drugs usually are not needed; sedation with midazolam reduces restlessness.
3. Check arterial puncture sites frequently; if a limb artery was used, check the circulation to that extremity.

Additional Possible Complications

In addition to the complications that may develop during administration of any anesthetic, some special problems may occur during neuroradiologic procedures.

1. Accidental extubation due to change in position of the patient
2. Hypothermia due to difficulty in keeping blankets and heating lamps in place during frequent changes in the patient's position
3. Acute rise in ICP, leading to coning of the brain stem. In this event:
   a. Hyperventilate the patient.
   b. Request that ventricular tap be performed as soon as possible.
   c. Give an osmotic diuretic (mannitol 2 g/kg or furosemide 0.6 mg/kg) and full doses of atropine to counter bradycardia.
4. Allergic reaction to contrast media. Recently, nonionic contrast media containing iodine have been introduced (e.g., iopamidol [Isovue]). Such agents have much less tendency to trigger adverse reactions. However, such a possibility must always be anticipated, especially in the patient with a history of allergy or asthma.

Reactions to Contrast Media

1. Reactions to intra-arterial contrast media are very rare in pediatric patients. However, the anesthesiologist must be prepared for this possibility.
2. Reactions are more common in patients with a history of asthma or other allergic phenomena.
3. Minor allergic reactions (e.g., skin rashes) may be treated with diphenhydramine 1 mg/kg IM.
4. Major anaphylactic shock (very rare) must be treated aggressively:
   a. Ventilation with oxygen; cardiopulmonary resuscitation as required.
   b. Epinephrine 10 µg/kg IV, followed by an epinephrine infusion 0.05–0.2 µg/kg/min.
   c. Hydrocortisone 10 mg/kg.
   d. Intravenous fluids as necessary to maintain the blood pressure.
5. Contrast media may cause sickling in patients with sickle cell disease.

Suggested Additional Reading

Strain JD: IV administered pentobarbital sodium for sedation in pediatric CT. Radiology 161:105–108, 1986.

RADIATION THERAPY

Infants and small children usually require general anesthesia or sedation to render them immobile for the period of radiotherapy. Treatments may have to be repeated daily or twice daily for many days. Therefore, a technique should be used that minimally interferes with the child's lifestyle and nutrition and causes the least emotional upset.

In the past general inhalation anesthesia was used, but more recently intravenous sedation with propofol has been demonstrated to be very effective.

Many children have a central venous line inserted for the duration of their therapy. Alternatively, an intravenous catheter should be painlessly introduced (using EMLA cream or Ametop) at the first treatment and maintained by the use of a splint and "Hep-lock" connection for use during subsequent sessions.

If the child is positioned and prepared with the parent in attendance, the treatment can sometimes be completed with a single bolus dose of propofol. Alternatively, an infusion should be used.

For radiotherapy to the head region, an immobilization frame that applies suction to the hard palate is commonly used. Surprisingly, this frame maintains the airway extremely well without the need for further interventions.

Monitoring by closed-circuit television and telemetry should be established during the treatments.

Recovery is very rapid after short procedures using propofol, and the child's appetite soon returns.

INVASIVE MEDICAL PROCEDURES

Children who need lumbar puncture, bone marrow aspiration, or other painful procedures should be provided with optimal sedation and analgesia. This is particularly important for the child with a malignant disease who requires repeated sessions; an optimal management plan should be instituted at the outset of treatment. Apart from the use of well-selected sedative and analgesic drugs, there are some other important considerations:

1. The child and the parents must be well prepared for the procedure and know exactly what to expect. Psychological preparation and behavioral training may be of value for the child.
2. The planned procedure should be performed in comfortable, pleasant surroundings. The parents should be encouraged to accompany the child. The area should be provided with oxygen, suction, and emergency equipment to deal with potential complications; this equipment can be discreetly covered but should be immediately available.
3. The procedure should be performed by the most skilled practitioner available. Junior medical staff should not be allowed to practice on these patients.

4. A suitable recovery area should be provided, and the parents should be allowed to remain with the child during awakening.

Suggested Routine

1. Guidelines for "nothing by mouth" (NPO), as used for general anesthesia, should apply.
2. If the child does not have an established intravenous route (e.g., Hickman line), prepare to establish one by placing EMLA cream or Ametop over a suitable vein as soon as the child arrives at the clinic.
3. The child should be fully assessed, and informed consent for the procedure should be obtained.
4. If the child is anxious, oral midazolam 0.5 mg/kg may be administered 20 minutes before the procedure.
5. Hypnosis for the procedure may be provided by intravenous propofol, supplemented, if necessary, by small doses of fentanyl or alfentanil. Frequently, if local analgesics are properly administered, propofol alone is adequate.
6. During the procedure, monitor by pulse oximetry, ECG, noninvasive blood pressure monitor, and precordial stethoscope.
7. Equipment to establish an airway and ventilate the patient should be immediately at hand.
8. Monitor ventilation carefully; when propofol is being used, the patient may be placed in a lateral position, or even prone on bolsters; usually a good clear airway is maintained without the need for intubation. Minor degrees of airway compromise usually can be corrected by insertion of an oropharyngeal airway, which is well tolerated during propofol anesthesia.

Gastrointestinal Endoscopy

Infants and children may require anesthesia during upper or lower endoscopy and for therapeutic procedures such as injection of esophageal varices and percutaneous endoscopic gastrostomy.

Colonoscopy

A propofol infusion usually provides satisfactory anesthesia for lower endoscopy, and, unless a special indication exists, endotracheal intubation is unnecessary. The extent of abdominal distention caused by insufflation of air into the bowel should be monitored. The endoscopist should be encouraged to remove all air possible before terminating the procedure.

Gastroduodenoscopy

Endotracheal intubation is usually recommended for upper endoscopy and therapeutic procedures. Many of these patients have a history of gastroesophageal reflux, and appropriate measures to ensure preoperative fasting, decrease gastric acidity, and rapidly secure the airway should be taken. If injection of varices is planned, a large-bore intravenous line should be inserted. The stomach should be aspirated at the end of the procedure before the endoscope is removed, and the patient should be awake before extubation.

Suggested Additional Reading

Cote CJ: Sedation for the pediatric patient. Pediatr Clin North Am 41:31–58, 1994.

Guidelines for monitoring and management of pediatric patients during and after sedation for diagnostic and therapeutic procedures. Pediatrics 89:1110–1115, 1992.

McFarlan CS, Anderson BJ, and Short TG: The use of propofol infusions in paediatric anaesthesia: a practical guide. Paediatric Anaesthesia 9:209–216, 1999.

Appendix I

Anesthesia Implications of Syndromes and Unusual Disorders*

This appendix contains brief descriptions of most of the syndromes that are commonly encountered in pediatric anesthesia practice and describes important considerations for the anesthesiologist. Many of the syndromes share features that make precise identification difficult, and the reader should consider all the information given in the description. If in doubt, the referenced literature should be consulted before an anesthesia technique is chosen.

There are now 10,000 medical syndromes recorded, so it is inevitable that this list is incomplete. Genetic studies have identified many new syndromes and increased our knowledge of old syndromes. Because the number of syndromes reported has increased and existing syndromes have become better understood, anesthesiologists may experience unreported difficulties and complications. When in doubt as to the identity and implications of a syndrome, the anesthesiologist should make preparations that take into account all possible associated disorders.

There are a number of recurring problems associated with these syndromes that influence the choice of an anesthetic technique, predominantly difficult airway management and the management of cardiac conditions. Cross-references to other chapters and pages in this text provide general advice on their management, which may be adapted to the particular syndrome presented and in accordance with the practice and experience of the anesthesiologist.

Classic descriptions of problems allow the reader to decide when newer drugs and techniques can be used safely in individual cases. Propofol and sevoflurane (see pages 48 and 51) are currently popular for pediatric anesthesia; a difficult airway may be managed by an algorithmic approach with assistance of a laryngeal mask airway or fiberoptic bronchoscopy techniques (see page 88); cardiac assessment and intraoperative management during cardiac surgery may be guided by echocardiography (see page 344), and intraoperative and postoperative pain relief are improved by the use of regional and epidural anesthesia (see page 137).

Invaluable sources of information are the latest editions of textbooks listed under *General Sources of Information*[1–14] at the end of this appendix and the *References* for the individual syndromes listed.[15–232] However, anesthesiologists must constantly bear in mind the possibility of overlap of syndromes and the confusion over their nomenclature.

---

*Adapted from Jones EP, Pelton DA: Can Anaesth Soc J 23:207, 1976 and extensively augmented and revised.

Name	Description	Anesthesia Implications
Achondroplasia[10-15]	Most common form of dwarfism. Defective fibroblastic growth factor (FGFR3) at chromosome 4. Defective bone formation with decreased rate of endochondral ossification leads to shorter tubular bones. Foramen magnum or spinal stenosis may occur. Sleep apnea may be related to brain stem compression. May need suboccipital craniectomy, laminectomy, or CSF shunts.	Intubation may be difficult but usually is not. Endotracheal tube size is best judged by weight (not age). Intravenous access is difficult owing to excess lax skin. High incidence of complications when operated on in the sitting position.
Acrocephalopolysyndactyly	See Carpenter syndrome.	
Acrocephalosyndactyly	See Apert syndrome.	
Adrenogenital syndrome[2, 3]	Inability to synthesize hydrocortisone; virilization of female.	All need hydrocortisone, even if not salt-losing. Check electrolytes preoperatively.[16]
Adrenoleukodystrophy	See Leukodystrophy.	
Alagille syndrome	Disorder of the bile ducts with cholestasis. May have cardiac, musculoskeletal, ocular, facial, and neurologic abnormalities. Variable presentation of an autosomal dominant inherited condition. Severe cases necessitate liver transplantation.	Bilirubin, coagulation profile, and vitamin K level should be checked preoperatively. Hepatosplenomegaly encourages regurgitation; a rapid-sequence induction may be necessary to prevent aspiration. Caution with drugs handled by the liver. Advisability of epidural anesthesia depends on clotting state.[17] **N.B.**
Albers-Schönberg disease[2] (marble bone disease; osteopetrosis)	Brittle bones: pathologic fractures. Anemia from marrow sclerosis; hepatosplenomegaly.	Care in positioning and use of restraints.[6] Limited mobility of joints.
Albright-Butler syndrome	Renal tubular acidosis, hypokalemia, renal calculi.	Renal impairment. Correct electrolytes to within normal limits.[18]

Disease	Description	Considerations
Albright hereditary osteodystrophy[1, 2] (pseudohypoparathyroidism)	Ectopic bone formation, mental retardation. Hypocalcemia: possible ECG conduction defects, neuromuscular problems, convulsions.	Check electrolytes, monitor ECG carefully for conduction defects. Do not use muscle relaxants.[19]
Aldrich syndrome	See Wiskott-Aldrich syndrome.	
Alexander disease	See Leukodystrophy.	
Alport syndrome[2]	Nephritis and nerve deafness; renal pathology variable. Renal failure in second to third decade.	Use caution with drugs excreted by kidneys.[20]
Alström syndrome[2]	Obesity, blindness by 7 years, hearing loss, diabetes after puberty, glomerulosclerosis. Renal impairment.	Diabetes and obesity require special consideration. Use caution with drugs excreted by kidneys.
Amaurotic familial idiocy	See Gangliosidosis GM2 (Tay-Sachs disease).	
Amyotonia congenita[2] (infantile muscular atrophy)	Anterior horn cell degeneration.	Sensitive to thiopental (due to reduced muscle mass) and respiratory depressants. Avoid muscle relaxants.[21-24]
Amyotrophic lateral sclerosis[2, 3]	Degeneration of motor neurons.	Do not use succinylcholine: possible K⁺ release and cardiac arrest. Use minimal doses of thiopental and relaxants; do not use respiratory depressants.[25]
Analbuminemia[2, 3]	Extremely low level of serum albumin (4-100 mg/dl).	Very sensitive to drugs that bind to protein (e.g., thiopental, curare, pancuronium).
Analphalipoproteinemia[2, 3]	See Tangier disease.	
Andersen disease[1-3] (glycogen storage disease type IV)	Deficiency of glucosyl transferase (brancher enzyme). Early severe hepatic cirrhosis; liver failure; splenomegaly; hemorrhagic tendency.	Check coagulation factors; treat excessive bleeding with fresh-frozen plasma. Possibility of hypoglycemia under anesthesia.

Table continued on following page

447

Name	Description	Anesthesia Implications
Anderson syndrome[1]	Severe midfacial hypoplasia → relative mandibular prognathism; abnormal structure and angle of mandible (triangular facies), kyphoscoliosis.	Possible airway problems; intubation may be difficult. Assess respiratory status.
Angioedema[1, 2, 10–14, 26–28] (hereditary angioneurotic edema)	Episodic brawny edema of extremities, face, trunk, airway abdominal viscera, lasts 4 hr to 1 wk. Mutation on chromosome 11 responsible. Onset in childhood differentiates this from idiopathic form. Etiology: (1) Deficiency of C1 esterase inhibitor, reduced to 20% normal levels or (2) normal levels of dysfunctional type of C1 esterase inhibitor. Accumulation of vasoactive substances → increased vascular permeability → edema. Usually painless; may have prodromal focal tingling or "tightness." Often induced by trauma or vibration. May have bouts of abdominal pain, diarrhea; hemoconcentration leading to hypotension, shock, pharyngeal edema (usually develops slowly). Most deaths from laryngeal edema; mortality rate up to 33%.[26] Treatment with anti-fibrinolytic and hormonal agents.	Check complement assay.[26, 27] Hct, fluid status, treatment history, previous drug reactions. Note voice change or dysphasia. *Prophylaxis* (e.g., for dental manipulation): EACA and/or fresh-frozen plasma for 1–3 days preoperatively. Continue EACA IV perioperatively and postoperatively. Danazol (androgen) is useful.[29] *Acute attack:* epinephrine, steroids, antihistamine (in case diagnosis is a true anaphylaxis), fresh-frozen plasma or purified C1 inhibitor. *If pharyngeal edema is imminent or develops:* endotracheal or nasotracheal intubation (leave in place for 24–72 hr); if this is not possible, perform tracheotomy.[26–31] *Anesthesia:* regional when possible. Otherwise, extreme care when instrumenting airway. *Preoperatively and postoperatively:* monitor vital signs closely.
Angio-osteohypertrophy	*See* Klippel-Trénaunay-Weber syndrome.	
Anhidrotic ectodermal dysplasia	*See* Christ-Siemens-Touraine syndrome.	

448

Antley-Bixler syndrome

Recessive condition with bony and cartilaginous abnormalities: craniosynostosis, midface hypoplasia, choanal atresia, and joint contractures. May have cardiac, gastrointestinal, and renal abnormalities. Need major cranial surgery as neonates to relieve craniosynostosis.

Potential respiratory problems and difficult intubation. Care with positioning. Extremity deformities may preclude easy vascular access.[32]

Apert syndrome[1, 2] (acrocephalosyndactyly)

Hypoplastic maxilla and exophthalmos. Craniosynostosis, possibly with increased ICP; mental retardation, syndactyly. CHD may be present.

If CHD is present, use antibiotic prophylaxis preoperatively. Intubation may be difficult.[33, 34] ICP may be increased.

Arachnodactyly

See Marfan syndrome.

Arima syndrome

Malformation of the brain stem with congenital amaurosis and psychomotor retardation. Renal dysfunction or failure due to polycystic kidneys. May also have hepatic failure.

Serum electrolytes should be checked preoperatively for abnormalities associated with chronic renal failure. Hyperkalemia during surgery can produce ECG changes necessitating treatment.[35]

Arthrogryposis multiplex[1, 2]

Multiple congenital contractures, stiffness of joints; CHD in about 10% of cases.

If CHD is present, use antibiotic prophylaxis preoperatively. Minimal thiopental required—muscles replaced by fat. Difficult intubation and airway problem due to limitation of mandibular movement.[36]

Asplenia syndrome[2]

Absent spleen; malposition of abdominal organs. Very complex cardiovascular anomalies; cyanosis and heart failure in many cases. Heightened susceptibility to overwhelming infection.

Antibiotic prophylaxis preoperatively; reverse isolation. Assess cardiovascular status carefully. Do not use cardiac depressants.[6]

Table continued on following page

449

Name	Description	Anesthesia Implications
Ataxia telangiectasia[1-3]	Cerebellar ataxia, skin and conjunctival telangiectasia; decreased serum IgA or IgE. Defective immunity → recurrent pulmonary and sinus infections; bronchiectasis. Severe anemia may be present. RES malignancy in about 10% of cases.[37]	Check Hb and Hct levels and pulmonary function if indicated. Treat anemia. Use antibiotic prophylaxis preoperatively. Use sterile technique (reverse isolation).
Bardet–Biedl syndrome[1, 2]	Mental retardation, pigmentary retinopathy, polydactyly, obesity, hypogenitalism. (Spastic paraplegia, typical in Laurence-Moon syndrome, is absent.) May have renal abnormalities and congenital heart defects.	Assess cardiac, renal, and fluid status.[38] If CHD is present, use antibiotic prophylaxis preoperatively.
Bartter syndrome[39, 40]	Hypokalemic, hypochloremic metabolic alkalosis. Normotensive but hypovolemic. Chloride reabsorption defect with urinary potassium loss. Juxtaglomerular cell hyperplasia, hyperaldosteronism, prostaglandin overproduction.	Check acid-base status: electrolyte abnormalities difficult to correct. Hemodynamic instability; invasive monitoring is recommended. Careful attention to electrolytes and volume status. Regional anaesthesia is suitable.[41]
Beckwith syndrome[1, 2] (Beckwith-Wiedemann syndrome, infantile gigantism)	Rare disease caused by genetic defect with variable inheritance patterns. Birth weight >4,000 g, macroglossia and exophthalmos. Visceromegaly, umbilical hernias and hypoglycaemia are common (see Neonatal hypoglycemia).	Airway problems and difficult intubation due to large tongue. Monitor blood glucose carefully and treat hypoglycemia by slow infusion of dextrose (bolus dose may cause rebound hypoglycemia).[42-45]
Behçet syndrome[46, 47]	Gross ulceration of mouth (usually first sign; may extend to esophagus) and genital area; uveitis, iritis, conjunctivitis, skin lesions, nonerosive arthritis. May have vasculitis, myocardial, and CNS involvement; risk of sepsis at sites of skin punctures, etc.	Use sterile technique. May have history of steroid therapy; nutritional status may be very poor. Intubation may be very difficult due to scarring in pharynx.[46, 47]

Binder syndrome[48]	Maxillonasal dysplasia; if severe, may be corrected surgically.	Advancement of maxilla and wiring of maxilla and mandible may cause airway problems perioperatively and postoperatively.
Blackfan-Diamond syndrome[2]	Congenital idiopathic RBC aplasia. Liver and spleen enlarged: hypersplenism, thrombocytopenia.	Do coagulation studies preoperatively; treat anemia and have platelets available for transfusion if necessary. Give additional steroids.[38]
Bland-White-Garland syndrome	Coronary artery malformation with left coronary arising from the pulmonary trunk. Myocardial ischemia leading to acute heart failure. Lethal if not corrected early.	Anesthesia as for coronary artery disease patients.[50]
Bowen syndrome	See Cerebrohepatorenal syndrome.	
Canavan disease	See Leukodystrophy.	
Cantrell pentalogy	Defect in the recti muscles of the abdominal wall above the umbilicus, agenesis of sternum and diaphragm, pericardial defect and cardiac malformations: cardiac septal and valvular defects present. Prone to develop severe respiratory distress.	Preoperative echocardiography to assess extent of cardiac anomalies. Treat arrythmias. Caudal epidural anesthesia during general anesthesia for noncardiac surgery has been employed successfully.[51]
Capillary angioma with thrombocytopenic purpura syndrome	See Kasabach-Merritt syndrome.	
Cardioauditory syndrome	See Jervell-Lange-Nielsen syndrome.	
Carpenter syndrome[1,2] (acrocephalopolysyndactyly)	Obesity, mental retardation, oxycephaly, peculiar facies, syndactyly, deformed extremities, CHD, hypogenitalism.	If CHD is present, use antibiotic prophylaxis preoperatively. Hypoplastic mandible may make intubation difficult.[33,34] Problems associated with heart disease.

Table continued on following page

451

Name	Description	Anesthesia Implications
Central core disease[2]	Muscular dystrophy; hypotonia without muscle wasting. Increased risk of malignant hyperpyrexia.[52]	Preoperatively, assess respiratory status carefully. Sensitive to thiopental and respiratory depressants: do not use muscle relaxants (postoperative ventilation may be required).[21-24] Do not give drugs that might trigger malignant hyperpyrexia (see page 172).
Cerebrohepatorenal syndrome[1, 2] (Bowen syndrome)	Hepatomegaly, neonatal jaundice, polycystic kidneys, muscular hypotonia. CHD may be present.	If CHD is present, give antibiotic prophylaxis preoperatively. Treat hypoprothrombinemia. Use extreme care with muscle relaxants and other drugs excreted by kidneys.[53]
Charcot-Marie-Tooth syndrome (peroneal muscular atrophy)	Hereditary polyneuropathy. Muscle weakness in legs and arms. Cardiac involvement: arrhythmias, conduction defects, cardiomyopathy.	Avoid succinylcholine: risk of hyperkalemic cardiac arrest. Possible increased risk of malignant hyperthermia. May be resistant to nondepolarizing muscle relaxants.[54]
CHARGE association	An association of coloboma, congenital heart disease, choanal atresia, ear defects, genitourinary abnormalities, and genital hypoplasia.	Difficult airway and intubation, congenital heart disease (prophylactic antibiotics), possible impaired renal function. Difficult intubation especially in older patients.[55]
Chédiak-Higashi syndrome[1-3]	Disorder of neutrophil function. Partial albinism, immunodeficiency, hepatosplenomegaly, recurrent bacterial infections. Neurologic disorders and mental retardation. Steroid therapy and cytotoxic drugs may be given to induce remission.	Use sterile technique (reverse isolation). Use disposable equipment. Repeated pulmonary infections may have impaired pulmonary function. Aggressive therapy to prevent postoperative complications is required. Give supplemental steroids. Thrombocytopenia may require platelet transfusions.[56]

Cherubism[1, 2]	Fibrous dysplasia of mandibles and maxillae with intraoral masses may cause respiratory distress.	Intubation may be extremely difficult; if there is acute respiratory distress, tracheotomy may be required. Profuse bleeding may occur during surgery.[57]
Chondroectodermal dysplasia	*See* Ellis-van Creveld syndrome.	
Chotzen syndrome[1, 2]	Craniosynostosis; associated renal anomalies.	Intubation may be difficult. Renal excretion of drugs may be impaired.[33]
Christ-Siemens-Touraine syndrome[1, 2] (anhidrotic ectodermal dysplasia)	Absence of sweating and tearing. Heat intolerance due to inability to control temperature by sweating. Poor mucus formation → persistent respiratory infections.	Hypoplastic mandible may make intubation difficult; monitor body temperature carefully and be prepared to institute cooling. Tape eyes closed. Use chest physiotherapy preoperatively and postoperatively.[58]
Chronic granulomatous disease[2]	Inherited disorder of leukocyte function: recurrent infections with nonpathogenic organisms; hepatomegaly in 95% of cases.	Poor pulmonary function. Use sterile technique (reverse isolation).[58]
Chubby puffer syndrome	Obesity, upper airway obstruction, daytime somnolence, and respiratory distress when sleeping. May be hyperactive and aggressive. Blood gases may show hypoxemia and hypercapnia. Cor pulmonale may develop.	May present for tonsillectomy. Avoid preoperative sedation. Monitor carefully postoperatively for airway obstruction. Avoid narcotic analgesics. Patients with severe obstruction may require tracheostomy.[59]
Cockayne syndrome	Dysmorphic dwarfism, mental retardation, and premature senescence; patients present in early childhood. Prominent maxillae, large teeth, and sunken eyes. Ataxia, peripheral neuropathy, and flexion contractures. Associated hypertension, arteriosclerosis, and renal disease. Survival beyond second decade is unusual.	Difficult intubation; use of the LMA before fiberoptic intubation is recommended. Subglottic stenosis; may require a small-diameter tube. May be difficult to position. Considerations of associated cardiovascular and renal disease.[60]

Table continued on following page

Name	Description	Anesthesia Implications
Collagen diseases[2] (dermatomyositis; polyarteritis nodosa; rheumatoid arthritis; systemic lupus erythematosus)	Systemic connective tissue diseases with variable systemic involvement. Osteoporosis, fatty infiltration of muscle, anemia, pulmonary infiltration with fibrosis. Renal involvement common. Frequently receiving steroid therapy.	Temporomandibular or cricoarytenoid arthritis may cause airway and intubation difficulties. Risk of fat embolism after osteotomy, fracture, or minor trauma. Supplement steroid therapy.[61, 62]
Congenital heart block	Comprises <1% of congenital heart disease. Defect of conduction between atrioventricular node and bundle of His, or within bundle of His. Supraventricular arrhythmias may occur, and up to 20% progress to congestive heart failure and Adams-Stokes attacks.	Because of possibility of arrhythmia or increased atrioventricular block, preoperative insertion of a temporary transvenous pacemaker is usually recommended.[63, 64]
Conradi syndrome[1, 2] (chondrodysplasia epiphysealis punctata; chondrodysplasia calcificans congenita; koala bear syndrome)	Chondrodystrophy with contractures, saddle nose, macroencephaly or microcephaly, mental retardation; dwarfing, congenital cataracts. CHD and renal anomalies in some other cases.	If CHD is present, use antibiotic prophylaxis preoperatively. Do not use drugs excreted by kidneys; assess cardiac status carefully.[65]
Cori disease	*See* von Gierke disease.	
Cornelia de Lange syndrome[66]	Short stature, microcephaly, mental retardation, hirsute. Short or dysmorphic extremities, hypoplastic nipples, rib and sternal defect. Low hairline, thin lips and downturned ("cod") mouth. Cry is low-pitched growl.	Intubation may be difficult, and airway obstruction develops easily.[67]

Cretinism[2,3] (congenital hypothyroidism)	Goiter; hypothyroidism secondary to defective synthesis of thyroxine. Large tongue. Respiratory center very sensitive to depression; CO_2 retention common. Hypoglycemia, hyponatremia, hypotension, low cardiac output.	Correct hypothyroidism and anemia preoperatively if possible. Airway problems due to large tongue. Monitor body temperature carefully. Use warming blankets if necessary. Do not use myocardial depressants. Transfuse carefully: overtransfusion is poorly tolerated because of myocardial flaccidity.[8]
Cri du chat[1,3]	Chromosome 5p abnormality causing mental retardation, abnormal cat-like cry, microcephaly, round face, hypertelorism. In some, ears abnormal, micrognathia, epiglottis and larynx small. CHD may be present.	If CHD is present, use antibiotic prophylaxis preoperatively. Airway problems: stridor, laryngomalacia. Intubation may be difficult; take care with choice of tube size.[33] Risk of postextubation airway obstruction.[68]
Crouzon syndrome[1,2,10–14]	Craniosynostosis, hypertelorism, parrot beak nose, hypoplastic maxilla, and exophthalmos due to chromosomal bony defect causing premature closure of cranial sutures, and intracranial hypertension.	Eye protection important. Possible difficult intubation.[33] Elective tracheostomy may be indicated.[69]
Cutis laxa[1–3]	Elastic fiber degeneration: pendulous skin, frequent pulmonary infections. Recurrent pulmonary infections, emphysema and cor pulmonale, arterial fragility.	Assess pulmonary status carefully. Use sterile technique. Difficulty maintaining IV line due to poor tissues. Excess soft tissues around larynx may cause respiratory obstruction.[5,70]
Dandy-Walker syndrome	See Hydrocephalus (see page 14).	
Dermatomyositis	See Collagen disease.	

Table continued on following page

Name	Description	Anesthesia Implications
DiGeorge syndrome[1-3, 10-14] (third and fourth brachial arch/ pharyngeal pouch syndrome)	Thymus and parathyroids absent, hypoparathyroidism, low serum Ca, tetany; stridor. Often associated with chromosome 22 defect. Immune deficiency: susceptibility to fungal and viral infections; recurrent chest infections. Treated by thymic transplants. Aortic arch abnormalities.	Use sterile technique (reverse isolation). Donor blood must be previously irradiated (30 Gy) to prevent graft-versus-host reaction. Check calcium levels—Ca^{++} infusion may be required.[71, 72]
Donohue syndrome	See Leprechaunism.	
Down syndrome[1-3, 10-14] (trisomy 21 syndrome, mongolism)	Most common congenital abnormality. Short stature, epicanthal folds, macroglossia, varying degree of mental retardation (and may surprise you!), hypotonia. Hypothyroidism common. Frequently have duodenal atresia and CHD (60%). Atlanto-occipital instability.	Large tongue and small mouth, possible difficult intubation.[73, 74] Airway obstruction occurs easily when sedated.[75] Subglottic narrowing is common—take care with choice of endotracheal tube. Risk of laryngeal spasm, especially on extubation. Do careful neurologic examination preoperatively in case of cervical dislocation and neck x-ray studies. Care with neck position at intubation. If CHD, give antibiotic prophylaxis. Anesthesia and surgery usually well tolerated.[76]
Duchenne muscular dystrophy[2, 3, 10-14, 77, 78]	Progressive pseudohypertrophy of muscles and cardiomyopathy in most cases. Succinylcholine may cause rhabdomyolysis and hyperkalemic cardiac arrest. Predominantly occurs in males; a milder form, Becker syndrome, in females. Genetic cause, X-linked recessive mutation in dystrophin gene at chromosome 21. May be subclinical until 2–6 yr and die before 20 yr of age.	Succinylcholine contraindicated. May be undiagnosed in infancy, leading to recommendation to try to avoid succinylcholine in children younger than 3–4 yr old in case of unexpected cardiac arrest. Respiratory depression occurs easily: use minimal drug dosage especially with cardiac depressants such as halothane, may require IPPV postoperatively.[79] Monitor cardiac status perioperatively. Give nondepolarizing muscle relaxants carefully.[79] Monitor cardiac status perioperatively. Use local analgesia whenever possible.

Dutch-Kentucky syndrome

See Trismus—pseudocamptodactyly.

EEC syndrome
(ectrodactyly, ectodermal dysplasia, and cleft lip and palate)

Congenital anomaly complex. Lobster claw deformity, dysplasia of all ectodermal elements (including central nervous system [CNS]), with disordered temperature control (hypohidrosis plus central defect). Decreased tearing, conjunctivitis, blepharitis. Cleft lip and palate, respiratory tract infections, genitourinary anomalies, malnutrition, and anemia. Mental retardation in 8%.

Assess nutrition and anemia. Preoperative chest physiotherapy advised; avoid atropine (effect on sweating). Extreme care with skin required; position and pad carefully. Protect eyes. Intubation may be difficult with cleft. Be prepared to manage temperature carefully using heating/cooling blankets, etc.[80]

Edwards syndrome[1]
(trisomy 18[E])

CHD in 95%, micrognathia in 80%, renal malformations in 50%–80%. Hypotonia. Most die in infancy.

Antibiotic prophylaxis preoperatively. Intubation may be difficult; use caution with drugs excreted by kidneys; assess cardiac status carefully.[9, 81]

Ehlers-Danlos syndrome[1–3, 82]
(cutis hyperelastica)

Collagen abnormality: hyperelasticity and fragile tissues; dissecting aneurysm of aorta, fragility of other blood vessels: ECG conduction abnormalities. Bleeding diathesis; hernias. May have heart, lung, and gastrointestinal malformations.

Difficult to maintain IV line; poor tissues and clotting defect may lead to hemorrhage. Spontaneous pneumothorax may occur. Monitor for ECG conduction abnormalities.

Eisenmenger syndrome

Association of high pulmonary vascular resistance, pulmonary hypertension, aortopulmonary, intracardiac or interarterial shunt. Dyspnea, fatigue, cyanosis, finger clubbing, and cardiac failure.

Often associated with Down syndrome. Need cardiac assessment. Polycythemia. Shunt reversal with hypoxia, hypercarbia, or acidosis. Inhalational agents are taken up slowly. Epidural anaesthesia has been used successfully.[83]

Table continued on following page

Name	Description	Anesthesia Implications
Elfin facies syndrome	*See* Williams syndrome.	
Ellis–van Creveld syndrome[1, 2] (chondroectodermal/ mesoectodermal dysplasia)	Ectodermal defects causing skeletal dwarfism, cardiac anomalies (50%), chest wall defects, and poor lung function. Short limbs, polydactyly, and hypoplastic nails. May have abnormal maxillae, cleft palate, cleft lip, hepatosplenomegaly. Patients often die in infancy.	Cardiorespiratory function assessment: if CHD is present, give antibiotic prophylaxis preoperatively. Intubation can be routine,[84] or airway problems may make intubation difficult.[85, 86]
Eosinophilic granuloma	*See* Histiocytosis X.	
Epidermolysis bullosa[1, 2, 10–14, 87, 88] (Herlitz syndrome)	Skin cleavage at dermal-epidermal junction, resulting in erosions and blisters from minor trauma to skin or mucous membrane. The disease occurs in several forms: *Simplex:* Dominant, maps to chromosome 17. Relatively mild with rapid healing and little scarring. *Lethalis:* Recessive, maps to chromosome 12. Junctional epidermolysis bullosa. Severe, presents at birth, leads to extensive scarring and death (often from sepsis) usually before 2 yr of age. *Dystrophic:* Recessive, maps to chromosome 12. Very rare but severe; lesions heal slowly with extensive scarring. Strictures may form and involve the pharynx, larynx, and esophagus. Digital fusion occurs ("mitten hand"). Nutritional deprivation leads to growth retardation and anemia. Infections are common.	Antibiotic prophylaxis preoperatively. Check history of steroid therapy. Use sterile technique (reverse isolation). Airway difficulty: oral lesions, adhesion of tongue. Avoid trauma to skin or mucous membranes; avoid intubation and/or instrumentation of the airway if possible; otherwise, lubricate tube and laryngoscope generously. Use insufflation or a well padded and lubricated mask for inhalation anesthesia or use ketamine. Do not use adhesive tape. Regional analgesia may be considered.[89]

Erythema multiforme	*See* Stevens-Johnson syndrome.
Eulenberg periodic paralysis	*See* Paramyotonia congenita.
Fabry disease[1–3] (angiokeratoma corporis diffusum)	X-linked lipid storage disorder. Lipid deposition in blood vessels causes periodic very severe pain and fever crises. Corneal opacities. Dark telangiectasia, particularly around genitals and buttocks; hypertension, myocardial ischemia, renal failure.	Hypertension and myocardial ischemia. Assess cardiorespiratory and renal function carefully; monitor ECG. Do not use drugs excreted by the kidneys.[90]
Familial dysautonomia	*See* Riley-Day syndrome.
Familial osteodysplasia	*See* Anderson syndrome.
Familial periodic paralysis	Periodic muscle weakness secondary to serum K^+ disturbance (hypokalemia or hyperkalemia). Muscle weakness in the hypokalemic variety is caused by massive uptake of K into muscles and thus decreased serum K.	Monitor serum K and ECG; prevent hyperglycemia or hypoglycemia. Do not use muscle relaxants; maintain body temperature. Avoid excessive glucose solutions.[91]
Fanconi syndrome[2, 3] (anemia with renal tubular acidosis)	Usually secondary to cystinosis, galactosemia. Proximal tubular defect: impaired renal function; acidosis, K loss, dehydration.	Treat electrolyte and acid-base abnormalities; do not use drugs excreted by kidneys. Be aware of possibility of other metabolic defects.[2, 3, 18, 92, 93]
Farber disease[2, 3] (lipogranulomatosis)	Sphingomyelin deposition: widespread visceral lipogranulomas, especially in CNS. General systemic involvement leading to cardiac, renal failure.	Assess cardiorespiratory and renal status carefully. Deposits in oral cavity, pharynx, and larynx; possible difficult intubation.[5, 94, 95]
Favism[2, 3] (glucose-6-phosphate dehydrogenase (G6PD) deficiency)	Diathesis for spontaneous/induced (drugs, fava beans, infection) hemolytic anemia.	Do not give drugs that cause hemolysis (e.g., acetylsalicylic acid, phenacetin, sulfonamides, quinidine, methylene blue). Anemia: transfuse if necessary.[94]

Table continued on following page

459

Name	Description	Anesthesia Implications
Fetal alcohol syndrome	Abnormalities of the infant due to maternal heavy alcohol consumption: growth retardation, intellectual impairment, craniofacial abnormalities (microcephaly, microphthalmia, hypoplastic upper lip, flat maxilla), cardiac defects (especially ventricular septal defect), renal abnormalities, and inguinal hernia.	If CHD is present, use antibiotic prophylaxis preoperatively. Difficult intubation. Problems of associated cardiac disease.[96–98]
Fibrodysplasia ossificans progressiva	*See* Myositis ossificans.	
Focal dermal hypoplasia[1, 2] (Goltz syndrome)	Multifarious features, including multiple papillomas of mucous membranes, skin.	Airway may contain papillomas.
Forbes disease (glycogen storage disease type III)	*See* von Gierke disease.	
Freeman-Sheldon syndrome[99] (whistling face)	Progressive congenital myopathy and dysplasia with autosomal or X-linked recessive inheritance. Increased tone and fibrosis of facial muscles. Hypertelorism, microstomia, and micrognathia. Leads to flexion contracture of limbs. Strabismus and inguinal hernia common. Later, kyphoscoliosis causes restrictive lung disease.	Very difficult intubation: tight facial muscles will not relax with neuromuscular blockade, and muscle rigidity may follow halothane or succinylcholine. Venous access difficult due to limb flexion contractures. Pulmonary function may be impaired (late). Insertion of an LMA has facilitated fiberoptic bronchoscopy and intubation.[100] Regional analgesia may be useful for postoperative pain.[100–105]
Friedreich ataxia[2, 3]	Progressive degeneration of cerebellum, lateral and posterior column of spinal cord; scoliosis; myocardial degeneration and fibrosis, leading to failure and arrhythmias.	Monitor ECG carefully. Care with cardiac depressant drugs.

Gangliosidoses[3]	Invariably fatal. Supportive measures only treatment.	Progressive neurologic loss leads to respiratory complications; assess pulmonary status carefully.[104]
GM1, type 1	*Acute onset in infancy*: Rapid neurologic decline, severe bone abnormalities; pulmonary infiltration common. Death by 2 yr of age.	
GM1, type 2	*Onset in early childhood*: Few somatic changes. Death from cardiopulmonary causes by 10 yr.	
GM2 (Tay-Sachs disease; Sandhoff disease)	*Onset in infancy*: Progressive psychomotor deterioration; blindness, seizures. Death by 5 yr (by 2 yr in most cases). *Rare juvenile variants*: same features; longer survival.	
Gardner syndrome[1-3]	Familial polyposis of colon; bone tumors, sebaceous cysts, fibromas.	No specific anesthesia problems described.[105]
Gaucher disease[2, 3]	Cerebroside accumulation in CNS, liver, spleen, etc. Serum acid phosphatase increased. Pulmonary disease from aspiration (pseudobulbar palsy); hepatosplenomegaly. Hypersplenism may cause platelet deficiency. If obvious neurologic signs: usually fatal in infancy. If more chronic: bone pain, fractures.	Assess pulmonary status carefully—beware of aspiration. Treat coagulation disorders and correct anemia.[104]
Glanzmann disease[2, 3] (thromboasthenia)	Abnormal platelet function, leading to mild thrombocytopenic purpura; abnormality of high-energy phosphate mechanisms.	No specific therapy for bleeding; platelet transfusion disappointing. May have history of steroid therapy;[106]

Table continued on following page

Name	Description	Anesthesia Implications
Glucose-6-phosphate dehydrogenase (G6PD) deficiency	*See* Favism.	
Glycogen storage disease[2, 3]		
Type I	*See* von Gierke disease.	
Type II	*See* Pompe disease.	
Type III (Cori disease; Forbes disease)	*See* von Gierke disease.	
Type IV	*See* von Gierke disease.	
Type V	*See* Andersen disease.	
Type VI (Hers disease)	*See* McArdle disease.	
Type VII	*See* Muscle phosphofructokinase deficiency.	
Type VIII	*See* Hepatic phosphorylase kinase deficiency.	
Goldenhar syndrome[1, 2] (oculoauriculovertebral syndrome)	Unilateral hypoplasia with mandibular hypoplasia; CHD in 20%. Embryonic malformation due to chromosome 22 trisomy.	If CHD is present, use antibiotic prophylaxis preoperatively. Airway problems; may be difficult to hold a mask in place and intubation may be very difficult. Have an LMA ready. Extubate awake. Problems of associated cardiac disease.[7]
Goltz syndrome	*See* Focal dermal hypoplasia and Gorlin-Goltz syndrome.	
Gonadal dysgenesis	*See* Turner syndrome.	
Gorham syndrome (disappearing bone disease)	Massive osteolysis and hemangiomatosis. Bony deformities: kyphoscoliosis.	Problems relate to bony involvement: cervical spine subluxation, thoracic deformity. Intubation may be difficult.[107]
Gorlin-Chaudhry-Moss syndrome[1, 2]	Craniofacial dysostosis, patent ductus arteriosus, hypertrichosis, hypoplasia of labia majora, dental and eye anomalies. Normal intelligence.	If CHD is present, use antibiotic prophylaxis preoperatively. Asymmetry of head—difficult airway. Problems associated with patent ductus arteriosus.[1]

Gorlin-Goltz syndrome[1,2] (basal cell nevus syndrome)	Multiple nevoid basal cell carcinomas, hypertelorism, mandibular prognathism, multiple jaw cysts and fibrosarcomas, kyphoscoliosis, incomplete segmentation of cervical and thoracic vertebrae; congenital hydrocephalus, mental retardation, etc.	Extreme care in positioning and intubating—cervical movement may be limited. Increased ICP may be unrecognized.
Groenblad-Strandberg syndrome[1,2] (pseudoxanthoma elasticum)	Degeneration of elastic tissue in skin, eye, and cardiovascular system; rupture of arteries, especially in gastrointestinal tract; hypertension; arterial calcification; occlusion of cerebral and coronary arteries.	Assess cardiovascular status carefully. Manage as for coronary artery disease. Difficult to maintain IV cannula.[5]
Guillain-Barré syndrome (acute [idiopathic] polyneuritis)	Acute polyneuropathy; progressive peripheral neuritis; usually involving cranial nerves; bulbar palsy with hypoventilation and hypotension. May require tracheotomy and intermittent positive-pressure ventilation (IPPV).	Do not use succinylcholine for at least 3 mo after onset of polyneuritis (K^+ release).[83,84] May have hemodynamic instability.
Hallervorden-Spatz disease	Autosomal recessive disorder of basal ganglia: dementia and dystonia with torticollis, scoliosis, and trismus.	Assess pulmonary status carefully. Inhalation induction of anesthesia leads to relaxation of abnormal posturing and trismus and facilitates intubation. Avoid succinylcholine (? hyperkalemic response[85]—may intensify rigidity) or rapid-sequence induction (in case of difficult intubation).
Hand-Schüller-Christian syndrome	*See* Histiocytosis X.	
Harlequin syndrome	Skin color changes with demarcation line bisecting the body. Benign in some premature infants or associated with heart disease. Hemifacial sweating and flushing due to surgical sympathectomy reported.	No contraindications to routine anesthesia. Hemifacial flushing may develop during neck surgery due to interference with sympathetic ganglia.[1,2]

Table continued on following page

Name	Description	Anesthesia Implications
Hecht-Beals syndrome	Arachnodactyly, kyphoscoliosis, and multiple congenital joint contactures.	Difficult airway—not obvious preoperatively.[113]
Hemangioma with thrombocytopenia	See Kasabach-Merritt syndrome.	
Hemolytic uremic syndrome	Usually occurs in 1- to 2-year-olds; prodromal (usually gastrointestinal) infection followed by sudden onset of renal failure, hemolytic anemia, and thrombocytopenia. All systems may be involved: *Cardiovascular system*—severe hypertension, myocarditis, and congestive cardiac failure; respiratory-pulmonary insufficiency. *Central nervous system*—depression progressing to drowsiness, seizures, and coma. Hepatosplenomegaly with hepatic dysfunction, seizures, and coma. Hepatosplenomegaly with hepatic dysfunction. *Coagulopathy*: thrombocytopenia, decreased platelet function, prolonged prothrombin time and bleeding time. Treatment is by blood transfusion, renal dialysis, and symptomatic therapy for other disorders.	Comprehensive cardiorespiratory assessment required. Correct electrolyte, acid-base, and coagulation as possible. May have full stomach (gastrointestinal dysfunction). Isoflurane and *cis*-atracurium agents of choice. Intensive continuous monitoring of biochemistry needed intraoperatively and postoperatively.[114]
Hepatic phosphorylase kinase deficiency[2, 3] (glycogen storage disease type VIII)	Hepatomegaly; increased liver glycogen concentration.	No anesthesia complications reported.
Herlitz syndrome	See Epidermolysis bullosa.	
Hermansky-Pudlak syndrome[2, 3]	Albinism: bleeding diathesis due to platelet abnormality.	May require platelet transfusion during surgery.

Hers disease	*See* von Gierke disease.	
Histiocytosis X[2] (eosinophilic granuloma: Hand-Schüller-Christian disease, Letterer-Siwe disease)	Lesions in bones and viscera (larynx, lungs, liver, and spleen). Clinical course similar to acute leukemia. Hypersplenism, pancytopenia, anemia, purpura, hemorrhage; hepatic involvement. Pulmonary—diffuse hilar infiltration: respiratory failure, cor pulmonale. Gingival inflammation and necrosis, with loss of teeth. Diabetes insipidus if sella turcica involved. Many die in first year of life.	Correct anemia and coagulation defects. Assess cardiorespiratory status carefully. Check electrolytes and fluid balance. May have history of steroid therapy. Laryngeal fibrosis, intubation may be difficult. Beware of loose teeth.[115]
Holt-Oram syndrome[2, 10–14] (heart-hand syndrome)	Upper limb abnormalities; CHD (usually atrial septal defect); possibility of sudden death from pulmonary embolus, coronary occlusion.	Antibiotic prophylaxis preoperatively. Problems of cardiac defect. No other anesthesia problem.[116]
Homocystinuria[1–3]	Thromboembolic phenomena due to intimal thickening; ectopia lentis, osteoporosis, kyphoscoliosis. Angiography may precipitate thrombosis, especially cerebral.	Give fluids to maintain urine output. Give dextran 40 to reduce viscosity and platelet adhesiveness and increase peripheral perfusion.[117]
Hunter syndrome[1–3] (mucopolysaccharidosis type II)	Similar, but less severe than Hurler syndrome.	As for Hurler syndrome. Difficult intubation due to large tongue. Attempts to secure airway using the LMA have not always been successful.[118] Delayed recovery from anesthesia reported.[119]

Table continued on following page

Name	Description	Anesthesia Implications
Hurler syndrome[1-3, 10-14] (mucopolysaccharidosis type I H; formerly classed as type I)	Mental retardation, gargoyle facies, deafness, stiff joints, dwarfing, pectus excavatum, and kyphoscoliosis. Abnormal tracheobronchial cartilages; severe coronary artery disease at early age, valvar and myocardial involvement. Hepatosplenomegaly. Most die from respiratory and cardiac failure before 10 yr; sudden death common after 7 yr of age.	*See* Mucopolysaccharidoses. Antibiotic prophylaxis and chest physiotherapy preoperatively. Give large doses of atropine preoperatively. Upper airway obstruction due to profuse lymphoid tissue infiltration. Hypoplasia of the odontoid; atlantoaxial subluxation may occur. Difficult intubation, especially in older children, due to micrognathia, short neck, and limited movement of temporomandibular joint. LMA may not relieve obstruction. Give anesthetic gases.[7, 120, 121]
Hurler-Scheie compound syndrome (type I HS)	*See* Scheie syndrome.	
Hutchinson-Gilford syndrome	*See* Progeria.	
Hyalinosis, cutaneous-mucosal	*See* Urbach-Wiethe disease.	
Hyperexplexia	*See* Stiff baby syndrome.	
Hyperpyrexia/hyperthermia, malignant	*See* page 172.	
I-cell disease (mucolipidoses)	Mental retardation, Hurler-type bone changes, severe joint limitation, chronic pulmonary disease; valvar insufficiency common. Death in early childhood (most by 1 yr of age).	Intubation and airway maintenance difficult—limited jaw movement, stiffness of neck and rib cage.

Idiopathic thrombocytopenic purpura	Autoimmune disease in which an antiplatelet factor is present, resulting in destruction of platelets in the spleen. May be acute or chronic. Resulting in thrombocytopenia and bleeding. Severe gastrointestinal and intracranial bleeding may occur. Treatment with steroids and γ-globulin. Splenectomy may be required.	May have history of steroid therapy. Platelet counts may be very low, but platelet transfusions are ineffective until the spleen is removed; therefore, infuse after splenectomy. Avoid intramuscular injections.
Ivemark syndrome	*See* Asplenia syndrome.	
Jervell-Lange-Nielsen syndrome (Romano-Ward syndrome)	Congenital deafness and cardiac conduction defects: arrythmias and syncopal attacks (may be misdiagnosed as epilepsy). ECG shows large T waves, prolonged Q-T interval. Sudden death may occur. Serious arrythmias (ventricular fibrillation) under anesthesia.[122]	Assess cardiac status carefully. General anesthesia may precipitate arrythmias; pretreat with β-blockers to decrease risk. Avoid atropine and halothane.[122-124] Stellate ganglion block recommended.[120, 125] Ventricular fibrillation may respond to lidocaine and defibrillation. Watch for hypoglycemia as a complication of β-blockade.[126, 127]
Juvenile hyaline fibromatosis	Autorecessive disease; multiple subcutaneous nodules, flexion contractures of large and small joints, radiolucent bone destruction (especially femur and humerus), hypertrophic gingiva. Systemic manifestations may involve pleura, lung, renal, and digestive system. Entrapment of nerves and vessels may occur. Intelligence normal.	Check preoperatively for evidence of other organ involvement. Difficult intubation due to gingival hyperplasia and limited motion at neck and temporomandibular joints. Careful positioning and padding required.[128]

Table continued on following page

467

Name	Description	Anesthesia Implications
Jeune syndrome[1, 2] (asphyxiating thoracic dystrophy)	Severe thoracic malformation; asphyxia. Cystic renal changes, progressing to failure.	Surgery to enlarge thorax may necessitate prolonged periods of assisted ventilation.[129] Care with drugs excreted by kidneys.
Joubert syndrome (Mohr syndrome variant, familial cerebellar vermis agenesis)	Rare autosomal recessive disorder. Cerebellar vermis dysplasia or agenesis and brain stem cysts. Hypotonia, ataxia, jerky eye movements, and tongue protrusion. Mental retardation. Abnormal respiration: alternating tachypnea and apneic spells. Lethal in early childhood.	Life-threatening respiratory problems perioperatively. Very sensitive to anesthetic agents and opioids. Inhalational induction, controlled ventilation and local or regional analgesia advised. Apnea monitoring postoperatively.[130]
Kartagener syndrome[1, 2]	Dextrocardia, situs inversus. Immotile cilia, deficient mucociliary clearance; sinusitis, bronchiectasis. Defective immunity.	Order physiotherapy preoperatively. Use sterile technique (reverse isolation). Assess respiratory status carefully.[131]
Kasabach-Merritt syndrome[1, 2, 132–134]	Hemangioma suddenly increases in size; thrombocytopenia, hypofibrinogenemia → purpura, bleeding, anemia, increased fibrinolytic activity. Treated by radiotherapy (surgery may precipitate disseminated intravascular coagulation). Recovery follows destruction of tumor.	Correct anemia, hypovolemia, and coagulation defects. Platelet transfusions required. Steroids may help.

Kawasaki syndrome (mucocutaneous lymph node syndrome)	Acute febrile exanthematous disease secondary to vasculitis with cardiac involvement (pancarditis, valvular dysfunction, arrythmias, and coronary artery vasculitis). Seen in infants and young children, endemic in Japan. Signs include fever, conjunctivitis, oral erythema, strawberry tongue, red hands and feet. Cardiac involvement in 20% of cases: ranges from asymptomatic ECG changes to severe congestive failure and massive myocardial infarction. Salicylates are used in treatment and may reduce coronary lesions. Biliary tract or bowel symptoms may require laparotomy. Hepatic involvement in 10% of patients.	Related to associated cardiac lesions. Assess cardiac state carefully. Avoid myocardial depressants and anesthetize as for a patient with coronary artery disease. Monitor for cardiac ischemic changes (V_5 and lead II). Be prepared with vasoactive and antiarrhythmic drugs.[135, 136] Sympathetic nerve blocks may improve ischemic limb circulation.[137] Sevoflurane induction and halothane anesthesia has been used satisfactorily.[44] Salicylates may increase surgical bleeding.
Kenny-Caffey syndrome	Dwarfism, macrocephaly, thoracic skeletal abnormalities, anemia, hypocalcemia, and can have mandibular hypoplasia.[138]	Intubation may be difficult. Use of the LMA is an option for securing the airway.[138]
Ketonuria, branched-chain	*See* Maple syrup urine disease.	
Klinefelter syndrome[1, 3] (gonosomal aneuploidy with tubular dysgenesis)	Tall; reduced intelligence; vertebral collapse due to osteoporosis. May have diabetes mellitus.	No anesthesia problem reported, except in diabetics. Position very carefully to avoid spinal cord damage.[9]
Klippel-Feil syndrome[1, 2]	Congenital fusion of two or more cervical vertebrae, causing neck rigidity.	Intubation may be very difficult: should be done awake if possible; otherwise inhalation induction without muscle relaxant. Have an LMA prepared. Do not extubate until fully awake.

Table continued on following page

Name	Description	Anesthesia Implications
Klippel-Trénaunay-Weber syndrome[1, 2] (angio-osteohypertrophy)	Hemangiomas with hypertrophy of adjacent bone; thrombocytopenia. AV fistulas and anemia lead to high cardiac output, with possible cardiac failure; thrombocytopenia in association with visceral hemangiomas.	Check cardiac status carefully, correct bleeding disorders.
Krabbe disease[2, 3] (globoid cell leukodystrophy)	*See* Leukodystrophy.	
Larsen syndrome	Multiple congenital dislocations: knees, elbows, hips. Characteristic facies, hydrocephalus, cleft palate, flat face, upturned nose. Connective tissue defect of cartilage of ribs, epiglottis, arytenoids, and tracheomalacia. Cervical spine abnormal, kyphoscoliosis, chronic respiratory problems, and cardiac anomalies.	Check for cardiac defects and respiratory status. Cervical spine instability. Intubation may be difficult and subglottic stenosis may be present. Possible increased ICP.[70, 139, 140]
Laurence-Moon syndrome[2]	Mental retardation, pigmentary retinopathy, hypogenitalism, and spastic paraplegia. (Polydactyly and obesity, typical in Bardet-Biedl syndrome, are absent.) May have renal abnormalities and CHD.	Assess cardiac, renal, and fluid.[141] If CHD present: Antibiotic prophylaxis preoperatively.
Leigh disease[142] (subacute necrotizing encephalomyelopathy)	May occur in infancy or childhood. Infants develop hypotonia, somnolence, optic atrophy, deafness, and pyramidal tract signs. Altered respiratory patterns may occur and may lead to sudden infant death syndrome. Older children present with acute neurologic deterioration and respiratory failure.	Monitor ventilation carefully in the perioperative period.

470

Leopard syndrome[1, 2]	Multiple large freckles; hypertelorism, eyelid ptosis, etc. CHD (pulmonary stenosis in 95%); ECG anomalies include aberrant conduction. Growth retardation common; pectus carinatum, kyphosis, etc., in some. Genitourinary anomalies (hypospadias cryptorchidism, ovarian hypoplasia, etc.).	If CHD is present, use antibiotic prophylaxis preoperatively. Assess cardiac status, lung function. Intubation may be difficult. Problems of associated cardiac disease; monitor ECG carefully.
Leprechaunism[1, 2] (Donohue syndrome)	Failure to thrive, endocrine disorders, severe mental retardation. Hypoglycemia due to hyperinsulinism from hyperplastic islets of Langerhans; renal tubular defects → impaired renal function. Most die before 1 yr of age.	Check metabolic status; monitor blood glucose. Do not use drugs excreted by kidneys.[143]
Lesch-Nyhan syndrome[1, 2]	Disorder of purine metabolism, occurs in males. Mental and growth retardation, malnutrition, choreoathetosis. Very aggressive with compulsive self-destructive behaior. Hyperuricemia leads to renal calculi, RBC damage, hypertension, and coronary artery disease. Renal failure by age 20 yr.	Avoid drugs excreted by the kidney. Beware of regurgitation, give metoclopramide. Diazepam, thiopental, isoflurane, and atracurium are recommended.[144] Caution with catecholamines.
Letterer-Siwe disease	*See* Histiocytosis X.	

Table continued on following page

Name	Description	Anesthesia Implications
Leukodystrophy[145] (Alexander disease, Canavan disease, Krabbe disease, Pelizaeus-Merzbacher disease, adrenoleukodystrophy, metachromatic leukodystrophy)	Inherited disorder of myelin formation. Progressive degenerative disease with spasticity, gait disturbance, poor motor development, seizures, extrapyramidal movements, and choreoathetosis. Disordered swallowing and gastroesophageal reflux lead to aspiration pneumonia. Malnutrition and anemia.	Assess pulmonary status and anticonvulsant medications. Copious oral secretion, use an antisialogogue. Danger of acid aspiration. Position and pad carefully. Avoid succinylcholine (central nervous system disease). Phenytoin therapy results in increased requirements for vecuronium and fentanyl. Maintain body temperature carefully. Extubate awake, monitor carefully postoperatively. **N.B.** Adrenal dysfunction in adrenoleukodystrophy; give steroids.[145]
Lipoatrophy with diabetes[1-3] (Seip syndrome)	Generalized loss of all body fat, fibrotic liver leading to failure, portal hypertension; splenomegaly, nephropathy, diabetes. May have renal failure.	Hypersplenism may lead to anemia and thrombocytopenia. Do not use drugs metabolized by liver. Check coagulation and renal function preoperatively. Take precautions as for diabetes.[104]
Lipogranulomatosis	See Farber disease.	
Lowe syndrome[2, 3] (oculocerebrorenal syndrome)	Affects males. Cataract, glaucoma, mental retardation; hypotonia, renal acidosis, proteinuria, osteoporosis, and rickets.	Check electrolyte and acid-base balance, and serum Ca (treated with vitamin D and Ca^{++}). Care with drugs excreted by kidneys.[18, 146]
Lupus erythematosus disseminatus	See Collagen diseases.	
Maffucci syndrome[1, 2]	Enchondromatosis and hemangiomas with malignant change. Pathologic fractures, gastrointestinal bleeding from hemangiomas, orthostatic hypotension.	Position carefully. May show orthostatic hypotension and be sensitive to vasodilator drugs.
Malignant hyperpyrexia/hyperthermia	See page 172.	

Mandibulofacial dysostosis

See Treacher Collins syndrome.

Mannosidosis[1–3, 147]
Type I (severe)
Type II (milder)

Primary metabolic deficiency of α-mannosidases A and B → lysosomal accumulation of mannose-rich substrates. Abnormal neutrophil immunologic function. Hepatosplenomegaly, severe recurrent infections, and early death. Hearing loss, mental retardation, Hurler-like skeletal changes, gargoyle-like facies, clumsy motor function, weak connective tissues.

Be alert for hepatic dysfunction, and for hypoventilation perioperatively and postoperatively.

Maple syrup urine disease[2, 3]
(MSUD; branched-chain ketonuria)

Inability to metabolize leucine, isoleucine, and valine. Severe neurologic damage and respiratory disturbances. Episodes of hypoglycemia. Treated by diet only; from birth; many die within 2 months. Acute, life-threatening episodes may require peritoneal dialysis or exchange transfusion.

Check acid-base balance, plasma amino acids preoperatively. Check serum glucose before, during, and after operation. Start glucose infusion (at least 10–15 mg/kg/min) preoperatively and continue until diet is re-established.[148]

Marfan syndrome[1–3, 10–14]
(arachnodactyly)

Tall, thin patients with long fingers, long face, and high arched palate. Mutant gene at chromosome 15 for fibrillin causes connective tissue disorder leading to joint instability and dislocation (including cervical spine), dislocation of lens, kyphoscoliosis, hernia, pectus excavatum, lung cysts. Aortic root dilation may lead to aortic incompetence or aneurysm; pulmonary artery or mitral valve may be diseased.

Antibiotic prophylaxis preoperatively. Intubation may be difficult. Laryngoscopy should be gentle to avoid cervical spine or temporomandibular joint damage. Position carefully to avoid dislocations. Avoid myocardial depressants, but do not allow the patient to become hypertensive (danger of aortic dissection). Beware of pneumothorax with controlled ventilation.

Table continued on following page

Name	Description	Anesthesia Implications
Maroteaux-Lamy syndrome[1-3] (mucopolysaccharidosis type VI)	Normal intellect. Kyphoscoliosis with poor lung reserve; chronic respiratory infections; hypersplenism, anemia, thrombocytopenia. Myocardial involvement; heart failure by 20 yr of age.	*See* Mucopolysaccharidoses. Check cardiac status, coagulation, respiratory function. Care with cardiac depressant drugs.[5, 94] Spinal cord compression may occur.[149] May require ventilation postoperatively.
Marshall-Smith syndrome	Skeletal dysplasia and dysmorphic facial features. Hypotonia and failure to thrive. Respiratory tract anomalies lead to complications.	Airway problems and difficult intubation. Association with laryngo- and tracheomalacia described: cause of failure to ventilate.[150]
Mastocystosis syndrome (urticaria pigmentosa)	Abnormal aggregates of histamine- and heparin-containing mast cells; skin lesion is a brownish-red maculopapular rash mainly on trunk. Mast cell degranulation with systemic histamine and heparin release may occur with trauma, temperature changes, alcohol, and drugs (including salicylates, opiates, curare, gallamine, papaverine, polymyxin, and atropine). Minor surgical procedures may lead to generalized anaphylaxis and death.	Avoid stimuli and drugs known to cause mast cell degranulation. Premedicate with an antihistamine. Inhalation anesthetics may be safely used, as may succinylcholine. Meperidine (Demerol) can be used as an analgesic. Bleeding secondary to heparin release may require protamine therapy.[151]
McArdle myopathy[2, 3] (glycogen storage disease type V)	Muscle phosphorylase deficiency; serum lactate not increased by exercise. Initially, increased fatigability; progresses to muscle cramps and weakness (all skeletal muscles affected), myoglobinuria. Myocardium may be involved; ECG abnormalities have been reported.[3]	Do not use tourniquets; maintain infusion of dextrose during surgery; do not use succinylcholine.[152] Care with cardiac depressant drugs; monitor ECG.
Meckel syndrome[1, 2] (dysencephalia splanchnocystica)	Microcephaly, micrognathia, and cleft epiglottis, CHD; renal dysplasia. Most die in infancy.	Antibiotic prophylaxis preoperatively. Assess cardiac status. Intubation may be difficult. Care with drugs excreted by kidneys.

Median cleft face syndrome[1]	Various degrees of cleft face; lipomas and dermoids over frontal bone.	Cleft nose, lip, and palate may cause intubation difficulties.
Menkes syndrome (kinky hair disease)	X-linked disorder of copper metabolism. Onset in first months of life; retarded growth and development, seizures, progressive cerebral degeneration. Gastroesophageal reflux commonly leads to pneumonia. Death from seizures or pneumonia in a few years.	Assess anticonvulsant therapy and optimize; continue therapy through perioperative period. Risk of acid aspiration; give ranitidine and metoclopramide. Prone to hypothermia. Avoid succinylcholine (neurologic disease). Phenytoin increases vecuronium requirements. Possibly use pancuronium. Postoperative ventilation may be required.[153]
Methylmalonyl-coenzyme A mutase deficiency	Autosomal recessive defect of protein metabolism. Protein metabolism leads to high plasma methylmalonic acid levels, producing lethargy, vomiting, dehydration, acidosis, ketonemia, and hyperammonemia. Treated by limiting protein intake, plus supplemental bicarbonate and cobalamin.[154]	Anesthesia and surgery may increase protein metabolism and lead to acidemia. Avoid excessive fasting or accumulation of blood in gastrointestinal tract. Maintain intravascular volume. Monitor blood gases, electrolytes, and ammonia level. Avoid nitrous oxide.[155]
Moebius syndrome[1, 2] (congenital oculofacial paralysis)	Congenital paralyses of sixth and seventh cranial nerves. Limb deformities, micrognathia. Feeding difficulties and aspiration may cause chronic pulmonary problems.	Assess respiratory status carefully. Intubation may be difficult.
Morquio syndrome[1–3, 10–14] Mucopolysaccharidosis type IV	*Normal intellect.* Severe dwarfing; aortic incompetence; kyphoscoliosis with poor lung function (cardiorespiratory symptoms by second decade). Unstable atlantoaxial joint leading to spinal cord compression; deafness. Inguinal hernia common.	*See* Mucopolysaccharidoses. Antibiotic prophylaxis preoperatively. Assess cardiorespiratory status; care with cardiac depressant drugs. Care with positioning and avoid excessive neck manipulation.[5, 94, 156]
Mucopolysaccharidosis type VII: β-glucuronidase deficiency)	*Severe mental retardation.* Skeletal anomalies similar to type IV.	Same as type IV.

Table continued on following page

Name	Description	Anesthesia Implications
Moschcowitz disease[3] (thrombotic thrombocytopenic purpura)	Hemolytic anemia and thrombocytopenia, arteriolar and capillary disease, neurologic damage, renal disease. Treatment: splenectomy and steroids.	Check coagulation studies and history of steroid therapy. Care with drugs excreted by kidneys.[106]
Moyamoya disease[157-159]	Severe carotid artery stenosis with a fine network of vessels around the basal ganglia. Cerebral ischemia leads to paroxysmal hemiplegia. Treatment is by surgical revascularization using scalp vessels.	Hypocapnia leads to severe cerebral ischemia: avoid hyperventilation, maintain normocapnia. Halothane or isoflurane may be useful as a cerebral vasodilator. Avoid hypothermia. Maintain cerebral perfusion pressure.
Mucolipidoses	See I-cell disease.	
Mucopolysaccharidoses[1-3, 149, 160] Type I H, I HS, II, VII Type III Type I S, IV, VI	Affects bones and intellect. Affects intellect only. Affects bones only. See Previous classifications: I H: Hurler syndrome. I S: Scheie syndrome; formerly classified as type V. HS: Hurler-Scheie compound (See Scheie syndrome). II: Hunter syndrome. III: Sanfilippo syndrome. IV: Morquio syndrome. V: Formerly Scheie syndrome. VI: Maroteaux-Lamy syndrome. VII: β-Glucuronidase deficiency (see Morquio syndrome).	All may be difficult to intubate. LMA may not relieve obstruction. Spinal cord compression may occur due to thickening of dura and odontoid hypoplasia; preoperative magnetic resonance imaging scans of spinal cord suggested.[149]

Multiple endocrine adenomatoses		
Type I	*See* Werner syndrome.	
Type II	*See* Sipple syndrome.	
Muscle, eye, brain disease (MEB)	Muscle dystrophy, eye disease (glaucoma, strabismus, nystagmus), and mental retardation. Severe muscle weakness, secretion retention, bedridden.	Caution with muscle relaxants: succinylcholine results in very high CK levels and is contraindicated.[161]
Muscle phosphofructokinase deficiency[2, 3] (glycogen storage disease type VII)	Reduced RBC life span (13–16 days).	No anesthesia complications have been reported.
Myasthenia congenita	Similar to myasthenia gravis in adults.[3] *See* page 309.	Do not use respiratory depressants or muscle relaxants; IPPV may be required postoperatively. Possibility of cholinergic crisis with anticholinesterase therapy.[162–164]
Myositis ossificans[2] (fibrodysplasia ossificans progressiva)	Bony infiltration of tendons, fascia, aponeuroses, and muscle. Thoracic involvement greatly reduces thoracic compliance: progressive respiratory failure.	Check respiratory function, history of steroid therapy. Airway and intubation problems if neck rigid and mouth fixed.[5]
Myotonia congenita[2, 3, 10–14] (Thomsen disease)	Decreased ability to relax muscles after contraction; diffuse hypertrophy of muscle (similar to myotonia dystrophica but more benign and nonprogressive.)	Do not use muscle relaxants or respiratory depressants. Postoperative respiratory complications common due to poor cough.[21–24]

Table continued on following page

477

Name	Description	Anesthesia Implications
Myotonia dystrophica[1-3] (myotonic dystrophy)	Weakness and myotonia; eyelid ptosis, cataracts, frontal baldness; cardiac conduction defects and arrhythmias; impaired ventilation; other systems may be involved. Has been reported in infancy.	Check respiratory function. Do not use succinylcholine (which causes myotonia in 50%). Nondepolarizing drugs do not produce good relaxation; neostigmine induces myotonia; halothane may cause shivering and myotonia postoperatively. Extremely sensitive to respiratory depressants—use regional or inhalational agents with IPPV postoperatively if necessary. Monitor ECG carefully. Anticipate postoperative pulmonary complications.[21-24, 167]
Nager syndrome	Micrognathia, fish-like face, cleft palate (similar to Treacher Collins), limb deformities. Tetralogy of Fallot may be associated.	Very difficult intubation. Upper airway obstruction may necessitate tracheostomy in the neonate. Mouth opening can be very limited and intubation only possible by a fiberoptic technique. Check cardiac status.[165, 166]
Nail-patella syndrome[2, 3] (arthrosteo-onychodysplasia)	Dysplasia of nails and absent or hypoplastic patellas. May have lilac horns, abnormality of elbows, nephropathy, increased mucopolysaccharide excretion.	Care with drugs excreted by kidneys.

Nemaline rod myopathy	Congenital myopathy, may be related to central core disease. Commonly present as neonates with hypotonia, weak cry, and poor feeding. Dysmorphic features, micrognathia, slender face, high arched palate. Motor development delayed, muscle weakness of trunk and limbs plus respiratory and pharyngeal; leads to respiratory failure, aspiration pneumonia. Congenital heart disease may be associated.	Assess airway and pulmonary status carefully. Preoperative physiotherapy and antibiotics for infection, intubation may be difficult. Brisk vagal responses noted; prescribe atropine. Possible central sensitivity to depressant drugs. Avoid succinylcholine (abnormal response); response to pancuronium is reported to be normal. Postoperative ventilation may be required. Link to central core disease suggests possibility of MH but not yet reported in nemaline myopathy.[168, 169]
Neonatal hypoglycemia, symptomatic	Symptomatic hypoglycemia in infants: (1) small for gestational age, (2) of diabetic mothers, (3) premature. If untreated—convulsions, lethargy, and mental retardation; no ketosis. Rarely, insulinoma or pancreatic hypertrophy requiring subtotal pancreatectomy. *See also* Beckwith syndrome.[1]	Start IV glucose infusion (5–10 mg/kg/min—no bolus) preoperatively and monitor blood glucose until condition stable postoperatively. (Boluses would precipitate rebound hyperglycemia.) Patient may be receiving steroids, diazoxide, and glucagon.[42]
Nevoid basal cell carcinoma syndrome	*See* Gorlin-Goltz syndrome.	

Table continued on following page

Name	Description	Anesthesia Implications
Niemann-Pick disease[2, 3]	Hepatosplenomegaly and accumulation of sphingomyelin and other lipids throughout body (*See also* Wolman disease.) Marrow, liver, and spleen involvement lead to anemia and thrombocytopenia. Diffuse foam cell infiltration of lungs leads to pulmonary insufficiency; pneumonia.	Check coagulation studies and cardiorespiratory function.[104]
Types A, C, D (onset in infancy)	Mental retardation. Epilepsy, ataxia. Death usually by third year (type A) to 15th year (type C).	
Type B	Normal intellect. Pulmonary disease (foam cells in alveoli). Not fatal.	
Noack syndrome[1, 2]	Craniosynostosis and digital anomalies; obesity.	Intubation may be difficult because of skull deformity.[33]
Noonan syndrome	Short stature, web neck, hypertelorism, mild mental retardation. Similar to Turner syndrome. Cardiac anomalies: usually pulmonary stenosis, hypertrophic cardiomyopathy Micrognathia, hydronephrosis, platelet dysfunction.	CHD, antibiotic prophylaxis. Possible difficult intubation.[170] Renal function tests and care with drugs excreted by kidneys.[5, 171, 172]
Oculoauriculovertebral syndrome	*See* Goldenhar syndrome.	
Oculocerebrorenal syndrome	*See* Lowe syndrome.	
Oculodento-osseous dysplasia (ODOD)	Microphthalmia and microcornea, small nose with anteverted nostrils, cleft palate, dental enamel dysplasia, plus a generalized defect of bony modeling; mandibular dysplasia, thick ribs, abnormal long bones.	Airway difficulties due to nasal, oral, and mandibular defects. Brittle teeth. Difficult intubation.[173]

Syndrome	Description	Anesthetic considerations
Oculofacial paralysis, congenital	*See* Moebius syndrome.	
Ollier syndrome[1, 2] (enchondromatosis with cavernous hemangioma)	Multiple chondromas within bones, usually unilateral; pathologic fractures. *See* Maffucci syndrome.	Position carefully. Hemangioma considerations as for Maffucci syndrome.
Opitz-Frias syndrome[174] (G syndrome, hypospadias, dysphagia syndrome)	X-linked or autosomal dominant, affects males more than females. Craniofacial and genital abnormalities. Dysphagia and recurrent aspiration, achalasia, hiatal hernia. Hypertelorism, micrognathia, and a high arched palate. Laryngeal malformations (including laryngotracheal cleft) and pulmonary hypoplasia. Bifid scrotum.	Difficult airway, small larynx (prepare small endotracheal tubes). Danger of regurgitation; empty stomach before induction.
Oral-facial-digital syndrome[1, 2]	Cleft lip and palate, lobed tongue, hypoplastic mandible and maxilla, digital anomalies; hydrocephalus, polycystic kidneys.	Airway problems and intubation may be difficult; possible renal impairment—do not use drugs excreted by the kidneys.
Osler-Rendu-Weber syndrome[1-3] (hemorrhagic telangiectasia)	Multiple capillary and venous dilation, most commonly of skin and nasal mucosa, but any organ may be affected. High incidence of pulmonary and hepatic AV fistula.	Anemia; internal hemorrhage may occur perioperatively. Blood loss difficult to control. Difficult to maintain IV due to fragile vessels. Check pulmonary status.[106]
Osteogenesis imperfecta[1-3, 10-14] (fragilitas ossium)	I. Congenita—Usually stillbirth or rapidly fatal. II. Tarda—Pathologic fractures, blue sclera, deafness. Osteoporosis → kyphoscoliosis → lung pathology. Fragility of vessels results in subcutaneous hemorrhage. Dentine deficiency results in carious, fragile teeth.	Use extreme care in positioning and intubating. Teeth are easily broken. Difficulty in maintaining IV due to fragile vessels.[175]
Osteopetrosis	*See* Albers-Schönberg disease.	

Table continued on following page

Name	Description	Anesthesia Implications
Paramyotonia congenita[2, 3] (Eulenberg periodic paralysis)	Myotonia on exposure to cold; paroxysmal weakness; serum K may be high or low	As for myotonic dystrophy; check serum K level.[21–24]
Patau syndrome[1, 3] (trisomy 13 syndrome)	Mental retardation, microcephaly, micrognathia, cleft lip or palate. May have cardiac anomalies (usually ventricular septal defect and/or dextrocardia). Patients die in infancy.	If CHD is present, use antibiotic prophylaxis preoperatively. Problems associated with heart disease.[9] Possible difficult intubation.[176]
Pelizaeus-Merzbacher disease	*See* Leukodystrophy.	
Pendred syndrome[2, 3]	Deafness and goiter; incomplete block of thyroxine production. May be euthyroid or hypothyroid.	Preoperatively ensure that patient is euthyroid; otherwise as for cretinism.[177]
Periodic paralysis	*See* Familial periodic paralysis and paramyotonia congenita.	
Phenylketonuria[2, 3]	Phenylalanine hydroxylase deficiency. Vomiting, CNS irritability, mental retardation, hypertonia, convulsions. Phenylalanine-deficient diet must be maintained.	Induction and maintenance by inhalation technique. Control ventilation. Give 10% dextrose infusion (tendency to hypoglycemia). Hypersensitive to narcotics and other CNS depressants. Do not use ketamine or enflurane; monitor body temperature carefully.[3] If patient has epilepsy, continue drugs.
Pierre Robin syndrome[1, 3, 10–14]	Cleft palate, micrognathia, glossoptosis due to first branchial arch embryologic defect. CHD in some. Neonates: respiratory obstruction may occur and can lead to cor pulmonale. Maintain airway by nursing prone on a frame: may require tongue suture, intubation, or tracheostomy. Airway may improve with growth.	If CHD is present, use antibiotic prophylaxis preoperatively. Intubation may be very difficult: use awake technique.[178] In skilled hands, fiberoptic intubation techniques under anesthesia may be used; an LMA may be inserted awake and used to induce anesthesia. Patient should be fully awake before extubation.[179, 180]

Plott syndrome	Vocal cord paralysis, psychomotor retardation, and sixth nerve palsy. Stridor at rest, respiratory distress and cyanotic or choking spells.	Anticipate airway obstruction and potential for aspiration perioperatively.[181]
Poland syndrome	Absent pectoral muscles with chest deformity. May have CHD, renal and gastrointestinal anomalies. Extreme form: Moebius syndrome has facial paralysis.	Lung herniation on crying: negative pressure on inspiration like open chest. Control ventilation.[182]
Polyarteritis nodosa	*See* Collagen disease.	
Polycystic kidneys[2]	Associated cysts in liver, pancreas, spleen, lungs, bladder, thyroid in one third; cerebral aneurysm in 15%.	Check renal status. Do not use drugs excreted by kidneys if renal function is impaired. Lung cysts may lead to pneumothorax. Prevent hypertension (possible cerebral aneurysm).[183]
Polyneuritis, acute	*See* Guillain-Barré syndrome.	
Polysplenia (bilateral visceral left-sidedness)	Complex cardiac anomalies are common: atrioseptal defect and endocardial cushion defects, usually not so complex as in asplenia.	If CHD is present, use antibiotic prophylaxis preoperatively. Do not use cardiac depressants.[64]
Pompe disease[2, 3] (glycogen storage disease type II)	Deposits of glycogen in muscles—severe hypotonicity; large tongue; massive cardiomegaly. Death from cardiorespiratory failure before 2 yr of age.	Extreme care: do not use respiratory or cardiac depressants or muscle relaxants. Large tongue may cause airway problem.[152]

Table continued on following page

Name	Description	Anesthesia Implications
Porphyrias[2, 3, 10–14]	Paralyses, psychiatric disorder, autonomic imbalance—hypertension, tachycardia; abdominal pain precipitated by drugs, infection, etc. High incidence of diabetes.	*Do not give* barbiturates (including thiopental), sedatives (including meprobamate, Librium, glutethimide, carbromal), hydroxydione (steroid anesthetic), nikethamide, hydantoin, derivatives, sulfonamides, antipyretics, or hypoglycemic agents. *The following have been used safely:* atropine, chloral, chlorpromazine, *d*-tubocurarine, ether, gallamine, morphine, N_2O, neostigmine, pentolium, pethidine, procaine, promazine, promethazine, propanidid, succinylcholine.[91]
Prader-Labhart-Willi syndrome[1–3, 183]	Sporadic mutation. Cytogenetic deletion at chromosome inherited from father (same genetic defect in Angelmann syndrome is inherited from mother.) Hypothalamic type "Pickwickian syndrome." Neonate: hypotonia, poor feeding, reflexes absent. Second phase: hyperactive, uncontrollable polyphagia, thermoregulation disturbed, mental retardation. Extreme obesity leading to cardiorespiratory failure.	Danger of hypoglycemia developing: monitor blood glucose carefully and infuse IV glucose solution before, during, and after operation.[185] Obesity makes venous cannulation difficult. Pyrexia in scoliosis, strabismus, or hernia surgery difficult to distinguish from malignant hyperthermia. Sleep apnea common: assisted or controlled ventilation may be necessary during and after operation, or apnea monitoring postoperatively.[186]
Progeria[1–3] (Hutchinson-Gilford syndrome)	Premature aging starts at 6 mo to 3 yr; cardiac disease—ischemia, hypertension, cardiomegaly. Death from coronary artery disease may occur before 10 yr of age.	Anesthesia as for adults with myocardial ischemia.[187]

Prune-belly syndrome[2]

Agenesis of abdominal musculature with renal anomalies. Poor cough; risk of postoperative atelectasis, respiratory infections, and respiratory failure.

Check renal status. Treat as for a full stomach: intubate and control ventilation. Avoid muscle relaxants and take care with drugs excreted by kidneys.[188] Thoracic epidural useful for postoperative analgesia and may avoid respiratory compromise.[189]

Pseudohypoparathyroidism

See Albright osteodystrophy.

Pseudoxanthoma elasticum

See Groenblad-Strandberg syndrome.

Pyle disease[1, 2]
(metaphyseal dysplasia)

Craniofacial abnormalities; enlarged mandible; cranial nerve paralyses.

Assess airway carefully.

Rett syndrome

Disabling neurologic disorder affecting only girls. Underweight, mental retardation, autism, seizures, scoliosis, abnormal pain sensation, cardiac arrythmias (long QT syndrome), marked irregular respiration: hyperventilation alternating with apneic spells.

Often spinal surgery for scoliosis. Severe risk of respiratory complications. Assess pulmonary and cardiac function carefully preoperatively. Apnea monitoring or IPPV needed postoperatively. Insensitive or hypersensitive to pain. Benzodiazepines to control seizures.[190]

Reye syndrome[2, 3, 191]

Severe encephalopathy and fatty degeneration of viscera (especially liver): hyperaminoacidemia; increased prothrombin time, blood ammonia, serum transaminases. Most reliable diagnosis is by liver biopsy. If untreated, increased ICP is usually fatal.

Anesthetize for investigation of and decompression of increased ICP. Patient may be receiving steroids and controlled hypothermia. Take care with drugs metabolized by liver. Do not give halothane (increased ICP; hepatic dysfunction). Control ventilation and continue hypothermia.

Rheumatoid arthritis

See Collagen diseases.

Rieger syndrome[1, 2]

Hypodontia, malformations of anterior chamber of eye, myotonic dystrophy. May have other developmental abnormalities including maxillary hypoplasia.

Anesthetic requirements dictated by muscle disease: *see* Amyotonia congenita, Myotonia congenita, Myotonia dystrophica.[15–18]

Table continued on following page

Name	Description	Anesthesia Implications
Riley-Day syndrome[1, 2, 146] (familial dysautonomia)	Recessive disorder of autonomic ganglia and sensory neurones found in Ashkenazi Jews. Deficiency of dopamine-β-hydroxylase: autonomic dysfunction and decreased sensation, paroxysmal hypertension and orthostatic hypotension. Emotional lability, absent lacrimation, abnormal sweating, poor sucking and swallowing. Recurrent aspiration pneumonia and chronic lung disease.	Premedication with diazepam and cimetidine. Atropine can be given. Need IV hydration; replace fluid losses carefully to maintain volume status. Sensitive to anesthetic agents: titrate inhalational agents to effect; can use barbiturates, narcotics, and relaxants. Respiratory center unresponsive to CO_2: narcotics given preoperatively may depress respiration and need to control ventilation. Risk of aspiration, postoperatively as well as at induction. Diazepam often controls an autonomic crisis.[193, 194] Epidural anesthesia was thought to be contraindicated but has been used uneventfully in a few cases with increased cardiovascular stability and superior analgesia reported.[195]
Robin Pierre syndrome	*See* Pierre Robin syndrome.	
Romano-Ward syndrome	*See* Jervell-Lange-Nielsen syndrome.	
Rubinstein-Taybi syndrome	Broad thumb and great toes, mental retardation, microcephaly. May have CHD (usually pulmonary stenosis), frequent chest infections, repeated aspiration leading to pneumonia and chronic lung disease.[6] Estimated frequency: 1 of every 500 institutionalized mentally retarded persons.	If CHD is present, give antibiotic prophylaxis preoperatively. Do not use respiratory depressants. Problems associated with heart disease.[6]
Russell-Silver syndrome	*See* Silver-Russell dwarfism.	
Sandhoff disease	*See* Gangliosidosis GM2.	

Sanfilippo syndrome[1–3] (mucopolysaccharidosis type III)	CNS malfunction in childhood progresses to mental retardation and dementia. Emotional disturbance and agitation. No hepatosplenomegaly, cardiac problems, or major bone problems.	*See* Mucopolysaccharidoses. No anesthesia problems described.[5, 92]
Scheie syndrome[1–3] (mucopolysaccharidosis type IS, formerly classified as type V)	Normal or almost normal intellect. Corneal clouding, hernias; joint stiffness, especially of hands and feet; aortic insufficiency. Sleep apnea may occur.	*See* Mucopolysaccharidoses. Monitor carefully for apnea. Give antibiotic prophylaxis preoperatively. Position with care. Problems associated with heart disease.[5, 92, 196]
Schwartz-Jampel syndrome	Dwarfism, micrognathia, myotonia.	Difficult intubation. Larynx may be anterior. Succinylcholine contraindicated because of possible hyperkalemia and association with malignant hyperthermia. Awake LMA-assisted fiberoptic intubation has been recommended.[197]
Scleroderma	Diffuse cutaneous stiffening. May have hemifacial atrophy. Plastic surgery required for contracture and constrictions. May have cardiac fibrosis or cor pulmonale.	Scarring of face and mouth—difficult airway and intubation. Chest restriction—poor compliance. Diffuse pulmonary fibrosis—hypoxia. Veins may be invisible, impalpable. Check history of steroid therapy.[198]
Sebaceous nevi, linear[2]	Linear nevi from forehead to nose; hydrocephalus, mental retardation; may have coarctation and hypoplasia of aorta.	If CHD is present, give antibiotic prophylaxis preoperatively. Problems associated with heart disease.[1]
Seip syndrome	*See* Lipoatrophy with diabetes.	

Table continued on following page

Name	Description	Anesthesia Implications
Shy-Drager syndrome	Orthostatic hypotension; diffuse degeneration of central and autonomic nervous systems; lability of pulse and blood pressure possibly due to defective baroreceptor response; decreased sweating; hypersensitivity to catecholamines and angiotensin.	Caution with potent inhalation anesthetics; use sevoflurane or halothane cautiously; use accurate fluid balance important; treat hypotension with IV fluids and phenylephrine. Use muscle relaxants with caution.[199, 200]
Silver-Russell dwarfism[1, 2]	Short stature, skeletal asymmetry, micrognathia. Low birth weight. Café au lait spots, endocrine abnormalities, hypogonadism. Wilms' tumor in 10%.	Possible difficult intubation.[7, 201]
Sipple syndrome[1, 2] (multiple endocrine adenomatosis type II)	Pheochromocytoma (bilateral in 75% of cases), medullary thyroid carcinoma, parathyroid adenoma, multiple endocrine enoplasia.	See Pheochromocytoma. See page 311. Problem of multiple endocrine disorders.[202]
Sleep apnea syndromes	See also Chubby puffer syndrome. Disorders of breathing during sleep, including the following; (1) Central sleep apnea, due to CNS immaturity (? sudden infant death syndrome), trauma, infections, or neoplasms, and primary central alveolar hypoventilation (Ondine's curse). Apnea occurs without evidence of respiratory muscle activity. (2) Obstructive sleep apnea due to obesity, adenoid hypertrophy, Pierre Robin syndrome, or any other condition causing chronic airway obstruction. Apnea occurs because of obstruction and is accompanied by increased respiratory muscle activity. (3) Mixed forms. Medical history may include daytime somnolence, loud snoring, restless sleep, insomnia, fatigue. Children may be hyperactive and aggressive.	Assess airway carefully. Avoid preoperative sedation. Intubate and ventilate during anesthesia. Beware of acute obstruction during induction of anesthesia. Intubation may be difficult. Avoid narcotic analgesics during and after anesthesia. Awaken patient completely during transfer to PACU. Monitor closely for apnea postoperatively.[203, 204]

Smith-Lemli-Opitz syndrome[1,2]	Microcephaly, mental retardation, genital and skeletal anomalies (including micrognathia), thymic hypoplasia, hypotonia; may have increased susceptibility to infection.	Use sterile technique. Airway and intubation problems.[7] Take care with muscle relaxants. Assisted or controlled ventilation may be necessary perioperatively and postoperatively.
Sotos syndrome[1,2] (cerebral gigantism)	Acromegalic features, dilated cerebral ventricles but normal ICP. Nonprogressive.	Possible airway problems due to acromegalic skull. No other problems reported.[7]
Stevens-Johnson syndrome[1] (erythema multiforme)	Urticarial lesions; erosions of mouth, eyes, genitalia. Possible hypersensitivity to exogenous agents (drugs, infections, etc.). If pleural blebs are present, pneumothorax may occur. Dehydration and malnutrition are common. May have myocarditis, pericarditis.	Use antibiotic prophylaxis preoperatively. Check cardiac and fluid status and pulmonary function. Use sterile technique (reverse isolation). Oral lesions—avoid intubation and insertion of esophageal stethoscope. Monitoring is difficult (because of skin lesions) but essential: danger of ventricular fibrillation. Temperature control—febrile episodes: IV infusion essential but do not use cutdown (possibility of infection). Ketamine is probably the best anesthetic agent.[205]
Stiff baby syndrome[206] (hyperexplexia, "startle disease")	Rare, genetic syndrome. Severe muscle rigidity appears at birth and persists for several years. Exaggerated startle response is present. Choking, vomiting, and difficulty swallowing may occur. EMG shows continuous muscle activity.	Use caution with relaxant drugs; monitor effects carefully. May be resistant to succinylcholine but have normal response to pancuronium.[207] Effect of neostigmine is normal.[207] Opioids increase rigidity.[208] Monitor for perioperative apnea.

Table continued on following page

489

Name	Description	Anesthesia Implications
Sturge-Weber syndrome[1,2]	Cavernous angioma over trigeminal nerve distribution, usually unilateral. Developmental mesodermal capillary defect. Glaucoma. Intracranial calcification, convulsions, mental retardation. Possible laryngeal and tracheal involvement.	No specific anesthetic problems.[209,210] Often have port wine stains treated. Care with instrumentation of larynx in case of undiagnosed angioma.
Supravalvar aortic stenosis with idiopathic infantile hypercalcemia	*See* Williams syndrome.	
Tangier disease[2,3] (analphalipoproteinemia)	Low plasma cholesterol; large orange tonsils; anemia and thrombocytopenia due to hypersplenism; peripheral neuropathy and abnormal EMG; premature coronary disease.	Check Hb and platelet count preoperatively. Use caution with muscle relaxants. Be alert for premature ischemic heart disease.[104]
Tay-Sachs disease	*See* Gangliosidosis GM2.	
Telangiectasis, hemorrhagic	*See* Osler-Rendu-Weber syndrome.	
Thalassemia major (Cooley anemia)	Hereditary disease—may affect any race, but most common in Mediterranean and SE Asia. Slow rate of Hb synthesis—high percentage of HbF is present. Low Hb levels require repeated transfusion leading to hemosiderosis. Heterozygous form (thalassemia minor) poses no special anesthesia problems.	Anemia may be severe. Hemosiderosis may affect heart and hepatic function. Facial deformity—overgrowth of maxilla may cause difficult intubation.
Thomsen disease	*See* Myotonia congenita.	
Thromboasthenia	*See* Glanzmann disease	

Thrombocytopenia with absent radius[2]	Episodic thrombocytopenia precipitated by stress, infection, surgery, etc. Platelets increase to normal by adulthood. CHD in 30% of cases.	If CHD is present, use antibiotic prophylaxis preoperatively. Platelet transfusion for surgery or bleeding. Avoid elective surgery in first year (35–40% die in first year from intracranial hemorrhage).[211]
Thrombocytopenia with eczema and repeated infections	See Wiskott-Aldrich syndrome.	
Thrombotic thrombocytopenic purpura	See Moschcowitz disease.	
Tourette syndrome	Complex neuropsychiatric disorder with onset in childhood. Attention deficit disorder progresses to spasmodic repetitious movements that may become powerful muscle jerks. Patient also may exhibit coprolalia (profane speech) and echolalia (repetitions). Treated with haloperidol, clonidine, or pimozide.	Establish rapport with patient and family. Continue medications. Sedate preoperatively. No specific anesthesia regimen is indicated, except that pimozine may cause prolonged Q–T interval syndrome and caution should be used with atropine or halothane.[212]
Treacher-Collins syndrome[1, 2] (mandibulofacial dysostosis)	Micrognathia, aplastic zygoma, microstomia, choanal atresia, coloboma of eyelids. Patients often have cleft palate and cardiac anomalies. Very like Pierre Robin syndrome.	If CHD is present, use antibiotic prophylaxis preoperatively. Possible airway and intubation difficulties (similar to Pierre Robin syndrome but less severe).[5] LMA can be useful in facilitating intubation.[213]
Trismus-pseudocamptodactyly[214] (Dutch-Kentucky syndrome)	Autosomal dominant condition. Decreased mouth opening due to enlarged coronoid process of the mandible and/or abnormal ligaments plus flexion deformity of the fingers when wrist is extended. Short stature and foot deformities may occur. May present for surgery to mandible.	Extremely difficult intubation. May require blind nasal or fiberoptic method.

Table continued on following page

Name	Description	Anesthesia Implications
Trisomies[1-3] Trisomy 13 Trisomy 18[E] Trisomy 21	See Patau syndrome. See Edwards syndrome. See Down syndrome.	
Tuberous sclerosis[1, 2]	Neurocutaneous condition with hamartoma growth in body. Multisystem disease: sebaceous adenoma of skin, epilepsy, mental retardation, intracranial calcification. May have tumors in lungs, heart, kidneys with pyelonephritis and renal failure.	Care with drugs excreted by kidneys. Possible cardiac arrythmia and rupture of lung cysts.[215] Anesthetic management depends on preoperative examination and limitations of organ functions found.[216]
Turner syndrome[1-3, 10-14] (gonadal dysgenesis)	XO females. Short stature, infantile genitalia, webbed neck; possible micrognathia, coarctation, dissecting aneurysm of aorta or PS. Renal anomalies in more than 50% of cases.	If CHD is present, use antibiotic prophylaxis preoperatively. Intubation may be difficult. Assess cardiovascular status. Care with drugs excreted by kidneys.[217]
Umbilical hernia in infancy	Be alert to possibility of Beckwith syndrome.	
Urbach-Wiethe disease[1, 2] (cutaneous mucosal hyalinosis)	Hoarseness or aphonia (hyaline deposits in larynx and pharynx) and skin eruption.	Establishing and maintaining airway may be difficult.[87]
VATER association (VACTERL association)	A nonrandom association of defects: V—vertebral anomalies (congenital scoliosis); A—anal atresia; C—cardiac disease; T—tracheoesophageal fistula; E—esophageal atresia; R—renal anomalies; L—limb defects.	Those of the individual lesions. Examine patient carefully for other congenital lesions, especially renal and cardiac abnormalities.[166]

Syndrome	Description	Anesthetic considerations
Velocardiofacial syndrome	Speech difficulties due to velopharyngeal anomalies, learning disability (mild), CHD (especially ventricular septal defect), and characteristic facies: large nose with broad nasal bridge, vertically long face, narrow palpebral fissures, and retruded mandible.	May present for pharyngoplasty, considerations of CHD. Obstructive sleep apnea may occur after pharyngoplasty and may cause death.[167, 168]
von Gierke disease[2, 3] Type I (glycocgen storage disease)	Hepatomegaly, renal hyperplasia; fasting causes hypoglycemia. Severe biochemical disturbances; unresponsive to epinephrine and glucagon. May have Fanconi syndrome also.	Continuous IV glucose infusion preoperatively and perioperatively. Monitor blood sugar and acid-base balance.[3, 116]
Type III (Cori disease; Forbes disease)	Similar to but milder than type I.	
Type VI (Hers disease)	Similar to but milder than type I.	
von Hippel-Lindau syndrome	Retinal angiomas and cerebellar hemangioblastomas; pheochromocytoma in some; may have pulmonary, pancreatic, hepatic, adrenal, renal cysts. Paroxysmal hypertension due to cerebellar tumor or pheochromocytoma.	Assess renal and hepatic function and investigate for pheochromocytoma (urinary vanillylmandelic acid). Hypertensive crises may occur.[153]
von Recklinghausen disease[1, 2] (neurofibromatosis)	Café au lait spots: tumors in all parts of the CNS (may be in larynx and right ventricular outflow tract); peripheral tumors associated with nerve trunks. Kyphoscoliosis in 50%. May have "honeycomb (cystic) lung." Pheochromocytoma and renal artery dysplasia (hypertension) common.	All these patients should be investigated for pheochromocytoma (urinary vanillylmandelic acid). Test response to neuromuscular drugs; effects of depolarizing and nondepolarizing muscle relaxants may be prolonged.[169] Check pulmonary, renal function. If kidneys are involved, care with drugs excreted by kidneys.[170, 171]

Table continued on following page

Name	Description	Anesthesia Implications
von Willebrand disease[3] (pseudohemophilia)	Prolonged bleeding time (decreased factor VIII activity leading to defective platelet adhesiveness) and capillary abnormality.	Bleeding can be controlled by transfusions of fresh blood or fresh-frozen plasma and/or cryoprecipitate. Do not use salicylates (effect on platelets, possible gastrointestinal bleeding).[106] Monitor factor VIII and bleeding time, maintain factor VIII at >50% activity.
Weber-Christian disease (chronic nonsuppurative panniculitis)	Necrosis of fat—in any situation, including the following: *Retroperitoneal tissue:* may cause acute or chronic adrenal insufficiency. *Pericardium:* leads to restrictive pericarditis. *Meninges:* causes convulsions.	Check cardiac and renal function. Avoid trauma to fat by heat, cold, or pressure. Maintain blood volume; do not use cardiac depressants.[224]
Welander muscular atrophy (late distal hereditary myopathy)	Initially involves distal muscles. Prognosis: for life good, for ambulation poor. *See also* Werdnig-Hoffman disease.	May require spinal fusion. Use extreme care with thiopental and muscle relaxants; do not use respiratory depressant drugs.[21-23]
Werdnig-Hoffman disease[2] (infantile muscular atrophy)	Earlier onset and more severe than Welander muscular atrophy. Feeding difficulties; aspiration of stomach contents. Chronic respiratory problems. Most patients die before puberty.	Minimal anesthesia required. Do not use muscle relaxants or respiratory depressant drugs. Ventilatory support may be required, and weaning from this may be difficult.[21-24]
Werner syndrome[173] (multiple endocrine adenomatosis type I)	Hyperparathyroidism, tumors of pituitary and pancreatic islet cells (hypoglycemia), gastric ulcer. Carcinoid tumors of bronchial tree are common. Renal failure due to stones.	Control blood sugar carefully. Take care with drugs excreted by kidneys.[225]

Syndrome		Management
Werner syndrome[1,3]	Premature aging; diabetes in 50%, mental retardation in 50%, early cataracts, osteomyelitis-like bone lesions, cardiac infarction and failure.	Anesthesia as for adult with myocardial ischemia and diabetes.[5]
Williams syndrome[1] (elfin facies syndrome)	Cardiac anomalies: supravalvular aortic stenosis, mental retardation, elfin facies. Fixed cardiac output and myocardial ischemia leading to dyspnea and angina. Hypercalcemia. Require low calcium diet, steroids, and cardiac corrective surgery.	Antibiotic prophylaxis preoperatively. Check steroid history. Monitor calcium levels perioperatively and avoid cardiac depressants.[226] Transesophageal echocardiography aids anesthetic management.[227]
Wilson disease[3] (hepatolenticular degeneration)	Decreased ceruloplasmin; copper deposits, especially in liver and CNS motor nuclei. Renal tubular acidosis; hepatic failure due to fibrosis.	Thiopental can be used in small doses. Muscle relaxants: succinylcholine—apnea rare, despite pseudocholinesterase reduction; d-tubocurarine—short action due to globulin binding. Care with drugs excreted by kidneys.[228]
Wilson-Mikity syndrome[176]	Prematurity (<1,500 g birth weight); severe chronic lung disease leading to generalized fibrosis with cystic areas, repeated chest infection, aspiration, right ventricular failure. Steroids may be given to try to prevent pulmonary fibrosis. Pathogenesis unknown; possibly a form of O_2 toxicity on lung tissue.	Check respiratory status carefully and assess cardiac function.[229,230] May have a history of steroid therapy.

Table continued on following page

Name	Description	Anesthesia Implications
Wiskott-Aldrich syndrome[2, 3]	Decreased production of platelets; hypersusceptibility to severe herpes simplex infections (disordered immune mechanism), eczema, asthma. May have RES malignancies. Most die before 10 yr of age, many from generalized herpes or opportunistic infection.	Use antibiotic prophylaxis preoperatively. Transfusions of blood and platelets may be required; bone marrow transplantation has been used. All blood products must be irradiated (30 Gy) to prevent graft-versus-host reaction. Use sterile technique (reverse isolation).[106]
Wolf-Parkinson-White (WPW) syndrome[2, 231]	Anomalous conduction path between atria and ventricles. ECG: Short P-R interval; prolonged QRS with phasic variation in 40%. Prone to paroxysmal supraventricular tachycardia (SVT). May have other cardiac defects. Infants, especially preterm, are very prone to SVT.[232]	If CHD is present, use antibiotic prophylaxis preoperatively. Prone to arrhythmias. Paroxysmal SVT on induction of anesthesia has been reported; treat with countershock. Avoid atropine, halothane, or pancuronium. Thiopental, isoflurane, and vecuronium are suitable agents. Avoid use of neostigmine.
Wolman disease[3] (familial xanthomatosis)	Failure to thrive due to xanthomatous visceral changes: adrenal calcification. Resembles Niemann-Pick disease, with hepatosplenomegaly, hypersplenism, and foam cell infiltration (of all tissues, including myocardium.) Death usually by 6 mo of age.	Treatment entirely supportive. Platelet transfusion successful only after splenectomy.[104]
Zellweger syndrome	See Cerebrohepatorenal syndrome.	

General Sources of Information

1. Gorlin RJ, Cohen MM Jr, and Levin LS (eds): Syndromes of the Head and Neck, 3rd ed. McGraw-Hill, New York, 1990.
2. McKusick VA: Mendelian Inheritance in Man, 10th ed. Johns Hopkins University Press, Baltimore, 1992.
3. Scriver CR (ed): The Metabolic and Molecular Bases of Inherited Disease. McGraw-Hill, New York, 1995.
4. Bewumof J (ed): Anesthesia and Uncommon Diseases, 4th ed. WB Saunders, Philadelphia, 1998.
5. McKusick VA: Heritable Disorders of Connective Tissue, 8th ed. Johns Hopkins University Press, Baltimore, 1988.
6. Buyse ML: Birth Defects Encyclopedia. Blackwell, Cambridge, MA, 1990.
7. Smith DW: Recognizable Patterns of Human Malformation, 4th ed. WB Saunders, Philadelphia, 1988.
8. Behrman BE, Kliegman RM, and Jensen HB (eds): Nelson Textbook of Pediatrics, 16th ed. WB Saunders, Philadelphia, 2000.
9. Rudolf AM, Hoffman J, and Rudolph CD (eds): Rudolph's Pediatrics, 20th ed. Appleton-Century-Crofts, East Norwalk, CT, 1996.
10. Katz J and Steward DJ: Anesthesia and Uncommon Pediatric Diseases, 2nd ed. WB Saunders, Philadelphia, 1993.
11. Weinberg GL: Genetics in Anesthesiology: Syndromes and Science. Butterwoth-Heinemann, Boston, 1996.
12. Magalini SI, Sabina C, and Magalini de Francisci G: Dictionary of Medical Syndromes, 3rd ed. JB Lippincott, Philadelphia, 1990.
13. Jablonski S: Jablonski's Dictionary of Syndromes and Eponymic Diseases, 2nd ed. Krieger Publishing, Malabar, FL, 1991.
14. Thoene JG and Smith DC (eds): Physicians' Guide to Rare Diseases. Dowden Publishing, Montvale, NJ, 1992.
15. Mayhew JF, Miner M, and Hall ID: Anaesthesia for the achrondroplastic dwarf. Can Anaesth Soc J 33:216, 1986.
16. Bongiovanni AM and Root AW: The adrenogenital syndrome. N Engl J Med 268:1283, 1963.
17. Choudry DK, Rehman MA, Schwartz RE, et al: The Alagille's syndrome and its anaesthetic considerations. Paediatr Anaesth 8:79, 1998.
18. Morris RC Jr: Renal tubular acidosis: mechanisms, classification and implications. N Engl J Med 281:1405, 1969.
19. Mann JB, Alterman S, and Hills AG: Albright's hereditary osteodystrophy, comprising pseudohypoparathyroidism and pseudo-pseudohypoparathyroidism: with a report of two cases representing the complete syndrome occurring in successive generations. Ann Intern Med 56:315, 1962.
20. Perkoff GT: The hereditary renal diseases. N Engl J Med 277:129, 1967.
21. Ellis FR: Neuromuscular disease and anaesthesia. Br J Anaesth 46:603, 1974.
22. Wislicki L: Anesthesia and postoperative complications in progressive muscular dystrophy: tachycardia and acute gastric dilation. Anesthesia 17:482, 1962.
23. Anesthetic problems in hereditary muscular abnormalities [Editorial]. N Y State J Med 72:1051, 1972.
24. Cobham IG and Davis HS: Anesthesia for muscle dystrophy patients. Anesth Analg 43:22, 1964.
25. Rosenbaum KJ, Neigh JL, and Strobel GE: Sensitivity to non-depolarizing muscle relaxants in amyotrophic lateral sclerosis: report of two cases. Anesthesiology 35:638, 1971.
26. Frank MM, Gelfand JA, and Atkinson JP: NIH conference. Hereditary angioedema: the clinical syndrome and its management. Ann Intern Med 84:580, 1976.

27. Hopkinson RB and Sutcliffe AJ: Hereditary angioneurotic oedema: treatment of angioedema. Anesthesia 34:183, 1979.
28. Gibbs PS, LoSasso AM, Moorthy SS, et al: The anesthetic and perioperative management of a patient with documented hereditary angioneurotic edema. Anesth Analg 56:571, 1977.
29. Gelfand JA, Sherins RJ, Alling DW, et al: Treatment of hereditary angio-edema with danazol. N Engl J Med 295:1444, 1976.
30. Ababa RP and Owens WD: Hereditary angioneurotic edema, an anesthetic dilemma. Anesthesiology 46:428, 1977.
31. Hopkinson RB and Sutcliffe AJ: Hereditary angioneurotic oedema. Anaesthesia 34:183, 1979.
32. LeBard SE and Thiemann LJ: Antley-Bixler syndrome: a case report and discussion. Paediatr Anaesth 8:89, 1998.
33. Andersson H and Gomes SP: Craniosynostosis: review of the literature and indications for surgery. Acta Paediatr Scand 57:47, 1968.
34. Davies DW and Munro IR: The anesthetic management and intraoperative care of patients undergoing major facial osteotomies. Plast Reconstr Surg 55:50, 1975.
35. Koizuka S, Nishikawa K-I, Nemoto H, et al: Intraoperative QRS-interval changes caused by hyperkalaemia in an infant with Arima syndrome. Paediatr Anaesth 8:425, 1998.
36. Friedlander HL, Westin GW, and Wood WL: Arthrogryposis multiplex congenita: a review of 45 cases. J Bone Joint Surg 50:89, 1968.
37. Peterson RDA and Good RA: Ataxia-telangiectasia. Birth Defects 4:370, 1968.
38. Bauman ML and Hogan GR: Laurence-Moon-Biedl syndrome. Am J Dis Child 126:119, 1973.
39. Gill JR Jr, Frölich JC, Bowden RE, et al: Bartter's syndrome: a disorder characterized by high urinary prostaglandins and a dependence of hyperreninemia on prostaglandin synthesis. Am J Med 61:43, 1976.
40. Bowden RE, Gill JR Jr, Radfer N, et al: Prostaglandin synthetase inhibitors in Bartter's syndrome: effect on immunoreactive prostaglandin E excretion. JAMA 239:117, 1978.
41. Kannan S, Delph Y, and Moseley HSL: Anaesthetic management of a child with Bartter's syndrome. Can J Anaesth 42:808, 1995.
42. Ehrlich RM and Martin JM: Diazoxide in the management of hypoglycemia in infancy and childhood. Am J Dis Child 117:411, 1969.
43. Filippi G and McKusick VA: The Beckwith-Wiedemann syndrome (the exophthalmos-macroglossia-gigantism syndrome): report of two cases and review of the literature. Medicine (Baltimore) 49:279, 1970.
44. Thomas ML and McEwan A: The anaesthetic management of a case of Kawasaki's disease (mucocutaneous lymph node syndrome) and Beckwith-Wiedemann syndrome presenting with a bleeding tongue. Paediatr Anaesth 8:500, 1998.
45. Suan C, Ojeda R, Garcia-Perla JL, et al: Anaesthesia and the Beckwith-Wiedemann syndrome. Paediatr Anaesth 6:231, 1996.
46. Chamberlain MA: Behçet's syndrome in 32 patients in Yorkshire. Ann Rheum Dis 36:491, 1977.
47. Turner ME: Anaesthetic difficulties associated with Behçet's syndrome. Br J Anaesth 44:100, 1972.
48. Henderson D and Jackson IT: Naso-maxillary hypoplasia—the Fort II osteotomy. Br J Oral Surg 11:77, 1973.
49. Diamond LK, Allen DM, and Magill FB: Congenital erythroid hypoplastic anemia: a 25-year study. Am J Dis Child 102:403, 1961.

50. Kleinschmidt S, Grueness V, and Molter G: The Bland-White-Garland syndrome: clinical picture and anaesthesiological management. Paediatr Anaesth 6:65, 1996.
51. Laloyaux P, Veyckemans F, and Van Dyck M: Anaesthetic management of a prematurely born infant with Cantrell's Pentalogy. Paediatr Anaesth 8:163, 1998.
52. Eng GD, Epstein BS, Engel WK, et al: Malignant hyperthermia and central-core disease in a child with congenital dislocating hips. Arch Neurol 35:189, 1978.
53. Bowen P, Lee CSN, Zellweger H, et al: A familial syndrome of multiple congenital defects. Bull Johns Hopkins Hosp 114:402, 1964.
54. Baraka A: Vecuronium muscular blockade in a patient with Charcot-Marie-Tooth syndrome. Anesth Analg 84:927, 1997.
55. Stack CG and Wyse RK: Incidence and management of airway problems in the CHARGE association. Anaesthesia 46:582, 1991.
56. Leader RW: The Chédiak-Higashi anomaly—an evolutionary concept of disease. Natl Cancer Inst Monogr 32:337, 1969.
57. Hammer JE III and Ketcham AS: Cherubism: an analysis of treatment. Cancer 23:1133, 1969.
58. Johnston RB and Baehner RL: Chronic granulomatous disease: correlation between pathogenesis and clinical findings. Pediatrics 48:730, 1971.
59. Stool SE, Eavey RD, Stein NL, et al: The chubby puffer syndrome: upper airway obstruction and obesity, with intermittent somnolence and cardio-respiratory embarrassment. Clin Pediatr 16:43, 1977.
60. Wooldridge WJ and Dearlove OR: Anesthesia for Cockayne's syndrome: contemporary solutions to an old problem. Pediatr Anaesth 4:191, 1994.
61. Jenkins LC and McGraw RW: Anaesthetic management of the patient with rheumatoid arthritis. Can Anaesth Soc J 16:407, 1969.
62. Drummond DS, Salter RB, and Boone J: Fat embolism in children: its frequency and relationships to collagen disease. Can Med Assoc J 101:200, 1969.
63. Diaz JH and Friesen RH: Anesthetic management of complete heart block. Anesth Analg 58:334, 1979.
64. Steward DJ and Izukawa T: Congenital complete heart block. Anesth Analg 59:81, 1980.
65. Tasker WG, Mastri AR, and Gold AP: Chondrodystrophia calcificans congenita (dysplasia epiphysealis punctata): recognition of the clinical picture. Am J Dis Child 119:122, 1970.
66. Smith DW: The compendium on shortness of stature. J Pediatr 70:463, 1967.
67. Corsini LM, Stefano G de, Porras MC, et al: Anaesthetic implications of Cornelia de Lange syndrome. Paediatr Anaesth 8:159, 1998.
68. Brislin RP, Stayer SA, and Schwartz RE: Anaesthetic considerations for the patient with cri du chat syndrome. Paediatr Anaesth 5:139, 1995.
69. Payne JF and Cranston AJ: Postoperative airway problems in a child with Crouzon's syndrome. Paediatr Anaesth 5:331, 1995.
70. Wooley MM, Morgan S, and Hays DM: Heritable disorders of connective tissue: surgical and anesthetic problems. J Pediatr Surg 2:325, 1967.
71. DiGeorge AM: Congenital absence of the thymus and its immunologic consequences: concurrence with congenital hypoparathyroidism. Birth Defects 4:116, 1968.
72. Flashburg MH, Dunbar BS, August G, et al: Anesthesia for surgery in an infant with DiGeorge's syndrome. Anesthesiology 58:479, 1983.

73. Benda CE: Down's Syndrome—Mongolism and its Management. Grune & Stratton, New York, 1969.
74. Whaley WJ and Gray WD: Atlanto axial dislocation and Down's syndrome. Can Med Assoc J 123:35, 1980.
75. Rautiainen P and Meretoja O: Intravenous sedation for children with Down's syndrome undergoing cardiac catheterization. Paediatr Anaesth 4:21, 1994.
76. Mitchell V, Howard R, and Facer E: Down's syndrome and anaesthesia. Paediatr Anaesth 5:379, 1995.
77. Sethna NF, Rockoff MA, Wonhen HM, et al: Anesthesia related complications in children with Duchenne muscular dystrophy. Anesthesiology 68:462, 1988.
78. Larsen UT and Hein-Sorensen O: Complications during anaesthesia in patients with Duchenne's muscular dystrophy (a retrospective study). Can J Anaesth 36:418, 1989.
79. Tobias JD and Atwood R: Mivacurium in children with Duchenne muscular dystrophy. Paediatr Anaesth 4:57, 1994.
80. Mizushima A and Satoyoshi M: Anaesthetic problems in a child with ectrodactyly, ectodermal dysplasia and cleft lip palate: the EEC syndrome. Anaesthesia 47:137, 1992.
81. Bailey C and Chung R: Use of the laryngeal mask airway in a patient with Edward's syndrome. Anaesthesia 47:713, 1992.
82. Dolan P, Sisko F, and Riley E: Anesthetic considerations for Ehlers-Danlos syndrome. Anesthesiology 52:266, 1980.
83. Lyons B, Motherway C, Casey W, et al: The anaesthetic management of the child with Eisenmenger's syndrome. Can J Anaesth 42:904, 1995.
84. Wu CL and Litman RS: Anaesthetic management for a child with the Ellis-van Creveld syndrome: a case report. Paediatr Anaesth 4:335, 1994.
85. Ellis RWB and van Creveld S: A syndrome characterized by ectodermal dysplasia, polydactyly, chondrodysplasia and congenital morbus cordis: report of 3 cases. Arch Dis Child 15:65, 1940.
86. Beahrs JO, Lillington GA, Rosan RC, et al: Anhidrotic ectodermal dysplasia: predisposition to bronchial disease. Ann Intern Med 74:92, 1971.
87. Reddy ARR and Wong DHW: Epidermolysis bullosa: a review of anaesthetic problems and case reports. Can Anaesth Soc J 19:536, 1972.
88. James I and Wark H: Airway management during anesthesia in patients with epidermolysis bullosa dystrophica. Anesthesiology 56:323, 1982.
89. Kaplan R and Strauch B: Regional anesthesia in a child with epidermolysis bullosa. Anesthesiology 67:262, 1987.
90. Wise D, Wallace HJ, and Jellinek EH: Angiokeratoma corporis diffusum. Q J Med 31:177, 1962.
91. Melnick B, Chang JL, Larson CE, et al: Hypokalemic familial periodic paralysis. Anesthesiology 58:263, 1983.
92. Joel M and Rosales RK: Fanconi syndrome and anesthesia. Anesthesiology 55:455, 1981.
93. Tobia JD: Anaesthesic implications of cystinosis. Can J Anaesth 40:518, 1993.
94. Gilbertson AA and Boulton TB: Anaesthesia in difficult situations: influence of disease on pre-op preparation and choice of anesthetic. Anaesthesia 22:607, 1967.
95. Asada A, Tatekawa S, Terai T, et al: The anesthetic implications of a patient with Farber's lipogranulomatosis. Anesthesiology 80:206, 1994.
96. Clarren SK and Smith DW: The fetal alcohol syndrome. N Engl J Med 298:1063, 1978.
97. Finucaine BT: Difficult intubation associated with the fetal alcohol syndrome. Can Anaesth Soc J 27:574, 1980.
98. Ashley MJ: Symposium: alcohol and the fetus. Can Med Assoc J 125:141, 1981.

99. Laishley RS and Roy WL: Freeman-Sheldon syndrome: report of three cases and the anaesthetic implications. Can Anaesth Soc J 33:388, 1986.

100. Munro HM, Butler PJ, and Washington EJ: Freeman-Sheldon (whistling face) syndrome: anaesthetic and airway management. Paediatr Anaesth 7:345, 1997.

101. Duggar RG, DeMars PD, and Bolton VE: Whistling face syndrome: general anesthesia and early postoperative caudal analgesia. Anesthesiology 70:545, 1989.

102. Jones R and Dolcourt JL: Muscle rigidity following halothane anesthesia in two patients with Freeman-Sheldon syndrome. Anesthesiology 77:599, 1992.

103. Vas L and Naregal P: Anaesthetic management of a patient with Freeman Sheldon syndrome. Paediatr Anaesth 8:175, 1998.

104. Fredrickson DS: Disorders of lipid metabolism and xanthomatoses. In Thorn GW, Adams RD, Braunwald E, et al. (eds.): Harrison's Principles of Internal Medicine, 8th ed. McGraw-Hill, New York, 1977, p 670.

105. Watne A: Gardner's syndrome. In Lynch HT (ed.): Skin: Heredity and Malignant Neoplasms. Medical Examinations Publishing Co., Flushing, NY, 1972, p 165.

106. Wintrobe M (ed.): Clinical Hematology, 7th ed. Lea & Febiger, Philadelphia, 1974.

107. Mangar D, Murtha PA, Aquilna TC, et al: Anesthesia for a patient with Gorham's syndrome: "Disappearing bone disease." Anesthesiology 80:466, 1994.

108. Beach TP, Stone WA, and Hamelberg W: Circulatory collapse following succinylcholine: report of a patient with diffuse lower motor neuron disease. Anesth Analg 50:431, 1971.

109. Smith RB: Hyperkalaemia following succinylcholine administration in neurological disorders: a review. Can Anaesth Soc J 18:199, 1971.

110. Roy RC, McLain S, Wise A, et al: Anesthetic management of a patient with Hallervorden-Spatz disease. Anesthesiology 58:382, 1983.

111. Padda GS, Cruz OA, Silen ML, et al.: Skin conductance responses in paediatric Harlequin syndrome. Paediatr Anaesth 9:159, 1999.

112. Nagata O, Tateoka A, Shiro R, et al.: Anaesthetic management of two paediatric patients with Hecht-Beals syndrome. Paediatr Anaesth 9:444–447, 1999.

113. Turco GR and Farber NE: Postoperative autonomic deficit: a case of harlequin syndrome. Anesthesiology 85:1197, 1996.

114. Johnson GD and Rosales JK: The haemolytic uraemic syndrome and anesthesia. Can J Anaesth 34:196, 1987.

115. Lieberman PH, Dargeon HWK, and Begg CF: A reappraisal of eosinophilic granuloma of bone: Hand-Schüller-Christian syndrome and Letterer-Siwe syndrome. Medicine (Baltimore) 48:375, 1969.

116. Lewis KB, Bruce RA, and Baum D, et al.: The upper limb-cardio-vascular syndrome: an autosomal dominant genetic effect on embryogenesis. JAMA 193:1080, 1965.

117. Crooke JW, Towers JF, and Taylor WH: Management of patients with homocystinuria requiring surgery under general anesthesia. Br J Anaesth 43:96, 1971.

118. Busoni P and Fognani G: Failure of the laryngeal mask to secure the airway in a patient with Hunter's syndrome (mucopolysaccharidosis type II). Paediatr Anaesth 9:153, 1999.

119. Kreidstein A, Boorin MR, Crespi P, et al: Delayed awakening from general anaesthesia in a patient with Hunter syndrome. Can J Anaesth 41:423, 1994.

120. King DH, Jones RM, and Barnett MB: Anesthetic considerations in the mucopolysaccharidoses. Anesthesia 39:1261, 1984.

121. Wilder RT, Belani KG: Fiberoptic intubation complicated by pulmonary edema in a 12 year old with Hurler syndrome. Anesthesiology 72:205, 1990.

122. Adu-Gyamfi Y, Said A, Chowdhary UM, et al.: Anaesthetic induced ventricular tachyarrhythmia in Jervell and Lange-Nielsen syndrome. Can J Anaesth 38:345, 1991.

123. Jervell A and Lange-Nielsen F: Congenital deaf-mutism, functional heart disease with prolongation of the Q-T interval and sudden death. Am Heart J 54:59, 1957.

124. Holland JJ: Cardiac arrest under anesthesia in a child with previously undiagnosed Jervell and Lange Nielsen syndrome. Anaesthesia 48:149, 1993.

125. Yanagida H, Kemi C, and Suwa K: The effects of stellate ganglion block on idiopathic prolongation of the Q-T interval with cardiac arrhythmia (the Romano-Ward syndrome). Anesth Analg 55:782, 1976.

126. Bush GH and Steward DJ: Severe hypoglycaemia associated with preoperative fasting and intraoperative propranalol. Paediatr Anaesth 6:415, 1996.

127. Baines DB and Murrell D: Preoperative hypoglycaemia, propranolol and the Jervell and Lange-Nielsen syndrome. Paediatr Anaesth 9:156, 1999.

128. Vaughn GC, Kaplan RF, Tieche S, et al.: Juvenile hyaline fibromatosis: anesthetic management. Anesthesiology 72:201, 1990.

129. Zelt BA and LoSasso AM: Prolonged nasotracheal intubation and mechanical ventilation in the management of asphyxiating thoracic dystrophy: a case report. Anesth Analg 51:342, 1972.

130. Habre W, Sims C, and D'Souza M: Anaesthetic management of children with Joubert syndrome. Paediatr Anaesth 7:251, 1997.

131. Miller RD and Divertie MB: Kartagener's syndrome. Chest 62:130, 1972.

132. Kasabach HH and Merritt KK: Capillary hemangioma with extensive purpura; report of a case. Am J Dis Child 59:1063, 1940.

133. Propp RP and Scharfman WB: Hemangioma—thrombocytopenia syndrome associated with microangiopathic hemolytic anemia. Blood 28:623, 1966.

134. Quick AJ: Hemorrhagic Diseases and Thrombosis, 2nd ed. Lea & Febiger, Philadelphia, 1966.

135. Melish ME: Kawasaki syndrome (the mucocutaneous lymph node syndrome). Annu Rev Med 33:569, 1982.

136. McNiece WL, Krishna C: Kawasaki disease—a disease with anesthetic implications. Anesthesiology 58:269, 1983.

137. Edwards WT and Burney RG: Use of repeated nerve blocks in management of an infant with Kawasaki's disease. Anesth Analg 67:1008, 1988.

138. Janke EL, Fletcher JE, and Lewis IH: Anaesthetic management of the Kenny-Caffey syndrome using the laryngeal mask. Paediatr Anaesth 6:235, 1996.

139. Stevenson GW, Hall SC, and Palmieri J: Anesthetic considerations for patients with Larsen's syndrome. Anesthesiology 75:142, 1991.

140. Lauder GR and Sumner E: Larsen's syndrome: anaesthetic implications. Six case reports. Paediatr Anaesth 5:133, 1995.

141. Banman ML and Hogan GR: Laurence-Moon-Biedl syndrome. Am J Dis Child 126:119, 1973.

142. Hommes FA, Polman HA, and Reerink JD: Leigh's encephalomyelopathy: an inborn error of gluconeogenesis. Arch Dis Child 43:423, 1968.

143. Kallo A, Lakatos I, and Szijarto L: Leprechaunism (Donohue's syndrome). J Pediatr 66:372, 1965.

144. Larson LO and Wilkins RG: Anesthesia and Lesch-Nyhan syndrome. Anesthesiology 63:197, 1985.

145. Tobias JD: Anaesthetic considerations for the child with leukodystrophy. Can J Anaesth 39:394, 1992.

146. Richards W, Donnell GN, Wilson WA, et al.: The oculo-cerebro-renal syndrome of Lowe. Am J Dis Child 109:185, 1965.

147. Desnick RJ, Sharp HL, Grabowski GA, et al.: Mannosidosis: clinical morphologic, immunologic, and biochemical studies. Pediatr Res 10:985, 1976.

148. Delaney A and Gal TJ: Hazards of anesthesia and operation in maple syrup urine disease. Anesthesiology 44:83, 1976.

149. Linstedt U, Maier C, Joehnk H, et al.: Threatening spinal cord compression during anesthesia in a child with mucopolysaccharidosis VI. Anesthesiology 80:227, 1994.

150. Antila H, Laito T, Aantaa R, et al: Difficult airway in a patient with Marshall-Smith syndrome. Paediatr Anaesth 8:429, 1998.

151. Coleman MA, Liberthson RR, Crone RK, et al: General anesthesia in a child with urticaria pigmentosa. Anesth Analg 59:704, 1980.

152. Cox JM: Anesthesia and glycogen-storage disease. Anesthesiology 29:1221, 1968.

153. Tobias JD: Anaesthetic considerations in a child with Menkes' syndrome. Can J Anaesth 39:712, 1992.

154. Rosenberg LE, Lilljeqvist AC, and Hsia YE: Methylmalonic acid-urea: an inborn error leading to metabolic acidosis, long chain ketonuria and intermittent hyperglycinemia. N Engl J Med 278:1319, 1968.

155. Sharar SR, Haberkern CM, Jack R, et al.: Anesthetic management of a child with methylmalonyl-coenzyme A mutase deficiency. Anesth Analg 73:499, 1991.

156. Birkinsaw KJ: Anesthesia in a patient with a unstable neck: Morquio's syndrome. Anaesthesia 30:46, 1975.

157. Bingham RM and Wilkinson DJ: Anesthetic management in moya moya disease. Anaesthesia 40:1198, 1985.

158. Brown SC and Lain AM: Moya moya disease—a review of clinical experience and anaesthetic management. Can J Anaesth 34:71, 1987.

159. Soriano SG, Sethna NF, and Scott RM: Anesthetic management of children with moya moya disease. Anesth Analg 77:1066, 1993.

160. Diaz JH and Belani KG: Perioperative management of children with mucopolysaccharidoses. Anesth Analg 77:1261, 1993.

161. Karhunen U: Serum creatine kinase levels after succinylcholine in children with "muscle, eye and brain disease." Can J Anaesth 35:90, 1988.

162. Davies DW and Steward DJ: Myasthenia gravis in children and an unaesthetic management for thymectomy. Can Anaesth Soc J 20:253, 1973.

163. Dalal FY, Bennett EJ, and Gregg WS: Congenital myasthenia gravis and minor surgical procedures. Anaesthesia 27:61, 1972.

164. Crawford J: A review of 41 cases of myasthenia gravis subjected to thymectomy. Anaesthesia 26:513, 1971.

165. Przylbo HJ, Stevenson GW, Vicari F, et al.: Retrograde fibreoptic intubation in a child with Nager's syndrome. Can J Anaesth 43:697, 1996.

166. Walker JS, Dorian RS, and Marsh NJ: Anesthetic management of a child with Nager's syndrome. Anesth Analg 79:1025, 1994.

167. Ravin M, Newark Z, and Saviello G: Myotonia dystrophica—an anesthetic hazard: two case reports. Anesth Analg 54:216, 1975.

168. Cunliffe M and Burrows FA: Anaesthetic implications of nemaline rod myopathy. Can Anaesth Soc J 32:543, 1985.

169. Asai T, Fujise K, and Uchida M: Anesthesia for cardiac surgery in children with nemaline myopathy. Anaesthesia 47:405, 1992.

170. Grange C, Heid R, Lucas SB, et al: Anaesthesia in a parturient with Noonan's syndrome. Can J Anaesth 45:332, 1998.

171. Schwartz N and Eisenkraft JB: Anesthetic management of a child with Noonan's syndrome and idiopathic hypertrophic subaortic stenosis. Anesth Analg 74:464, 1992.

172. Campbell AM and Bousfield ID: Anaesthesia in a patient with Noonan's syndrome and cardiomyopathy. Anesthesiology 47:131, 1992.

173. Colreavy F, Colbert S, and Dunphy J: Oculodento-osseous dysplasia: a review of anaesthetic problems. Paediatr Anaesth 4:179, 1994.

174. Bolsin SN and Gillbe C: Opitz-Frias syndrome: a case with potentially hazardous anesthetic implications. Anaesthesia 40:1189, 1985.

175. King JD and Bobechko W: Osteogenesis imperfecta. J Bone Joint Surg 53:72, 1471.

176. Pollard RC and Beasley JM: Anaesthesia for patients with trisomy 13 (Patau's syndrome). Paediatr Anaesth 6:151, 1996.

177. Fraser GR, Morgans ME, and Trotter WR: The syndrome of sporadic goitre and congenital deafness. Q J Med 29:279, 1960.

178. Jones SEF and Derrick GM: Difficult intubation in an infant with Pierre Robin syndrome and concomitant tongue tie. Paediatr Anaesth 8:510, 1998.

179. Freeman MK and Manners IM: Cor pulmonale and the Pierre-Robin's anomaly. Anesthesia 35:282, 1980.

180. Baraka A and Muallem M: Bullard laryngoscopy for tracheal intubation in a neonate with Pierre-Robin syndrome. Paediatr Anaesth 4:111, 1994.

181. McDonald D: Anaesthetic management of a patient with Plott's syndrome. Paediatr Anaesth 8:155, 1998.

182. Sethuraman R, Kannan S, Bala I, et al.: Anaesthesia in Poland syndrome. Can J Anaesth 45:277, 1998.

183. Epslein FH: Cystic diseases of the kidneys. In Thorn GW (ed.): Harrison's Principles of Internal Medicine, 8th ed. McGraw-Hill, New York, 1977, p 1470.

184. Dunn HG: The Prader-Labhart-Willi syndrome: review of the literature and report of nine cases. Acta Paediatr Scand (Suppl) 186:3, 1968.

185. Palmer SK and Atlee JL: Anesthetic management of the Prader-Willi syndrome. Anesthesiology 44:161, 1976.

186. Dearlove OR, Dobson A, and Super M: Anaesthesia and Prader-Willi syndrome. Paediatr Anaesth 8:267, 1998.

187. Chapin JW and Kahre J: Progeria and anesthesia. Anesth Analg 58:424, 1979.

188. Hannington-Kiff JG: Prune-belly syndrome and general anesthesia: case report. Br J Anaesth 42:649, 1970.

189. Heisler DB, Lebowitz P, and Barst SM: Pectus excavatum repair in a patient with prune belly syndrome. Paediatr Anaesth 4:267, 1994.

190. Dearlove OR and Walker RWM: Anaesthesia for Rett syndrome. Paediatr Anaesth 6:155, 1996.

191. Haller JS: The enigmatic encephalopathy of Reye's syndrome. Hosp Pract 10:91, 1975.

192. Axelrod FB, Donenfeld RF, Danziger F, et al.: Anesthesia in familial dysautonomia. Anesthesiology 68:631, 1988.

193. Inkster JS: Anaesthesia for a patient suffering from familial dysautonomia (Riley-Day syndrome). Br J Anaesth 43:509, 1971.

194. Meridy HW and Creighton RE: General anaesthesia in eight patients with familial dysautonomia. Can Anaesth Soc J 18:563, 1971.

195. Challands JF and Facer EK: Epidural anaesthesia and familial dysautonomia (the Riley-Day syndrome): three case reports. Paediatr Anaesth 8:83, 1998.

196. Perks WH, Cooper RA, Bradbury S, et al.: Sleep apnea in Scheie's syndrome. Thorax 35:85, 1980.

197. Theroux MC, Kettrick RG, and Khine HH: Laryngeal mask airway and fiberoptic endoscopy in an infant with Schwartz-Jampel syndrome. Anesthesiology 82:605, 1995.

198. Birkhan J, Heifetz M, and Haim S: Diffuse cutaneous scleroderma: an anaesthetic problem. Anaesthesia 27:89, 1972.

199. Cohen CA: Anesthetic management of a patient with the Shy-Drager syndrome. Anesthesiology 35:95, 1971.

200. Malan MD and Crago R: Anesthetic implications in idiopathic orthostatic hypotension and the Shy-Drager syndrome. Can Anaesth Soc J 26:322, 1979.

201. Dinner M, Golden EZ, Ward R, et al: Russell-Silver syndrome: anesthetic implications. Anesth Analg 78:1197, 1994.

202. Steiner AL, Goodman AD, and Powers SR: Study of a kindred with pheochromocytoma, medullary thyroid carcinoma, hyperparathyroidism and Cushing's disease: multiple endocrine neoplasia type 2. Medicine (Baltimore) 47:371, 1968.

203. Chung F and Crago RR: Sleep apnea syndrome and anesthesia. Can Anaesth Soc J 29:439, 1982.

204. Phillipson EA: Control of breathing during sleep. Am Rev Resp Dis 118:909, 1978.

205. Cucchiara RE and Dawson B: Anesthesia in Stevens-Johnson syndrome: report of a case. Anesthesiology 35:537, 1971.

206. Lingham S, Wilson J, and Hart EW: Hereditary stiff baby syndrome. Am J Dis Child 135:909, 1981.

207. Cook WP and Kaplan RF: Neuromuscular blockade in a patient with stiff baby syndrome. Anesthesiology 65:525, 1986.

208. Doolittle GM and Greiner AS: Anesthetic complications in an infant with hyperexplexia. Anesthesiology 73:181, 1990.

209. Alexander GL and Norman RM: The Sturge-Weber Syndrome. Wright, Bristol, 1960.

210. Batra RK, Gulaya V, Madan R, et al.: Anaesthesia and the Sturge-Weber syndrome. Can J Anaesth 41:133, 1994.

211. Hall JG, Levin JP, and Kuhn JP, et al.: Thrombocytopenia with absent radius. Medicine (Baltimore) 48:411, 1969.

212. Morrison JE and Lockhart CH: Tourette syndrome: anesthetic implications. Anesth Analg 65:200, 1986.

213. Inada T, Fujise K, Tachibana K, et al.: Orotracheal intubation through the laryngeal mask airway in paediatric patients with Treacher-Collins syndrome. Paediatr Anaesth 5:129, 1995.

214. Vaghadia H and Blackstock D: Anesthetic implications of the trismus pseudocamptodactyly (Dutch-Kentucky or Hecht-Beals) syndrome. Can J Anaesth 35:80, 1988.

215. Lagos JC and Gomez MR: Tuberous sclerosis: reappraisal of a clinical entity. Mayo Clin Proc 42:26, 1967.

216. Schweiger JW, Schwartz RE, and Stayer SA: The anaesthetic management of the patient with tuberous sclerosis complex. Paediatr Anaesth 4:339, 1994.

217. Strader WJ III, Wachtel HL, and Landberg GD Jr: Hypertension and aortic rupture in gonadal dysgenesis. J Pediatr 79:473, 1971.

218. Quan L and Smith DW: The VATER association, vertebral defects, anal atresia, tracheoesophageal fistula with esophageal atresia, radial dysplasia. Birth Defects 8:75, 1972.

219. Shprintzen RJ, Goldberg RB, Lewin ML, et al: A new syndrome involving cleft palate, cardiac anomalies, typical facies and learning disabilities: velocardio-facial syndrome. Cleft Palate J 15:56, 1978.

220. Kravath RE, Pollask CP, Borowieki B, et al: Obstructive sleep apnea and death associated with surgical correction of velopharyngeal incompetence. J Pediatr 96:645, 1980.

221. Yamashita M, Matsuki A, and Oyama T: Anaesthetic considerations on von Recklinghausen's disease (multiple neurofibromatosis): abnormal response to muscle relaxants. Anaesthetist 26:317, 1977.

222. Brasfied RD and Das Gupta TK: von Recklinghausen's disease: a clinicopathological study. Ann Surg 175:86, 1972.

223. Gibbs NM, Taylor M, and Young A: von Recklinghausen's disease in the larynx and trachea of an infant. J Otolaryngol 71:626, 1957.

224. Spivak JL, Lindo S, and Coleman M: Weber-Christian disease complicated by consumption coagulopathy and microangiopathic hemolytic anemia. Johns Hopkins Med J 126:344, 1970.

225. Wermer P: Endocrine adenomatosis and peptide ulcer in a large kindred: inherited multiple tumors and mosaic pleiotropism in man. Am J Med 35:205, 1963.

226. Fay JE, Lynn RB, and Partington MW: Supravalvular aortic stenosis, mental retardation and a characteristic facies. Can Med Assoc J 94:295, 1966.

227. Kawahito S, Kitahata H, Kimura H, et al.: Anaesthetic management of a patient with Williams syndrome undergoing aortoplasty for supravalvular aortic stenosis. Can J Anaesth 45:1203, 1998.

228. Trachtenberg HA: Anesthesia for patient with hepatic disease. Int Anesthesiol Clin 8:437, 1970.

229. Wilson MG and Mikity VG: A new form of respiratory disease in premature infants. Am J Dis Child 99:489, 1960.

230. Northway WH Jr, Rosan RC, and Porter DY: Pulmonary disease following respirator therapy of hyaline-membrane disease: bronchopulmonary dysplasia. N Engl J Med 276:357, 1967.

231. Hannington-Kiff JG: The Wolff-Parkinson-White syndrome and general anesthesia. Br J Anaesth 40:791, 1968.

232. Richmond MN and Conroy PT: Anesthetic management of a neonate born prematurely with Wolff-Parkinson-White syndrome. Anesth Analg 67:477, 1988.

Appendix II

Cardiopulmonary Resuscitation, Including Neonatal Resuscitation

Cardiopulmonary resuscitation (CPR) is concerned with the restoration of pulmonary, cardiovascular, and neurologic function. Initially it consists of artificial ventilation and artificial circulation by whatever means are immediately available. This is termed *basic life support*. Its object is to prevent clinical death from progressing to biologic death before other remedial measures (i.e., *advanced life support*) can be instituted to restore and maintain cardiopulmonary function.

As in adults, heroic resuscitative efforts may not be indicated in children with lethal terminal disease. This is a decision that should be made in advance and clearly documented and communicated.

The success rate for pediatric CPR is possibly worse than for adults, especially if success is defined as long-term survival without neurologic deficit. A possible reason is that many cases of cardiac arrest in pediatric patients are a result of hypoxemia. In such patients it must be assumed that by the time the heart has suffered hypoxia enough to stop it, the brain has also suffered hypoxia enough to severely damage it. This being so, every effort must be directed at detecting and treating any respiratory compromise before it leads to serious hypoxemia.

PREVENTION OF CARDIAC ARREST

Awareness of precipitating factors is essential in preventing cardiac arrest in children, in whom the primary cause is usually extracardiac.

Common causes include:

1. Failure of ventilation:
   a. Due to central depression, airway obstruction, or primary pulmonary disorders
   b. Secondary to regurgitation and vomiting
   c. As a result of neurologic and neuromuscular disorders
2. Hypovolemia
3. Toxicity (drugs, poisons, toxins)
4. Primary cardiac disorders. (These account for only a small percentage of cardiac arrests on the general wards of a pediatric hospital.)

Prevention requires:

1. Recognition of potential causes, which may be multiple
2. Constant surveillance
3. Early recognition of respiratory failure

Special Hazards for Pediatric Patients

Anesthesiologists should constantly be aware of factors that may be insignificant in the adult but may rapidly become life-threatening in small patients.

At any time, the upper airway may become obstructed by

1. Small amounts of mucus or blood
2. Hypertrophied adenoidal tissue
3. The relatively large tongue, associated with
   a. Muscle flaccidity in the anesthetized patient
   b. Inadvertent displacement or compression of submental soft tissue and tongue by the anesthesiologist's fingers
   c. Inadequate head extension
   d. Inadequate elevation of jaw
   e. Premature removal of an artificial airway
4. Regurgitated stomach contents—a common occurrence because of the frequency of feedings

In addition, ventilation may be compromised if the stomach becomes inflated, usually a result of

1. An inflation pressure that is too high
2. Partial obstruction of airway

Use a no. 10 or 12 suction catheter to aspirate the stomach, after protecting the airway with an endotracheal tube to reduce the possibility of aspiration.

Remember: Infants are primarily nose-breathers. If the nasal airway is inadequate, an oral airway should be inserted.

Routine Precautions

Preoperative

1. Be prepared to give atropine to all young patients if they are to be intubated or to receive cholinergic drugs (e.g., halothane, succinylcholine).
2. Always give 100% O_2 before intubating the child. (Desaturation occurs much more rapidly in children, particularly infants, than in adults.) Intubate as quickly and smoothly as possible.
3. Select the endotracheal tube size carefully, secure it firmly, and check its position. Confirm the end-tidal carbon dioxide trace and listen to both sides of the chest. Arrange and support the tube so that it cannot possibly kink. (These procedures are critical in children.)

Perioperative

1. Maintain a patent airway and adequate ventilation.
2. Monitor the following constantly:
   a. Heart and lung function by stethoscope
   b. Pulse oximeter and end-tidal carbon dioxide
   c. Body temperature
   d. Blood losses
3. Measure carefully all gases, vapors, and drugs.
4. Measure fluid losses accurately and replace as quickly as possible. (Even a small loss is significant in a small child.)
5. Avoid unintentional pressure on the chest and abdominal wall from dressings, hands, surgical assistants leaning on drapes, and so on.
6. If problems arise, advise other members of the team (especially the surgeon) immediately.

Postoperative

Note: Cardiac arrest in the postanesthesia care unit is as likely as in the operating room.

1. All infants and all seriously ill patients: do not extubate unless and until patient is reacting vigorously.
2. If possible, all children should be taken to the postanesthesia room in the lateral position, with the upper leg flexed at the hip and knee and the neck moderately extended.
3. In the postanesthesia room:
   a. Do not leave until you have handed over care of your patient to a nurse

    b. The patient's position is maintained.
        i. Order humidified O_2 by mask until the child is responding well.
       ii. Ensure that vital signs are recorded and reported to you.
    c. Some neonates and infants need to be disturbed frequently to stimulate respiration.
    d. Before assigning the child back to a ward, ensure that the danger of drug-induced respiratory depression has passed and that the child is fully conscious.
    e. All preterm infants of less than 45 weeks' conceptual age and those with a history of chronic respiratory disease should be monitored on an apnea alarm for at least 24 hours.

RESUSCITATION

Basic Life Support

N.B. For basic life support in hospitals, recommendations regarding mouth-to-mouth ventilation for initial resuscitation are replaced by advice to use an interposed plastic airway (e.g., the Brook airway) or bag and mask to avoid risk of infection to hospital personnel. Make sure that such equipment is provided to all patient-care areas.
    Do not leave the patient. Call for help!
    Begin with the ABCs:

A: Airway: check
B: Breathing (four ventilations)
C: Cardiac activity: check

    When called to resuscitate a child, assess the situation immediately according to the following priorities:

A. Check Ventilation

1. *If there are respiratory movements:*
    a. Position the patient to provide a clear airway.
    b. Give O_2 by mask as soon as it becomes available.
2. *If there are respiratory movements but there is evidence of airway obstruction* (breath sounds absent, intercostal retraction, flaring of lateral chest margins, cyanosis):
    a. Pull the tongue or lower jaw forward and remove any foreign matter from the pharynx, keeping the mouth slightly open.
    b. Give O_2 by mask.
    c. Check for improved chest movement and breath sounds.

B. If There Is No Respiratory Movement or Ventilation Appears Inadequate

1. Begin positive-pressure ventilation at once.
2. Ventilate directly, mouth to mouth, until resuscitation equipment is placed in your hand. (The small infant face necessitates application

of your mouth to the patient's mouth and nose). An infant's tidal volume is small (8–10 ml/kg); therefore, only puffs are necessary.

As soon as possible begin ventilation using a bag and mask with oxygen.

C. If the Pulse Is Undetectable by Femoral, Carotid, or Brachial Artery Palpation

1. Start external cardiac compression at once:
   a. The site of compression in an infant is one finger-breadth below the intermammary line; in a child, it is one finger-breadth above the xiphisternum.
   b. Depth of compression: one-third to one-half of the anteroposterior diameter of the chest.
   c. Rate of compression: infants, 100–120 breaths/min, depth 1.5–2.5 cm; children, 80–100 breaths/min, depth 2.5–4.0 cm; adolescents, 80 breaths/min.
   d. Rate of ventilation: Having selected the appropriate rate for cardiac compression, maintain the same ratio of ventilation to cardiac compressions regardless of age or size:
      i. Two-person technique: 1 ventilation to 5 compressions
      ii. Single-person technique: 2 ventilations to 15 compressions
      iii. In small infants, one person may be able to maintain a 1:5 ratio, because the resuscitator does not have to move from mouth to chest.
      iv. For anesthetized patients who are already intubated, a ratio of 1 cardiac compression to 2 ventilations with 100% O_2 should be initiated immediately.
   e. If possible, and especially if the patient is on a soft bed, apply cardiac compressions to infants by encircling the chest with your hands (Fig. II–1). This method results in a larger cardiac output than anterior sternal compression.
   f. Cardiac compression should occupy 50% of the cycle.
2. After the initial 1 minute and at subsequent 5-minute intervals:
   a. Check for pulse.
   b. Note pupil size.
   c. Resume resuscitation within 10 seconds.

N.B. All anesthesiologists should have perfected this skill enough to meet the International Heart Association standards by practice with expert coaching on a manikin.

Advanced Life Support

The foregoing provides only basic interim resuscitation. Most children also require:

1. Ventilation with O_2 as soon as it is available. Ventilation and oxygenation are the first line of therapy for the acidosis that accompanies cardiac arrest.

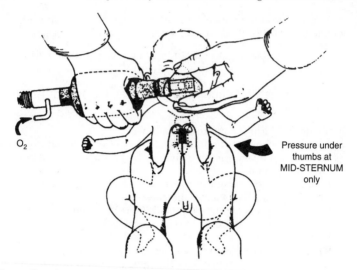

O₂

Pressure under
thumbs at
MID-STERNUM
only

Figure II-1. Two-handed method of external cardiac compression. Note how both hands encircle the chest and how both thumbs are used for cardiac compression. (From Todres D, Rogers MC: Method of external cardiac massage in the newborn infant. J Pediatr 86:781, 1975, with permission.)

2. Protection of the airway by insertion of an endotracheal tube. (The laryngeal mask airway may be useful in some instances).
3. Definitive electrocardiographic diagnosis of cardiac activity and defibrillation if indicated (*see below*).
4. Supportive drugs, beginning with epinephrine (*see below*).
5. Further pharmacologic and medical treatment, including fluid replacement, as indicated.
6. Consideration of the possibility of lung injury by aspirated acidic stomach contents.
7. Early assessment of neurologic function—plan early and continue treatment to minimize and prevent further hypoxic-ischemic brain damage.

Initial Drug Therapy

Choice and Dose of Initial Drug

Although subsequent drug therapy is necessarily individualized, a standard initial protocol is advantageous.

1. Epinephrine: To be maximally effective, it must be given intravenously (preferably into a central vein).
   a. Initial dose: 0.01 mg/kg (0.1 ml/kg of a 1:10,000 solution).
   b. Subsequent doses for refractory asystole: 0.1 mg/kg (0.1 ml/kg of a 1:1,000 solution). In some cases doses as high as 0.2 mg/kg

have proved successful in refractory arrest. This may be repeated every 5 minutes, as necessary.

   c. Epinephrine infusion 20 μg/kg/min may be used in place of repeated boluses for the treatment of refractory arrest.

   d. Epinephrine infusion 0.1–1 μg/kg/min may be used to maintain circulation once cardiac action is restored; titrate to achieve desired effect.

   e. Epinephrine by the intratracheal route is less predictable; use a dose of 0.1 mg/kg if this is the only available route.

2. Dopamine infusion may be required for continued hypotension and poor tissue perfusion; 5–20 μg/kg/min may be titrated to achieve the desired effect.

3. Sodium bicarbonate administration should be considered in prolonged cardiac arrest for documented continuing severe metabolic acidosis despite adequate ventilation, oxygenation, and chest compressions.

N.B. Administration of excessive doses of sodium bicarbonate produces hyperosmolarity, hypernatremia, hypokalemia, decreased ionized calcium, impaired cardiac action, and possibly severe alkalosis after recovery.

   a. Titration of bicarbonate dosage with serial blood gas analysis is ideal. Failing this:

   b. If initial response to resuscitation is lacking despite adequate ventilation and oxygenation, 1 mEq/kg of sodium bicarbonate may be given and may be repeated every 10 minutes during prolonged cardiac arrest.

4. Calcium: The use of calcium during resuscitation is being questioned, because intracellular calcium accumulation is known to accompany cell death. However, the use of calcium has occasionally appeared to have had a good effect in some refractory pediatric cases. It should be given to patients with suspected low levels of ionized calcium that are contributing to continued poor cardiac action. It may also have a place in the treatment of prolonged persistent asystole in children. It is also used in the urgent treatment of hyperkalemia.

   a. Indications: poor cardiac action, hyperkalemia

   b. Dose: 20 mg/kg IV

5. Glucose: Documented hypoglycemia should be treated by glucose infusions. Otherwise, avoid any glucose administration, because hyperglycemia may compromise neurologic outcome after a hypoxic event.

Route of Administration of Drugs

Inject epinephrine into a central line, if one is available; otherwise, use a peripheral intravenous line. Epinephrine may be administered into the trachea via the endotracheal tube if no intravenous route is present.

   Intracardiac injections should not be made except as a last resort.

Damage to the heart and coronary arteries and/or a pneumothorax may result.

Calcium should be injected via a central line if possible. Severe skin necrosis may result from superficial extravasation.

Fluid Replacement

1. Insert a large-bore intravenous cannula as soon as possible:
   a. To provide a route for drug therapy.
   b. For rapid replacement of fluid. (In cardiac arrest, hypoxic capillaries leak rapidly, diminishing the circulating blood volume.)
2. Replace losses initially with clear fluid and later with colloid (plasma or blood) as indicated. **N.B.:**
   a. Even a child previously in congestive heart failure needs infusions totaling at least 10% of the expected blood volume (EBV; equal to approximately 1% of body weight).
   b. With recovery, the extravasated fluid returns slowly to the vascular compartment, giving time for assessment of fluid volume and a decision as to whether diuretic therapy is necessary.
3. Avoid the use of dextrose-containing solutions. They may cause hyperglycemia, which may compromise cerebral survival. If hypoglycemia is suspected, it should be confirmed by blood glucose determination and treated accordingly.

Defibrillation

Ventricular fibrillation is rare in infants and children: asystole is usual. If ventricular fibrillation is present, proceed with defibrillation as soon as equipment is available.

1. For infants and children weighing less than 20 kg, use pediatric defibrillator plates (diameter of 4.5 cm for infants and 8 cm for children).
2. Set the machine to deliver shocks appropriate to the patient's size (to maximize the chance of success and minimize the danger of electrically induced myocardial damage); 2 joules (watt-seconds)/kg should be the initial setting. If this is unsuccessful, the dose should be doubled.
3. Patients who are digitalized should be treated with the lowest power settings initially; then the power setting is gradually increased. Normal doses of countershock may cause irreversible cardiac arrest in the presence of bound digitalis in the heart muscle.

Continuing Care

After successful cardiac resuscitation, attention must be directed to the need for further care, especially that needed to ensure maximal cerebral recovery.

1. Transfer the patient to a pediatric intensive care unit.
2. Continue artificial ventilation until the patient is fully conscious and capable of normal spontaneous ventilation.
3. Monitor cardiac status closely and arrange for therapy as indicated (e.g., inotropic drugs, antiarrhythmic agents).
4. If cerebral status is in doubt, nurse the patient in a 30° head-up position, and
   a. Continue with controlled ventilation to produce an arterial carbon dioxide pressure ($PaCO_2$) of 30–35 mmHg.
   b. Continue to ventilate with 100% O_2 to ensure the best possible cerebral oxygenation.
   c. Maintain blood pressure at normal or slightly elevated levels to ensure optimal cerebral perfusion; treat hypotension.
   d. Maintain normothermia—prevent the hyperthermia that usually follows a cerebral insult.
   e. Restrict fluid replacement: avoid large infusions of crystalloid solutions once cardiovascular stability is ensured.
   f. Treat seizure activity with phenobarbitone and/or phenytoin (Dilantin).
   g. Obtain an early neurologic consultation.

N.B. There have been many controversial issues and many unanswered questions remain in pediatric CPR. Recommendations concerning techniques for CPR and drug doses (especially for epinephrine) have varied considerably. The foregoing section represents a standard approach based on published guidelines.

Suggested Additional Reading

Chameides L, Brown GE, Raye JR, et al.: Guidelines for defibrillation of infants and children. Circulation 56(Suppl):502A–503A, 1977.

Feinberg WM and Ferry PC: A fate worse than death. Am J Dis Child 138:128–130, 1984.

Patterson MD: Resuscitation update for the pediatrician. Pediatr Clin North Am 46:1285–1303, 1999.

Redmond AD: Post resuscitation care. Br Med J 292:1444–1446, 1986.

Standards and guidelines for cardiopulmonary resuscitation and emergency cardiac care. Part VI: pediatric basic life support. JAMA 268:2251–2261, 1992.

Standards and guidelines for cardiopulmonary resuscitation and emergency cardiac care. Part VI: pediatric advanced life support. JAMA 268:2262–2275, 1992.

Young KD and Seidel JS: Pediatric cardiopulmonary resuscitation: a collective review. Ann Emerg Med 33:195–205, 1999.

Zideman DA: Resuscitation of infants and children. Br Med J 292:1584–1588, 1986.

NEONATAL RESUSCITATION

The anesthesiologist is frequently called upon to assist at or manage the care of the newborn immediately after birth.

Neonatal resuscitation must be based on a detailed knowledge of the normal physiologic changes that occur during transition to extrauterine life (*see* Chapter 2) plus a recognition of the pathologic processes in the mother or the fetus that may affect the infant at this time.

Many infants require little help. Some, however, require rapid intervention if serious sequelae are to be avoided. Preexisting maternal or fetal disease and events during labor may affect the newborn infant after delivery. Frequently, infants at risk may be recognized before birth; preparations can then be made for their immediate resuscitation on delivery. However, some infants who have demonstrated no antenatal signs of distress need urgent intervention after birth.

Immediate Assessment of the Newborn

A rapid assessment must be made to determine the extent of treatment required. The heart rate is the first and most useful index; the Apgar score is also a most useful guide. A heart rate of less than 100 beats/min dictates the need for immediate intervention. A low 5-minute (or later) Apgar score may indicate poor prognosis for long-term neurologic outcome.

Procedures for Neonatal Resuscitation

Routine Measures for All Infants

The mouth, pharynx, and nares should be suctioned as the head presents before delivery of the chest and initiation of the first breath. After delivery, the infant is held at the level of the uterus until the cord stops pulsating and is clamped. Elevation of the infant above or below this level may affect blood distribution between the infant and the placenta and result in hypovolemia or hypervolemia, respectively.

The infant should be dried, moved to a warm environment, and carefully examined to confirm the immediate status and detect any anomaly.

Artificial Ventilation

Infants with apnea, bradycardia (heart rate less than 100 beats/min), or cyanosis should be given immediate bag and mask positive-pressure ventilation using 100% O_2. A rate of 40–60 breaths/min is recommended; air entry should be monitored by auscultation and observation of the chest wall movement. High pressures (40 cmH$_2$O) may be required initially.

If bag and mask ventilation is unsuccessful in achieving good ventilation, immediate endotracheal intubation should be performed. (In some instances a laryngeal mask airway may be useful as an alternative.)

The heart rate should now be checked:

1. If the heart rate is more than 60 beats/min and rising, continue with positive-pressure ventilation.
2. If the heart rate is less than 60 beats/min or between 60 and 80

beats/min and not rising, chest compressions should immediately be commenced (*see below*).

Infants with Thick Meconium in the Amniotic Fluid

Meconium aspiration is a leading cause of morbidity and mortality.

If thick meconium ("pea soup") is present, it should be suctioned from the pharynx, hypopharynx, and trachea before the onset of breathing.

As soon as the head is delivered, suction the nose, mouth, and pharynx using a large-bore catheter. If thick particulate meconium is present once the baby is delivered, or if the baby is depressed, laryngoscopy should be performed. The trachea should be intubated, and controlled suction (meconium aspirator) should be applied to the endotracheal tube as it is immediately withdrawn. This should be repeated as necessary to clear the trachea of all meconium, if possible, before it becomes imperative to ventilate.

All infants should then be well oxygenated, have the stomach aspirated, and be closely observed for development of further respiratory problems (e.g., air-leak syndromes, persistent pulmonary hypertension).

Vigorous infants with thin meconium should be suctioned as soon as the head is delivered but may not require endotracheal intubation.

The Preterm Infant

Some special considerations are necessary for the very small infant:

1. Special care must be taken to prevent heat losses; immediately dry and place the infant on a warm mattress under a heating lamp. Use humidified oxygen.
2. Infants weighing more than 1,000 g should be given O_2, suctioned, and stimulated.
3. Infants weighing less than 1,000 g are very likely to require early intubation and ventilation. Be prepared to intervene rapidly unless the infant obviously is in satisfactory condition.
4. Any preterm infant displaying respiratory difficulty should be intubated to provide for optimal ventilation and oxygenation.

Continued Resuscitation

Patients who need continued ventilation should have their airway pressure monitored to prevent pressures higher than 25 cmH$_2$O. In addition, they should have:

1. A blood gas sample from the umbilical artery taken for analysis
2. A radial artery sample taken if there is no rapid response to therapy
3. Correction of respiratory acidosis by ventilation
4. Blood pressure monitoring and correction of hypovolemia
5. A blood glucose determination, and therapy for levels lower than 40 mg/dl

Chest Compression

Patients with a low heart rate despite ventilation with 100% O_2 should be treated with chest compressions.

1. The chest-encircling method is preferred because it may produce more effective cardiac output. Two thumbs are placed at the midsternum with hands encircling chest (*see* Fig. II–1). Avoid the lower sternum and xiphoid, because compression there may damage abdominal organs.
2. The sternum should be depressed 1/2 to 3/4 inch with each compression.
3. The recommended sequence is three compressions followed by a pause for ventilation, with a combined rate of 120 per minute (i.e., 90 compressions and 30 ventilations per minute). (Faster rates may be effective in smaller infants.)

Correction of Hypovolemia

Establish an intravenous route. The umbilical vein is easily cannulated; pass a 3.5F catheter to just below the skin level until a free return of blood is obtained; 10 ml/kg of blood, albumin, or lactated Ringer's solution should be given to treat persistent hypotension. *In an emergency, blood can be withdrawn from the mother and transfused into the baby (provided the mother has no significant diseases.)*

Drug Therapy

Drug therapy should be begun if the heart rate remains lower than 80 beats/min despite ventilation and chest compressions; epinephrine is the drug of first choice.

Epinephrine: 10–30 µg/kg (0.1–0.3 ml/kg of 1:10,000 solution) for asystole or slow heart rate despite all other efforts. Give the drug intravenously preferably, or alternatively via the endotracheal tube. The latter route is less predictable and produces lower plasma concentrations; every effort should be directed at obtaining an intravenous route.

Naloxone: when treating recognized narcotic depression, 0.1 mg/kg IV. Monitor the child carefully, because the duration of action of naloxone may be shorter than that of the narcotic drug. **N.B.** Naloxone may induce a withdrawal reaction in the infant of a narcotic addict.

Other drugs are very rarely indicated:

Calcium gluconate: 0.1 ml/kg of 10% solution—to correct hypotension that persists despite volume replacement and correction of acidosis.

Glucose: 4 ml/kg/hr of 10% solution—to treat documented hypoglycemia based on blood glucose measurement. Avoid causing hyperglycemia, which may compromise cerebral resuscitation.

Sodium bicarbonate: to correct metabolic acidosis that persists during prolonged resuscitation despite oxygenation and correction of respiratory acidosis. This should be given preferably in a dose based on current acid-base studies. Administer in dilute solution (0.5 mEq/ml), slowly, to prevent the danger of intracerebral bleeding caused by the hyperosmolar solution. Remember that sodium bicarbonate may cause hypotension due to vasodilation and a reduction in ionized Ca^{++}.

Postresuscitation Care

After successful neonatal resuscitation, the infant must be cared for in an intensive care area. Close nursing observation should be maintained and appropriate medical therapy continued to treat persisting derangements. Careful notes should be made to document the infant's condition and the therapeutic procedures undertaken.

Suggested Additional Reading

Frand MN, Honig KL, and Hageman JR: Neonatal cardiopulmonary resuscitation: the good news and the bad. Pediatr Clin North Am 45:587–598, 1998.

Guidelines for cardiopulmonary resuscitation and emergency cardiac care. Part VII: neonatal resuscitation. JAMA 268:2276–2281, 1992.

Ting P and Brady JP: Tracheal suction in meconium aspiration. Am J Obstet Gynecol 122:767, 1975.

Todres ID and Rogers MC: Methods of external cardiac massage in the newborn infant. J Pediatr 86:781–782, 1975.

Wiswell TE and Bent RC: Meconium staining and the meconium aspiration syndrome. Pediatr Clin North Am 40:955–981, 1993.

Appendix III

Drug Doses

PREOPERATIVE PERIOD

N.B. Avoid giving drugs intramuscularly if possible. Intramuscular injections are painful and children do not like them! If intramuscular drugs are necessary and more than one has to be given, combine them in the same syringe whenever possible.

Drugs for Premedication

Anticholinergics

Atropine: IV—0.02 mg/kg at induction (maximum dose, 0.4 mg);
    IM—0.02 mg/kg 30–60 minutes preoperatively (maximum, 0.6 mg).
    PO—same dose, 60–90 minutes preoperatively.
Glycopyrrolate: 0.01 mg/kg IV or IM.

Sedatives

Midazolam (Versed): 0.5–0.75 mg/kg PO, or 0.2 mg/kg intranasally, or
    0.3 mg/kg PR, or 0.08 mg/kg IM, or 0.1 mg/kg IV (in a monitored
    area).
Lorazepam (Ativan): for adolescents, 1–2 mg PO.
Fentanyl Oralet: up to 15 μg/kg.

Antacids, H$_2$-Histamine Blocking Agents

Cimetidine: 10 mg/kg PO, or 30 mg/kg PR, or 5 mg/kg IV.
Ranitidine: 2.0 mg/kg PO, or 1.0 mg/kg IV or IM.
Sodium citrate: 0.4 ml/kg PO.

Drugs to Speed Gastric Emptying

Metoclopramide: 0.15 mg/kg IV. (**Note:** Atropine blocks the effect of
    metoclopramide and should be withheld until induction of
    anesthesia.)

INTRAOPERATIVE PERIOD

Induction Agents

Thiopental sodium (Pentothal): neonates (younger than 1 month), up to
    3–4 mg/kg; infants (1 month–1 year), up to 7–8 mg/kg; children,
    up to 5–6 mg/kg.
Methohexital: up to 2 mg/kg IV or 15 mg/kg PR (1% solution).
Propofol (Diprivan): 2.5–3.5 mg/kg.
Ketamine: 2 mg/kg IV or 4–8 mg/kg IM.

Drugs for Intubation

Succinylcholine: infants, 2 mg/kg IV; older children, 1 mg/kg IV or 2
    mg/kg IM.
Mivacurium: 0.2 mg/kg IV.
Rocuronium: 1 g/kg IV.
Vecuronium: 0.1 mg/kg IV.

(**Note:** Do not inject rocuronium or vecuronium immediately after
thiopental; the resulting precipitate may block the needle.)

Cis-*Atracurium:* 0.1 mg/kg.
Pancuronium: 0.1 mg/kg.
Topical lidocaine for laryngeal spray: total dose, up to 4 mg/kg.

Maintenance

Fentanyl: 1–2 µg/kg IV to supplement analgesia or as an intravenous
infusion for major surgery; loading dose 5 µg/kg, infusion at 2–4
µg/kg/hr.
Meperidine (Pethidine, Demerol): 0.2–0.4 mg/kg IV or 1.5 mg/kg IM.
Morphine: 10–30 µg/kg IV or intravenous infusion (for children older
than 5 years of age); loading dose 100 µg/kg over 5 minutes,
infusion at 40–60 µg/kg/hr.

Neuromuscular Blocking Drugs

1. Give these drugs intravenously.
2. Give initial and repeat doses preferably as indicated by nerve
   stimulator, especially for infants (whose response to these drugs is
   extremely variable).
3. Remember that potent volatile agents (especially isoflurane) reduce
   the dose requirement of nondepolarizing drugs.
4. Infusion rates are given as a guide only and should be modified as
   indicated by neuromuscular blockade monitoring.

Cis-*Atracurium:* initial dose 0.1 mg/kg, repeat dose 0.03 mg/kg, or by
infusion—loading dose 0.1 mg/kg, infusion at 2–3 µg/kg/min.
d-*Tubocurarine:* initial dose 0.3–0.5 mg/kg; repeat doses should not
exceed half of the initial dose.
Mivacurium: 0.2 mg/kg, incremental dose 0.1 µg/kg, infusion rate
15–30 µg/kg/min.
Pancuronium: initial dose 0.06–0.1 mg/kg; repeat doses should not
exceed one-sixth of the initial dose.
Rocuronium: initial dose 0.6–1 mg/kg, incremental doses 0.15 mg/kg;
infusion rate 10–12 µg/kg/min.
Vecuronium: loading dose 0.1 mg/kg, incremental doses 0.02 mg/kg.

Antagonism of Neuromuscular Blockade

Atropine 0.02 mg/kg or *glycopyrrolate* 0.01 mg/kg mixed with *neostigmine*
0.05 mg/kg—administer slowly; use a nerve stimulator to monitor
effect; **OR**
Atropine 0.02 mg/kg, followed by *edrophonium* 1 mg/kg.

POSTOPERATIVE PERIOD

Analgesics

Acetaminophen (Tylenol): 10–40 mg/kg PO or PR. (Do not exceed 100
mg/kg/24 hr).

Codeine (useful for minor surgery): 1–1.5 mg/kg IM. (Note: Codeine must not be given intravenously.)
Meperidine (Demerol, Pethidine): 1–1.5 mg/kg IM, 0.2–0.5 mg/kg IV.
Morphine, IM or IV: children, 0.05–0.1 mg/kg; infants, 0.05 mg/kg.
Morphine infusion: children, 10–40 μg/kg/hr. To prepare the solution, mix:

0.5 × the patient's weight in kilograms × 3 mg morphine in 50 ml

The solution then contains 10 mg/kg/ml. Infuse at 1–4 ml/hr (equivalent to 10–40 μg/kg/hr).
For infants, give 5–15 μg/kg/hr.

Epidural morphine (preservative free): 50–75 μg/kg single-shot.
Spinal morphine (preservative free): 10 μg/kg single-shot.

Narcotic Antagonist

Naloxone (Narcan): 0.01–0.1 mg/kg IV or IM. This drug should be titrated slowly until undesired narcotic effects are reversed. Rapid administration of an excessive dose results in loss of analgesia, pain, and extreme restlessness.

Antinausea Drugs

Dimenhydrinate (Gravol, Dramamine): 1 mg/kg IV or 2 mg/kg PR.
Droperidol: up to 75 μg/kg IV (may cause excessive sedation).
Metoclopramide: 0.15 mg/kg.
Ondansetron: 0.15 mg/kg infused slowly.
Prochlorperazine (Stemetil, Compazine): 0.05–0.1 mg/kg IV. (Do not give to infants younger than 2 years of age; avoid if possible in those younger than 5 years.)

ANCILLARY DRUGS

Antibiotics

The dose given is that for a single intraoperative intravenous administration. The lower dose should be given to neonates under 1 week (limited neonatal liver and renal function). The usual maximum daily dose for children is given in parentheses. Antibiotics should be infused over a period of minutes, rather than by "push" technique, to minimize the possibility of adverse reactions. Some must be given over a longer period (e.g., vancomycin). Regimens for antibiotic prophylaxis against subacute bacterial endocarditis are listed on page 386.

Ampicillin*: 50–100 mg/kg (300 mg/kg).
Cefazolin: 20–40 mg/kg (100 mg/kg).

---

*Use caution in patients with renal failure.

Cefoxitin: 20–40 mg/kg (160 mg/kg).
Cefuroxime: 20–50 mg/kg (240 mg/kg).
Clindamycin: 5–10 mg/kg (30 mg/kg).
Cloxacillin: 12–25 mg/kg (100 mg/kg).
Erythromycin: 2.5–5 mg/kg (20 mg/kg).
Gentamicin: 2.0 mg/kg (7.5 mg/kg).
Benzyl penicillin*: 30,000–50,000 IU/kg (250,000 IU/kg).
Vancomycin*: 10 mg/kg (60 mg/kg) (must be given over a period of at least 1 hour).

Adrenocorticosteroids

Dexamethasone (Decadron): 0.2–0.5 mg/kg IV (maximum, 10 mg).
Methylprednisolone (Solu-Medrol): 5–25 mg/kg IV slowly over 10 minutes.
Hydrocortisone sodium succinate (Solu-Cortef): 1–5 mg/kg IV over 8–10 minutes.

Cardiovascular Drugs

Adenosine: 50–100 μg/kg.
Amiodarone: loading dose 5 mg/kg (over 30–60 minutes).
Amrinone: loading dose 0.75 mg/kg; infusion 3–5 mg/kg/min in neonates, 5–10 mg/kg/min in children.
Calcium chloride: 5 mg/kg.
Calcium gluconate: 10 mg/kg.
Dopamine: 5–15 μg/kg/min infusion.
Dobutamine: 2–20 μg/kg/min infusion.
Epinephrine: 0.1–1 μg/kg/min infusion.
Esmolol: 100–500 μg/kg IV, 50–200 μg/kg/min infusion.
Hydralazine: 0.1–0.2 mg/kg IM, IV.
Isoproterenol (Isuprel): 0.025–0.1 μg/kg/min infusion.
Lidocaine: 1–2 mg/kg.
Nitroglycerin: 1–10 μg/kg/min infusion.
Phenoxybenzamine: loading dose 0.25 mg/kg × 4 over 2–4 hours; maintenance, 0.25 mg/kg q6h.
Phentolamine: 0.2 mg/kg IV.
Procainamide: 3–6 mg/kg IV.
Propranolol: 0.01–0.1 mg/kg IV over 10 minutes.
Prostaglandin E_1: 0.05–0.1 μg/kg/min.
Sodium nitroprusside: 0.5–4 μg/kg/min.
Verapamil: 0.1–0.3 mg/kg IV. (Do not give to infants younger than 1 year of age.)

Diuretics

Ethacrynic acid: 0.5–1 mg/kg.
Furosemide (Lasix): 1 mg/kg.
Mannitol: 0.5–2.0 g/kg.

Anticonvulsants

Diphenylhydantoin (Dilantin): loading dose 15–20 mg/kg IV slowly;
     maintenance, 2.5–5 mg/kg bid IV or PO.
Phenobarbital: loading dose 10 mg/kg IV; maintenance, 1.5–2.5 mg/kg
     bid IV.

Bronchodilators

Salbutamol (Ventolin): loading dose 5–6 μg/kg IV; infusion 0.1–1.0 μg/
     kg/min; inhaled aerosol 100 μg dose q6h.
Aminophylline: loading dose 5 mg/kg over 30 minutes; infusion 1 mg/
     kg/hr (if no recent doses). Monitor blood levels (therapeutic range,
     10–12 μg/ml).

Local Anesthetics

Recommended safe maximum doses:

Lidocaine plain: 5 mg/kg.
Lidocaine with epinephrine: 10 mg/kg.

N.B. The maximum recommended dose of epinephrine to be infiltrated during halothane anesthesia is 10 μg/kg.

Bupivacaine: 3 mg/kg.
Ropivacaine: 3 mg/kg.
Tetracaine, spinal: children, 0.2 mg/kg; infants, 0.4–0.6 mg/kg.

DRUG INFUSIONS FOR INFANTS AND SMALL CHILDREN*

These formulas are designed to permit medications to be infused without
the need to administer excessive fluid volumes. Weight = the patient's
weight in kilograms.

Dopamine or dobutamine:
     Weight × 30 mg of drug in 100 ml
     1 ml/hr = 5 μg/kg/min
Epinephrine:
     Weight × 0.6 mg of drug in 100 ml
     1 ml/hr = 0.1 μg/kg/min; *dose 0.1–1.0 μg/kg/min*
Sodium nitroprusside or nitroglycerin:
     Weight × 6 mg drug in 100 ml
     1 ml/hr = 1 μg/kg/ min
Isoprenaline:
     Weight × 0.15 mg drug in 100 ml
     1 ml/hr = 0.025 μg/kg/min; *dose 0.025–0.1 μg/kg/min*

---

*Mix in 5% dextrose solution.

Prostaglandin:
   Weight × 60 μg in 20 ml
   1 ml/hr = 0.05 μg/kg/min; *dose 0.05–0.1 μg/kg/min*

OTHER INFUSIONS FOR CARDIAC PATIENTS

Desmopressin: May improve platelet function and reduce bleeding in some platelet diseases. Dose: 0.3 μg/kg by slow infusion over 20 minutes after weaning from cardiopulmonary bypass. Monitor cardiovascular parameters carefully during infusion.

ε-*Aminocaproic acid (Amicar):* Used to treat fibrinolytic states. May reduce postoperative bleeding, especially in cyanotic children. Should be administered before sternotomy. Loading dose: 100–200 mg/kg diluted and infused slowly over 1 hour.

Aprotinin: A serine protease inhibitor. Beware—may cause severe anaphylactoid reaction. Concentration: 1.4 mg/ml (10,000 KIU/ml). Test dose: 1 ml (1.4 mg) should be given via a central line; wait 10 minutes for possible adverse reaction (i.e., rash, bronchospasm, hypotension). Full loading dose: 240 mg/m^2 (maximum, 280 mg); give via a central line over 20–30 minutes. Maintenance infusion: 56 mg (40 ml)/m^2/hr (maximum, 70 ml/hr); continue until end of surgery.

Index

Note: Page numbers in *italics* refer to illustrations; page numbers followed by the letter t refer to tables.